PRINCIPLES

AND METHODS

OF PHARMACY

MANAGEMENT

PRINCIPLES AND METHODS OF PHARMACY MANAGEMENT

HARRY A. SMITH, Ph.D.

Professor of Pharmacy Administration,
College of Pharmacy,
University of Kentucky,
Lexington, Kentucky

THIRD EDITION

LEA & FEBIGER *Philadelphia* 1986

Lea & Febiger
600 Washington Square
Philadelphia, PA 19106-4198
U.S.A.
(215) 922-1330

First Edition, 1975
  Reprinted, 1977
Second Edition, 1980
Third Edition, 1986

Library of Congress Cataloging in Publication Data

Smith, Harry A. (Harry Alcide), 1925–
  Principles and methods of pharmacy management.

  Includes bibliographies and index.
  1. Pharmacy management. I. Title. [DNLM: 1. Pharmacy Administration.
QV 704 S649p]
RS100.S57   1986   615.1'068   86-7304
ISBN 0-8121-1040-4

Printed in the United States of America

Print Number: 4   3   2   1

DEDICATION

To my wife, Norma,

who has assisted me untiringly in this effort and
provided encouragement when needed.

Preface

The third edition is a complete and expanded revision of the previous editions. The book is now divided into five sections: Perspectives, Planning, Organization, Directing and Controlling. There are four chapters in each of the first three sections, five chapters in the fourth section and three chapters in the final section.

Because of the renewed emphasis on social and managerial aspects of pharmacy, a new approach and philosophy have been taken in the third edition. Also, pharmacy management is unique in comparison to general business management as a result of the blending of major managerial and professional functions. It is because of this unique blending of two sets of different, yet compatible, functions that it seemed to be relevant and useful to include the section on perspectives. These four chapters provide pharmacists with a basis for a better understanding of their future vocation in order to better manage their professional and business affairs, as well as those of their colleagues who may be placed under their supervision or management. Thus, the concepts and principles of this section should be useful to every pharmacist whether in a managerial role or not.

The historic chapter relates briefly how and why pharmacy evolved into the unique social institution it occupies in our society. The chapter on social roles within this institution provides further insight and appreciation of the unique nature of pharmacy and its functions. The chapter on the scope of pharmacy practice elaborates on this general theme.

The section culminates with a managerial perspective. Every pharmacist will manage at some level and do it either well or poorly. This chapter and the remainder of the book are designed to provide pharmacists with the tools to do a superior job of management.

Management-by-objectives is the reference frame for much of this book; not because it is a panacea, but because it provides an excellent framework for participatory management (which is well suited for managing professionals and managers) while retaining appropriate management control.

I have assumed a positive entrepreneurial posture in this third edition for the following reasons. Proprietorship provides the environment that promotes autonomy, innovation and professional satisfaction. It also provides the only means presently available whereby the pharmacist can receive remuneration for *any* and *all clinical services,* either directly or indirectly through increased patronage, in proportion to quantity and quality of services delivered. In this respect, the private practice of pharmacy can provide the highest standards of practice, and simultaneously it can provide the highest level of income of any form of practice.

Following the perspective section, the remainder of the text material is organized into the four major functions of management. This division provides a basis for integrating, to a degree, related material as study units. The book with selective additional readings can be used as a text for a two-semester, or two-quarter course, or it can be used as a comprehensive text for a four-semester-hour course.

In addition to the new arrangement, considerable new materials have been included in the third edition. These include social roles in Chapter 2, additional material on the scope of pharmacy practice in Chapter 3, new material on planning in Chapter 5, new material on capital planning in Chapter 8, much new material on macro- and micro-organization in Chapters 9 and 10, a new approach to computing the professional fee in Chapter 15, as well as updating the information in other chapters.

I appreciate the suggestions that several of my colleagues have passed along to me. Many of these have been incorporated into this edition. I welcome continuing suggestions, and these will be considered for future revisions. No textbook is ever as good as it can be, and it is because of this fact that I continue to look for ways to improve this textbook. I appreciate the support of fellow pharmacy management teachers.

Lexington, Kentucky   Harry A. Smith

Contents

Section III ORGANIZATION

SECTION IV DIRECTING

13. Purchasing

14. Inventory Control

15. Pricing and Professional Fees

SECTION V CONTROLLING

SECTION **I**

PERSPECTIVES

This first section provides four perspectives or views of pharmacy practice and management. Although this is primarily a book on management, many of the concepts, principles and methods have implications for the professional functions as well. Pharmacy is constituted as a professional institution *and* a business enterprise, and these are integrated into one social entity or institution. Pharmacy is not "just a business," neither is it "just a profession." That is why pharmacy management is not simply business management, but instead, it is a unique discipline that treats a wide range yet unique set of problems and challenges. Also social and economic forces and technological advances affect the entire practice simultaneously. Thus, these perspectives provide the pharmacist with insights into the challenges encountered in pharmacy practice and management.

1 | Historic Perspective

The general purpose of this chapter is to provide the pharmacy student with a sociohistoric perspective of his profession, in order that he may better understand the diversities of practices and organizations and the conflicts of vested interests, as well as personal or internal conflicts, and thus be better prepared to make sound choices as he pursues his life's work. Sufficient reason for including this brief historic sketch of the pharmacy profession in a course in pharmacy management can be seen in the following quote from the preface of *Kremers and Urdang's History of Pharmacy.*[1]

> The history of pharmaceutical science and technology has the cumulative, progressive quality that characterizes the history of science at large; the history of the pharmaceutical profession shows the character of social history, with its unforeseen regressive turns of events, its conflicts of interests, and their resolution by trends and forces that would elude comprehension solely in terms of science, or conviction, or effort, circumscribed by a given time or group.

Origin of Pharmacy

Pharmacy, as well as other professions and sciences, had a common origin in primitive civilizations. The witch doctor possessed the only perceived source of help in solving all of the problems that beset mankind. This concentration of power was the direct result of ignorance and superstition, which were prevalent among primitive people. As civilizations progressed, the various areas of authority and sources of help were divided among various "specialists." The priests were sought for religious matters; physicians were the source of healing; and wise men or judges were given political power and authority to dispense justice. In most societies, these three groups of authority and sources of ministration were combined into a single politicoreligious system or order at the early stages of development. With the advancement of knowledge and specialization within the priesthood, these three major areas of human endeavor were separated and came to be known as the three learned professions.

Up to a point in time, pharmacy and medicine were not separate occupa-

3

tions. In fact, after the two professions became separated, the practice of medicine resembled the early practice of pharmacy more than it did the practice of medicine as we know it today. During the ninth to the thirteenth centuries, much of the Arabian contribution to medicine was more pharmaceutical than medical in its contents and techniques. However, it was not until the edict of Frederick II, the German Emperor, in 1240, that pharmacy was recognized officially as a profession separate from medicine.[1]

Separation of Pharmacy from Medicine

The edict of Frederick II contained three regulations that provided the legal basis for the separation of pharmacy as an independent branch of health services: (1) separation of the pharmaceutical profession from the medical profession; (2) official supervision of pharmaceutical practice; and (3) obligation by oath to prepare drugs reliably, according to skilled art, and in a uniform, suitable quality.

The first regulation is self-explanatory. The second provided the historic and legal basis for the control of the practice of pharmacy and the enactment of our various pharmacy laws. The third regulation provided the basis for official pharmacopeias.

Two other principles of the edict greatly affected the future practice of pharmacy in many European countries, but had negligible effect on the practice in Anglo-Saxon countries, especially the United States: (1) the limitation of the number of pharmacies within a designated geographic and political entity; and (2) the fixing of the prices of drugs by the government. Both principles have been adopted in several countries in which health care is under the control of government. The second principle, but not the first, is applied in England and, with the advent of third-party payment arrangements and the fixing of dispensing fees, is becoming fairly common in the United States.

English Conflicts and Organizations

A brief sketch of the history of English pharmacy has been included because American pharmacy was influenced more directly by English practices than by those of any other single country. The development of English pharmacy was different from that of European countries and, thus, the same is true of American pharmacy. The separation of pharmacy from medicine did not occur early or by direct edict or regulation. It evolved slowly through much conflict, negotiation, civil suits, and, finally, regulation and legislation. The delayed separation of the two professions paralleled the slow development of both professions. This slow development was the result of the various conquests of England, the slow amalgamation of the various peoples with different cultural backgrounds, the relatively small percentage of educated people, and, probably most importantly, the philosophy of *laissez faire*.

In the beginning no distinction was made between the physician, the apothecary, and the surgeon. Over the years a trade developed in spices, peppers, herbs, and other items of small weight but great value. Those dealing in these wares at the retail level were known as "spicers," and at the wholesale level as "peppers." Their stock in trade was called "spicery." Gradually the wholesalers developed a guild, known as the Grocers' Company, for their social and economic protection. Meanwhile, the spicers developed unique skills and knowledge in the preparation of their wares and became known distinctively as "apothecaries."

The first regulation defining the functions of the physician and the apothecary was issued by Henry VIII in 1511. After the formation of the College of Physicians (later known as the Royal College of Physicians) in 1540, the apothecaries were placed under the direct regulation of the College. This did not last long, and by 1543, an act was passed giving the right of "every person being the King's subject having knowledge and experience of the nature of herbs, roots and waters to use and minister, according to their cunning, experience, and knowledge."[1] Later the apothecaries enjoyed the protective benefits of the Grocers' Company as a division of the guild, with official status, but not independence, granted by King James I in 1607. In 1617 they finally formed the separate Society of the Art and Mysteries of the Apothecaries.

It was common practice for the apothecaries to practice as "minor physicians" and for the physicians not only to dispense medication, but to operate dispensaries. Under the authority of the 1543 Act, many people with less training practiced both medicine and pharmacy within certain limits. The major reason for the development was the small number of trained, certified physicians.

The feuds continued for centuries. By the eighteenth century, the dealers in herbs, spices, and medical remedies came to be known as "druggists" and "chemists," the chemists performing certain operations of a pharmaceutical nature. Ironically, the chemists took the place in the Grocers' Company formerly occupied by the apothecaries. As a result of the Great Plague (1665 to 1666), during which most physicians died or fled London, the apothecaries gained official sanction to practice medicine when the House of Lords overruled a court decision in 1703. The fight did not end, but continued for many more years. Finally, apothecaries became the general practitioners of medicine and the chemists became the pharmacists. After many attempts, adequate laws were passed to regulate the practice of pharmacy and that of medicine. The Pharmaceutical Society of Great Britain became the official organization of pharmacists and ultimately became the licensing and regulating agency. Pharmacists were usually called chemists by the public. The pharmacies, or drugstores as we sometimes call them, were known as chemists' shops in England. The transformed apothecaries-physicians retained the Royal College of Physicians as their official organization and regulatory agency.[1]

Pharmacy in the Colonies

The brief historic sketch of pharmacy in England is similar to the development of pharmacy in the United States, with perhaps less direct legal confrontation among the various interests in the United States. The early settlers, and most immigrants, came to this country for political, economic, and religious freedom. They came from many different countries. As in the early history of Great Britain, there were (1) an amalgamation of people with varied cultural backgrounds, (2) a small percentage of educated people trained in the "arts and mysteries" of pharmacy or medicine, and (3) certainly people who subscribed to the philosophy of *laissez faire*. The primary consideration of the settlers was survival, which meant basically food, clothing, and shelter.

At the outset, the early settlers borrowed heavily from the Indians for remedies to treat the various and numerous illnesses. In fact, Indian drugs contributed nearly as much to European medicine as European medicine contributed to medicine in the New World. The settlers did bring with them some of their favorite recipes and materia medica (and seeds) to supplement the Indian remedies. This led to the fundamental principle of the "right to self-medicate." When people trained in the arts of physicks began to immigrate, it was much more practical to encourage those who were trained in both the arts of the apothecary and of the physician than to encourage those trained in only one art. Why pay the fare for two people when a single person would suffice?

During the first 200 years of colonization, medicine and pharmacy were practiced by housewives, barbers, governors, the clergy, and educators, in addition to trained apothecaries, surgeons, and physicians who were in the minority. As a result of this intrusion into the practice of pharmacy and medicine, when larger numbers of apothecaries and physicians later arrived in the New World many were forced to seek a livelihood in other occupations, such as teachers, ministers, or politicians.

The first apothecary to immigrate to North America was Louis Hebert, landing first in Nova Scotia in 1604 and later moving to Quebec in 1617.[1] He pursued husbandry in addition to providing his pharmaceutical skills and drugs to the members of the fur company. The first pharmacist in America was William Davice, who established a pharmacy in 1646.[1] One of the earliest American drugstores on record, actually a general store with a stock of drugs, was established in the colonies by a Dutch surgeon, Gysbert van Imbroch, in Kingston, New York, in 1663.[1]

There were letters sent to the Virginia Company with headquarters in London requesting "foure honest and learned Ministers, two Surgeons, two Druggists," indicating a need for educated people in the colonies. A later letter asked the Company to "send them some Phisitians and Apothecaries of which they stand much in need of."[1] A few, perhaps three, apothecaries came to the colonies during the seventeenth century. According to Blanton,[1] a medical historian, "there is no further record of apothecaries living in the colony in this century, the physician being for the most part his own apothecary.'' This represented the dominant factor influencing the development of pharmacy throughout the period of colonization.

There were at least four significant events during the eighteenth century that began to influence the development and practice of pharmacy in the United States. First, there was a great influx of English "patent medicines" into the colonies. These were widely advertised with greatly exaggerated claims, a practice that continued after the passage of the United States Patent Act and still exists under considerably more regulation today. These remedies provided an economical means to ameliorate diseases in view of the shortage of qualified physicians, and apothecaries, and nourished the practice of self-medication.

Second, the first hospital pharmacy was established in the Pennsylvania Hospital founded on the initiative of Benjamin Franklin. Jonathan Roberts, the pharmacy's first apothecary, was directed to compound medicines and make up prescriptions of physicians only, and this pharmacy was one of the early concrete examples of the separation of pharmacy and medicine in the colonies.

Third, Robert's successor, John Morgan, resigned after only one year to study medicine. After becoming a physician, Morgan was a strong advocate of the separation of the two professions and of restriction of the practice of those trained in the respective professions.

Fourth, an Act was passed in Virginia in 1736 to regulate and restrict the practice of medicine.

However, the progress toward the professionalization of pharmacy was slow, following the precedent set in England.

Early American History and Competition

THE REVOLUTIONARY WAR

The Revolutionary War caused pharmacy to be recognized officially as a separate and distinct profession when Andrew Craigie was appointed Apothecary-General. Much credit for this distinction of pharmacy goes to John Morgan, the Director General of the military hospitals and Chief Physician of the Army. Sonnedecker summarized the significance of the War:

> Eight years of successful pharmaceutical activity, separate from medicine but equally recognized and given the same official status; the first known American manufacture of pharmaceutical products on a large scale; the first practical attempt at a uniform and obligatory formulary as a basis for satisfactory and reliable pharmaceutical work (in this case, military pharmacy); and the meeting of American pharmacists with European colleagues who were more advanced professionally.[1]

INTERWAR PERIOD

With the end of the Revolutionary War, the colonists enjoyed a newly found freedom and an opportunity to develop a new society not tied to a monarchy or any oppressive political code or system. This climate was conducive to experimentation and rapid technologic and economic growth. It also deterred the enactment of laws that greatly restricted trade and the professions. However, one important law, the Patent Act, fostered the development of a flourishing trade in "patent medicines" or proprietary drugs independent of medicine. In addition, it provided the legal foundation for several medical practices such as the "Thomsonian," "Eclectic," and "Homeopathic" branches of medicine. Special remedies were developed and patented, based on the theories and practices of these various branches of medicine. The practical significance of the patent law was to promote a degree of monopoly for the various medical practices, including the dispensing of their special remedies. Also, the general public generally was ignorant of the nature of the various patented remedies and purchased these remedies wantonly in the hope of miraculous cure perpetrated by the vendors, physicians included.

Sonnedecker[1] named three classes of people involved in the drug field at this point in history:

1. Persons who had served a more-or-less lengthy apprenticeship with a medical practitioner, and had learned to compound prescriptions; not infrequently, these people seem to have had a greater interest in their commercial talents and prospects than in their medical accomplishments.

2. Those who had trained as apothecaries, chemists, or druggists, and all who had pharmaceutical education, such as the apothecaries or Apotheker in their native countries. However, most of these people preferred medical practice combined with dispensing.

3. Storekeepers who specialized in drugs to some extent without having any special pharmaceutical training.

To this list should be added the dispensing physicians and physicians operating their own apothecary shops or dispensaries. And as the people migrated westward, the competition of the storekeepers was provided first by the proprietors of the trading posts and later the general stores. The competitive condition was enhanced by the itinerant peddlers and medicine shows selling their dubious remedies. Thus, not unlike their English counterparts, the trained American apothecaries or pharmacists faced vigorous competition from both ends of the professional-commercial spectrum—the physicians at the professional end who had a distinctive monopolistic advantage, and the ordinary storekeepers and peddlers at the commercial end, who also had the advantage of being less scrupulous in making exaggerated claims for the drugs they sold. Both categories of competition far outnumbered the true apothecary shops until the latter part of the nineteenth century.

The legitimate pharmacists were forced to sell many lines of goods other than drugs to make a livelihood. Other commodities included spices, tobacco, pigments, paints, brushes, oils, glass, and various chemicals. Some, especially during the early years, became drug and spice importers and wholesalers providing raw materials to physicians, other apothecaries, and even general stores—especially those in the rural areas. Some of these pharmacists became manufacturers, for example Schieffelin, Wm. S. Merrell, and Smith Kline and French.

On the brighter side was the gradual development of professional pharmacy. Local associations were organized and many of them established colleges of pharmacy, the first being the Philadelphia College of Pharmacy in 1821. By 1860, six colleges were established and each organization later became an educational institution. In 1852 the American Pharmaceutical Association (APhA) was organized. It fostered the organization of state associations, which in turn, with the assistance of the APhA, enacted state pharmacy laws. The APhA adopted a code of ethics and sponsored a number of national pharmaceutical associations, including the National Association of Retail Druggists and the American Society of Hospital Pharmacists. Ironically, the latter group and the APhA disaffiliated by a series of individual actions in late 1972 and early 1973. The Pharmacopoeia of the United States was published in 1820 by "authority of the medical societies and colleges." Pharmacists were utilized in the first revision, and by 1860 pharmacists constituted one-half of the Revision Committee.

Meanwhile, several truly professional apothecary shops were established, principally in the large cities—Boston, New York, Philadelphia, Cincinnati, Louisville, St. Louis, and New Orleans. This development was fostered by the European trained physicians, both immigrants and United States citizens, who were trained to write prescriptions to be compounded by professional apothecaries. The greater number of pharmacies, however, were the traditional type, selling various nondrug commodities. Some drugstores were closer in character to general stores than they were to pharmacies, especially in the frontier towns.

THE CIVIL WAR

The Civil War had a dramatic effect on the political, social, and economic structure of our society and provided the impetus for the rapid industrialization of our country. This industrialization affected all trades and industries, including pharmacy, and had a direct effect on American pharmacy.

First, the development of the textile industry reduced the demand for dyestuffs in the drugstores since the production of clothing was shifted from the home (and drugstore purchases) to the factory. Similarly, the paint, glass, and oil trade was shifted to the building trade industry. Retailers in paint, general building materials, and/or hardware absorbed much of this business, which had previously belonged to the general store or drugstore. The third direct effect on pharmacy was the gradual shifting of the compounding function from the drugstore to the emerging pharmaceutical industry. As Sonnedecker observed,[1] the shifting of the preparation of drugs to large manufacturers in the early years had a lesser effect in the United States than it did in Europe because most of the prescriptions were compounded by physicians or their apprentices. However, competition in the form of dispensing by physicians and physician ownership of pharmacies continued well into the twentieth century and still exists to a significant degree in several locales. According to a recent article, this practice is increasing.[2]

Deterrents to Professionalization

The question may be asked why pharmacy did not seize the opportunity to develop a strictly professional type of practice as the sale of several of the traditional lines of goods was transferred to other trades. The answer is manifold: The deterrents to professionalization of pharmacy include: (1) the demise of the general store, (2) competition of various types, (3) the introduction of the soda fountain, (4) inadequate regulations and education, (5) prohibition, (6) Fair Trade laws, and (7) the economic philosophy of *laissez faire*.

DEMISE OF THE GENERAL STORE AND TRANSFER OF STOCK

As indicated earlier, the general stores and the drugstores were similar in the frontier towns; however, the typical pharmacy in the larger cities was quite different and was distinctly a different institution. It was not as highly specialized and professional as the German Apotheke, but was more specialized than the larger diversified general store, a true *American institution*. As the country became more settled and urbanized, the general stores gradually faded from the scene, although they still can be found in rural areas today. Other lines of trades absorbed certain lines common to the general store, for example, clothing in the dry goods store and tools and nails in the hardware stores. Because of their accessibility and convenience—large numbers and long hours—the drugstores were the logical choice to carry many of the smaller items common to the general stores. These items collectively came to be referred to as "sundries." These include chemicals used as pesticides, veterinary drugs and implements, needles and thread, stationery and writing accessories, magazines and books, tobacco and accessories, toiletries, and confectioneries. Spices, extracts both flavoring and medical, and preservatives had been a part of the pharmacist's stock all along. It should be realized that the greatest motivation for stocking these sundry items was economic survival in the face of the competitive conditions facing pharmacy.

Table 1–1.   Early Drugstore Chains

Date Founded	Name	Location
1850	Schlegal Drug Stores	Davenport, Iowa
1852	Meyer Brothers Company	Fort Wayne, Indiana
1879	T.P. Taylor & Company[a]	Louisville, Kentucky
1879	Jacobs Pharmacy Company	Atlanta, Georgia
1883	Read Drug & Chemical Co.	Baltimore, Maryland
1884	Marshall Drug Co.	Cleveland, Ohio
1885	Skillern's Drug Stores	Dallas, Texas
1889	Cunningham Drug Stores[b]	Detroit, Michigan
1890	Bartell Drug Company[a]	Seattle, Washington
1892	Owl Drug Company	San Francisco, Calif.
1898	Eckerd Drug Stores[a]	Erie, Pa.
1899	Standard Drug Stores[a]	Cleveland, Ohio
1901	Walgreen Drug Co.[a]	Chicago, Illinois
1907	Louis K. Liggett Co.	New York City

Source: Lebhar, G.M.: *Chain Stores in America, 1859–1962,* 3rd ed. New York: Chain Store Publishing Corp., 1963, pp. 43–44.
[a]Still in business under the same name or a variation of it.
[b]Now known as the Quael Corporation.

COMPETITION AND DIVERSIFICATION

Competition can assume several forms. Basically these are the number and types of business units or establishments vying for patronage with price and services. It should be obvious that the latter two forms, price and services, derive from the first, the large numbers of establishments competing for the consumer's patronage and dollars.

Competition through diversification may be classified into two categories: within the drug trade and from outside the drug trade. This distinction is difficult to make today because of mergers. Recently, supermarkets, variety chains, and mass merchandisers have entered the pharmaceutical business. Historically, competition has always come from both within and outside the traditional pharmaceutical businesses. During the early years, competition came from the general stores and physicians' dispensaries, which have been discussed already. As the general stores faded from the scene, mail order houses, beginning with Montgomery and Ward in 1872, provided considerable competition, especially in the rural areas. Meanwhile, drugstore chains were being established as indicated in Table 1–1.

According to the *NASCS-LILLY DIGEST,*[3] chain drugstores in 1983 derived an average of 23.7 percent of their total revenue from prescriptions. In contrast, independent pharmacies derived an average of 58.5 percent of their revenue from prescriptions.[4] It is estimated that the typical independent pharmacy realizes 70 percent of its total sales from health-related goods and activities.[5]

The department store, which is an organization of many single-line stores under one roof and management, naturally would sell many products in competition with the traditional drugstore. To provide a historic perspective, Macy's, one of the biggest and best-known department stores, was established in 1858.[6] However, recently Macy's has discontinued some of its pharmacy departments. Some department stores have professional pharmacies located within their establishments.

In the year 1859 the Great Atlantic and Pacific Tea Company (A&P) was founded. Later the Kroger Company was established in 1882. Although these chain grocery companies provided little real competition in the beginning, after World War II, the health and beauty aid departments of the grocery stores began to compete significantly with the drugstores. These departments were stocked with limited lines and sizes with a high turnover rate. The competition became more direct and vigorous when Kroger established its SuperX Drug Corporation in 1961.[7] This period marked the vigorous expansion of price reduction and advertising of selected prescription drugs. This practice was not restricted to any one company, but it became prevalent among many drug chains and large discount stores with prescription departments.

The variety, or "Five and Dime," stores provided a degree of competition for the traditional drugstore from the inception of the variety stores. Woolworth, the first variety store chain, was established in 1879. Woolworth was followed by McCrory in 1881, Kress in 1896, and S.S. Kresge in 1899. The J.C. Penney Co., which was established in 1902, was somewhat unique in that it combined some of the features of both dry goods and variety stores, a sort of junior department store. Its real significance relative to drugstore competition is that the company has recently entered the pharmaceutical business with its Thrift Drug Company, Treasury Drugs, and leased prescription and drug departments.

Some of the most persistent and effective competitors were the "pine-board drugstores." Their origin dates from the early part of this century.[8] They were characterized by : (1) location in low-rent areas; (2) furnishings of inexpensive fixtures—usually pine boards nailed to the wall or placed on bricks which supported them; (3) stock limited to fast-selling products and popular sizes; and (4) sale prices of products at low gross margins. The "pine-board drugstore" flourished during the early part of the Great Depression and had its counterpart in the grocery trade.

It appears that the "pine-board drugstores" were forerunners of the so-called "discount stores." The "pine-board drugstore" disappeared from the scene by the end of World War II. Although some form of discount merchandising had existed throughout history, the large, vigorously merchandised discount stores really began to develop and grow in the 1950s. The discount stores differed from the "pine-board stores" in the following aspects: (1) the discount stores were much larger and carried a greater variety of merchandise lines; (2) their fixturing was better and more attractive, but still not expensive; (3) they were located along a high traffic street or highway, but usually not in major shopping centers; and (4) they advertised vigorously and attempted to establish the one-stop-shop concept in the minds of the public—a "shopping center" under one roof. Of course, drugs and prescription departments were included and were used as "loss leaders" to promote greater traffic and sales volume.

Competition in pricing is as old as commerce itself, and it certainly is as old as pharmacy in this country. T.W. Dyatt is considered to have been the "father of price-cutting" in American pharmacy when he established a patent medicine warehouse in Philadelphia in 1806. The George A. Kelly Company, which later became Beckham and Kelly, was the forerunner of the chain drugstore concept in this country. The Company operated four drugstores in Pittsburgh around 1860, which used the sign "Cut-rate Drugstores."[1]

Price-cutting, a practice used by certain independents even more than the older chains, became prevalent in certain cities by the 1880s, and several steps were taken to combat this practice.

First, pharmacists began to manufacture, or have manufactured for them, exclusive private label drugs with controlled distribution and prices. Several of these co-ops were organized, but they gradually faded from the scene. Approximately six of these cooperative ventures existed over a period of fifty years. One such company, the United Drug Company, under the leadership of L.K. Liggett, became a permanent national organization. It began as a manufacturer of proprietary drugs and toiletries under the label of "Rexall" for franchised independent pharmacies, serving about 10,500 pharmacies by 1960. Meanwhile, the Company established a chain of drugstores reaching a total of 550 units, the largest drug chain in the United States in 1947.[1] This large diversified organization demonstrated that the economic interests of the chain drug industry and the independent pharmacists can merge. The Walgreen Drug Company represents a similar type of organization, which developed in the reverse order. The Company first organized a chain of drugstores and then established a large number of franchises among independent pharmacists to obtain a wider distribution of the Company's private label drugs and other products. Now, the Walgreen Drug Company is one of the largest drug chain organizations.

Another attempt to combat price-cutting was the formation of mutual wholesale drug companies. Beginning as buying groups, some of these were initiated by pharmacists, while others were organized by regular wholesalers to establish a system of franchise dealers to promote and sell a controlled line of drugs and other products.

THE SODA FOUNTAIN AND PHARMACY

The soda fountain had a significant impact on the practice of pharmacy in the United States and became an integral part of the typical pharmacy in this country. "Soda water" was used as a medicinal preparation in the latter part of the eighteenth century. The first soda fountain probably was operated in Philadelphia around 1825. Soda fountains became common by 1860 to the extent that some were adorned with ornate fixtures. The soda fountain came into its own in the 1880s when the anti-whiskey movement resulted in the passage of local prohibition laws. This movement culminated in the Volstead Act in 1919 and the soda fountain reached its peak of popularity.

The impact of the soda fountain on pharmacy practice was dramatic and is hardly debatable, but the value to the professional practice of pharmacy *is* debatable. The extra income derived from fountains was significant and saved many proprietors from economic failure. It also revolutionized the nature of the drugstore, changing it from a sober professional-business institution to one that emanated a relaxed atmosphere where people gathered to "indulge" in a refreshing drink or repast, to share local news or gossip, or to consult with "Doc" privately about matters of a more serious nature. The latter purpose may not always have been health related. This feature, together with the diversified merchandising practice, has caused several writers to observe that "the American Drugstore is a unique social institution" peculiar to the United States.

There were other concrete changes in the characteristics of the drugstore brought about by the complementary effects of the soda fountain and diversified merchandising.

1. The size of the drugstore increased to accommodate the increased merchandise and activities.

2. The business hours of the drugstore increased to take advantage of attracting patrons to the soda fountain in the evenings.

3. The location of the drugstore shifted from the lower-rent sites to the high-rent, busy-corner locations, again to maximize traffic, sales, and profits.

4. All of the above changes increased investment and operating expenses, thereby increasing the capital and risk of establishing a pharmacy practice.

5. Overall, the practice of pharmacy became more a commercial venture and less a professional venture. Of course, this was not always the case. One must keep in mind that the practice of pharmacy in the United States had been commercially oriented from the earliest years.

The positive financial results of the combined merchandising and soda fountain activities are shown in Table 1–2.

There was a sharp decline in the number of soda fountains during World War II. It has been reported that one out of every six stores closed their fountains during the war because of the shortage of personnel and materials, especially sugar and syrups.[9] In a survey of approximately 1700 pharmacies conducted by the National Association of Retail Druggists and *The Saturday Evening Post,* the percentage of pharmacies operating fountains showed a decrease from 81.5 percent to 74.8 percent.[10] Some of the fountain closings during the War may have been temporary, but a permanent trend of closing

Table 1–2. Relationship of Sales Volume to Presence of Soda Fountain

Item	Pharmacies with fountain			Pharmacies without fountain			All pharmacies		
	1939	*1935*	*1929*	*1939*	*1935*	*1929*	*1939*	*1935*	*1929*
No. of pharmacies	39,452	38,431	34,844	18,451	17,966	23,414	57,903	56,697	58,258
Total sales millions of $	1,205	950	1,149	357	282	541	1,563	1,233	1,690
Avg. yearly sales in $	30,542	24,528	32,695	19,362	16,253	23,111	26,983	21,740	29,015
Avg. daily sales in $	84	67	89	53	44	63	74	60	80

Source: Publications of the Bureau of the Census.

fountains coincided with the large-scale remodeling of pharmacies after World War II. Today, a small percentage of the pharmacies operate soda fountains.

INADEQUATE REGULATIONS AND EDUCATION

There was a definite parallel between the formation of state pharmaceutical associations and the passage of state pharmacy laws, with the laws usually following the associations by a few years. The major failing in the early pharmacy acts and regulations was their trade or product orientation in contrast to a professional and personal orientation. Had more thought and effort been directed toward certifying highly competent pharmacists and less effort toward regulation of the drug trade, pharmacy would have benefited from self-regulation via an enforced code of practice.

Pharmacy was about three decades behind in the passage and amendment of the pharmacy acts. For example, if a college degree had been a requisite for licensure as a pharamcist by 1900, the flooding of the market with poorly trained graduates of the "cram schools" could have been avoided. This would have reduced the severe competition, elevated the practice of pharmacy to a higher plane, and caused physicians to accept pharmacists as co-equal colleagues in providing health services. Many of the conflicts within the ranks of pharmacy could have been avoided by a more enlightened body of practitioners. Comradeship would have largely replaced predatory competition. Given the nature of pharmacy even under nearly ideal conditions, wholesome competition probably would have existed.

Just as pharmacy laws and regulations lagged in their personal and professional orientation, so did pharmaceutical education. This is understandable, given the manipulative and technologic nature of pharmacy throughout much of its history. Pharmacy *was* preparing drugs. Much of the educational content of pharmacy curricula was the *art* of preparing drugs. Later, as pharmacy moved toward requiring a bachelor degree for licensure in the 1930s, the emphasis shifted to the *science* of preparing drugs, although most drugs were no longer prepared by pharmacists in pharmacies. It was not until the latter part of the 1960s that pharmaceutical education began to direct its attention and educational effort toward serving people.

Pharmacy administration as a discipline in pharmacy emerged in the 1950s. Some of the criticism directed toward the teachers of pharmacy administration was their preoccupation with the place of practice, the pharmacy, but their orientation paralleled those of the pharmaceutical scientists, who were preoccupied with chemicals, test tubes, and drugs. It is a credit to most of the pharmacy administration professors who, among other members of pharmacy faculties, were the early advocates of *people-oriented,* clinically based pharmaceutical education in the 1960s.

It is only recently that pharmaceutical laws and regulations have been directed toward the concerns of people—patient medication (profiles) records, patient consultation, and experimental programs of pharmacists' prescribing for self-limiting illness. As in the past, regulations generally follow education.

PROHIBITION AND PHARMACY

The Volstead Act, previously alluded to in the context of its influence on an increase in fountain patronage, also had other effects on pharmacy. During the prohibition era, the pharmacy was the only legitimate source for alcoholic beverages. This, of course, provided yet another source of revenue for proprietors of drugstores. The incentive was such that some people were induced to establish pharmacies primarily for that purpose. Some, no doubt, were induced to study pharmacy in order to obtain a license to practice and dispense prescriptions, including those for whiskey. As a consequence, the number of pharmacies rose to an all-time high of 58,258 in 1929—before the stock market crash, the depression of the thirties, and the *repeal of prohibition*.

During the prohibition era, a pharmacy could be found at nearly every major intersection in the large cities. Many drugstores continued their liquor departments after prohibition. Considerable numbers of pharmacies sell liquor today. A 29 percent subsample of *Lilly Digest* Pharmacies reported liquor sales in 1983. The wisdom of maintaining a liquor department may be questionable since those pharmacies reporting liquor sales of less than 5 percent of total sales reported a net profit of 2.6 percent of sales, whereas those with more than 5 percent liquor sales reported 1.0 percent net profit.[11] The net profit for the total sample was 2.9 percent of sales. However, these data should be viewed cautiously since there was only 43 pharmacies in the "more than 5 percent liquor sales" subsample. On balance, the so-called great American experiment (prohibition) did little, if anything, to further professional pharmacy; some pharmacists contend that it even exerted a negative effect.

"FAIR TRADE" LAWS

"Fair Trade" laws represented the greatest concerted effort to combat price-cutting. Earlier efforts to maintain prices had failed for various reasons. The Campion plan, a rebate for not undercutting the regular retail price, failed for a lack of an enforcement mechanism. The tripartite plan was a mutual agreement among the National Association of Retail Druggists (NARD), the National Wholesale Druggists Association (NWDA), and the Proprietary Association (PA). This plan, in essence, was to limit the distribution and sale of many of the nationally known products to those drugstores who maintained the suggested retail price. This plan was declared illegal under the Sherman Antitrust Law in a United States Circuit Court in Indiana in 1907.

It was not until the 1930s, when the Great Depression caused many business failures, that public sentiment turned in favor of laws and regulations to preserve American business, especially small businesses. The National Recovery Act (NRA), which was later declared unconstitutional, was a significant measure for this very purpose. Beginning with California in 1931, many states passed "fair trade" laws with the assistance of the NARD. By 1949, all of the states except Texas, Missouri, and Vermont had enacted fair trade laws. It should be noted that the old-line chain drugstores supported fair trade completely.

It would assist in the understanding of fair trade laws and some of the socioeconomic aspects of pharmacy if we briefly reviewed the social and legal bases for the fair trade laws. The social theory of fair trade supported the concept of pure or perfect competition. This is a classic economic theory that perfect competition can exist only when there are numerous small suppliers and buyers, and both have a complete knowledge of the market relative to price, quality, and other factors. The price is determined by the market through the interactions of the suppliers and purchasers. Fair trade laws helped to maintain a large number of small suppliers; there were numerous small buyers (consumers); and the price of a fair trade product became familiar to most purchasers even though it was fixed by the manufacturer and not by the market. The main purpose, however, was the preservation of small businesses.

The legal basis for fair trade was quite different. It was based on the protection of property rights, the good will associated with trademarked or branded products. The product had to meet the following three criteria: (1) the product had to be in free and open competition with products of the same general class (use); (2) the product had to have a trademark or a trade name identifiable with the producer; and (3) the producer had the option of establishing the minimum resale price. It should be noted that price maintenance was legally binding vertically and not horizontally (among retailers) and enforceable only by the producer. Three conditions when the minimum resale price could be disregarded were: (1) if the product was damaged or deteriorated; (2) if the product was sold by order of a court; and (3) if the product was sold in a genuine closing-out sale.

The first fair trade laws did not contain the so-called "nonsigner" clause, which meant that each retailer had to sign a contract with each supplier and/ or manufacturer. These early laws were amended, and the later laws incorporated the "nonsigner" clause, which caused the fair trade law to be binding on all retailers provided one retailer signed a fair trade contract in each state.

The fair trade laws were fortified by two legal developments at the federal level. The United States Supreme Court in 1936 upheld the constitutionality of the Illinois Fair Trade Act.[12] The Miller-Tydings Federal Enabling Act amended the Sherman Anti-trust Act, which enabled states to pass fair trade laws applicable to interstate commerce without being in violation of the Anti-trust Laws.

The fair trade laws received a severe setback in the famous Schwegman case.[13] The United States Supreme Court ruled the "nonsigner" clause unconstitutional for interstate commerce. This defect was quickly remedied with the passage of the McGuire Amendment to the Federal Trade Commission

Act in 1952, and the "nonsigner" clause was reinstated for interstate commerce. From this point in time, fair trade laws lost ground rapidly, primarily through court decisions at the state level. It was mostly the "nonsigner" clause that was declared invalid; however, in some states the entire law was invalidated. Also, manufacturers became weary of enforcing the fair trade contracts. Today fair trade laws are of little or no effect except in the liquor and milk trades.

The fair trade laws had a favorable economic impact upon pharmacy by decreasing the number of business failures, and the laws, obviously, were construed favorably by a number of practitioners. However, the fair trade laws had a negative aspect from a strictly professional viewpoint. The net effect was a reduced sales volume per pharmacy for prescriptions and health-related products reflecting reduced revenues from professional activities. As late as 1939, Nolen reported that prescriptions accounted for only 13 percent of the total sales and 19.3 percent of the gross margin of sales.[14] Under these conditions, pharmacists were forced to offer a wider variety of products and services, and as a result pharmacy became more commercial than professional in character.

INFLUENCE OF LAISSEZ FAIRE

The French term *laissez faire* literally means "allow (them) to do." It quite simply is the doctrine that government should not interfere with commerce. It is one of two center pieces of the doctrine of the modern day American Libertarian party, the other being a similar doctrine on other noneconomic, social issues. The doctrine of *laissez faire* was quite natural for the early settlers and immigrants to the United States because they came to get away from oppressive laws and policies. Given the combined business-professional nature of pharmacy, there was little sentiment for passing strict laws regulating the practice of pharmacy or the drug trade. The *laissez faire* philosophy fostered the attitude of allowing most anyone to enter the pharmacy business, physicians to dispense their own drugs or own and operate their own dispensaries.

Summary

All of the influences discussed in this chapter combined, perhaps synergistically, to shape the American pharmacy into a unique social institution, one that is a combination of a business and professional enterprise. In this respect, it is different from Western European pharmacy only in the extent of diversification of goods and services offered for sale. Again, the same comparison holds for other professions. More on this particular aspect of pharmacy will be discussed in the next chapter on pharmacists' roles.

The typical American pharmacy is a place where the public expects to have their prescriptions dispensed professionally with adequate advice on how to best use the medication and what to expect from its use, to be able to purchase nonprescription drugs and medical accessories from personnel with expertise (including the involvement of the pharmacist PRN), to purchase toiletries and cosmetics for the maintenance of a healthy and more attractive appearance and to purchase many other convenient items that make life easier, if not better, and sometimes more interesting. Looking at pharmacy from the consumer's perspective, it isn't necessarily bad, but good that Mrs. Jane Q. Public can purchase all of the various items and services available in most pharmacies.

REFERENCES

1. Sonnedecker, R.: *Kremers and Urdang's History of Pharmacy,* 3rd ed. Philadelphia: J.B. Lippincott Co., 1963.
2. Siegelman, S.: Editorial, *Am. Druggist. 191*(3):1, 46, 48, March, 1985.
3. *NACDS—Lilly Digest,* Indianapolis: Eli Lilly & Co., 1984.
4. *The Lilly Digest,* Indianapolis: Eli Lilly & Co., 1984.
5. The estimate was derived from references 3 and *Drug Topics, Chain Edition,* June 1, 1979, pp. 22–28.
6. Lebhar, G.M.: *Chain Stores in America 1859–1950.* 1st ed. New York: Chain Store Publishing Corporation, 1952, p. 13.
7. Fletcher, F.M.: *Market Restraints in the Retail Drug Industry.* Philadelphia: University of Pennsylvania Press, 1967, p. 175.
8. Sonnedecker, *op cit.,* p. 271.
9. *Drug Topics' Drug Trade Marketing Guide.* New York, 1961, p. 57.
10. *The Independent Druggist, Report #1.* NARD and Curtis Publishing Company, 1945, p. 64.
11. Deiner, C.H.: The impact of liquor and tobacco sales on community pharmacy operatiuons. *The Kentucky Pharmacist, 48*(4):125, 126, 1985.
12. *Old Dearborn Co. v. Seagram Corp.* 299 U.S. 183, 1936.
13. *Schwegman Bros. v. Calvert Distillers.* 341 U.S. 384, 1951.
14. Nolen, H.C., and Maynard, H.H.: *Drug Store Management.* New York: McGraw-Hill Book Co., 1941, p. 7.

REVIEW

1. Explain why pharmacy and medicine did not begin as separate professions.

2. What were the regulations of the edict of Frederick II?

3. Identify the three socioeconomic factors that deterred the early development of pharmacy in both England and the United States.

4. What were the two pre-Revolutionary War factors and the one post-Revolutionary War factor that promoted the principle of self-medication in the United States?

5. Discuss the influence of the Revolutionary War on the development of pharmacy, and name the two important men involved.

6. Describe the three classes of drug vendors and their manner of competing for the drug business during the early history of this country.

7. Discuss the effects of the Civil War on the practice of pharmacy.

8. Discuss the three major professional developments in pharmacy during the early part of the nineteenth century.

9. Discuss in detail how each of the following deterred the professionalization of pharmacy: demise of the general store; competition and diversification; the soda fountain; inadequate regulations; prohibition; fair trade laws; and *laissez faire*.

10. Discuss the positive effects, if any, of the seven factors enumerated in Question 9.

11. Describe the economic impact of the early drugstore chains and the pine-board drugstores in pharmacy.

12. Contrast and explain the social and legal theories or bases of the fair trade laws.

2 | Social Perspective: Pharmacy Roles

In order for any profession or occupational group to be fully successful, there must be general congruency between the expectations of the group and the expectations of the rest of society. When there is a consensus of these expectations, they become the social norm. In this manner, social order and a degree of social stability are maintained. These expectations or norms develop over a long period of time as a culture develops from a tribal society into a complex social organization, a developed society. This social process is dynamic, even after attaining a high level of maturity, with social norms and boundaries ever shifting. New institutions, social groups and roles emerge while older ones become extinct.

Social Roles

The concept of social roles is one of great utility. Banton in his comprehensive treatment of social roles stated: "The role concept is one of great generality. It is one of the very few concepts that can help in the analysis of any kind of conscious behavior and is of potential utility to psychologists, sociologists, and anthropologists."[1] Banton then defines *role* "as a set of rights and obligations, that is, as an abstraction to which the behavior of people will conform in varying degree."[1] Social scientists have not, over the years, agreed upon one simple definition of roles because the concept of role has evolved from two other social concepts, status and position. It is beyond the scope of this text to trace the changes in the definitions of the various related terms or to unravel conflicting points of view. It is useful, however, to dissect the definition into three complementary components and then to restate the definition. It is generally agreed that behavior can be related to a social position (not necessarily a job or work position) in a social structure, and that actual behavior can be related to the individual's own ideas of what is appropriate *(role cognition)*, or to other people's ideas about what he *will* do (*expectations*), or to other people's ideas about what he *should* do *(norms)*. Thus, social role may be defined as a set of *norms, expectations,* and *rights* applied to the incumbent of a particular *social position.*

There are two major classes of roles, ascribed and achieved. *Ascribed* roles are those roles that are bestowed upon an individual, often at birth, e.g., sex, babyhood, prince and others. *Achieved* roles are those roles that are earned. In primitive societies, most roles were based on sex, age and kinship. In modern day societies, social roles are structured as complex systems with many new criteria for distributing roles, especially earned roles. It is not uncommon for a pharmacy student, for example, to occupy many roles, several of each class: male or female, young adulthood, and possibly majority age, student, spouse, parenthood, employee, leader as a class president, sick role, and the list is not exhaustive. Every social transaction (or interaction) involves a pair of roles, each one different from the other but not necessarily so.

ROLE STRAIN

Early theory of social roles postulated that social stability was based on the normative, consensual commitment of the individuals of the society and the integration of the norms held by those individuals into their daily life.[2,3] Goode, in 1960, developed the notion that role strain, i.e., the difficulty of fulfilling the demands of various roles, is the norm and that an individual organizes his own system (or set) of roles through the process of bargaining with those with whom he has social relationships. The individual does this in order to minimize role strain and to achieve the greatest long-term, net benefit from those relationships.[3] There are, of course, constraints provided by institutions, social norms and economics, which constitutes the social-economic context for all behavior. Thus Goode's theory of role strain provided us with a practical view of role theory, which generally is consistent with our ordinary view of society and with the basic foundation of Parson's general social theory of action systems.[4]

Most of the earliest studies of professional roles were predicated on the structural-functional model of social theory, and on either Hughes' personality-type approach to the theory of occupations,[5] or Greenwood's attribute theory of professions,[6] or a combination of these.

Studies of Pharmacy Roles

Thorner, in 1942, applied the social role concept to pharmacy in one of the earliest social studies of pharmacy.[7] Other early studies of roles in pharmacy focused on various aspects of the profession:

1. "students' disenchantment as they progress through college and their reluctance to enter the role of retail practice;"[8]

2. students' perception of pharmacy which the researcher labeled the "druggist's dilemma" of entering a "marginal occupation;"[9]
3. an analysis of pharmacists' roles and major efforts of the A Ph A to professionalize the occupation;[10]
4. how pharmacists facing potential role conflict adjust to structured occupational role strain,"[11] and;
5. whether the occupational role structure of pharmacy and the resulting role strain of pharmacists can explain their deviant behavior of violations of pharmacy regulation.[12]

All of these studies addressed the same perceived problem in pharmacy—two divergent roles, one professional and the other business.

Denzin and Mettlin[13] patterned their research of pharmacy roles after the Hughesian approach to occupations and Greenwood's attribute theory of professions, but they departed from the structure—functionalists' notion of the homogeneity of professional groups. They cited pharmacy's lack of control over the social object, drugs, as one of its major failings.

Harvey's research on pharmacy roles[14] was guided by Rosenberg's work value orientation theory[15] as the underlying factor on which people make vocational choices. Harvey used a set of 12 items to evaluate 4 types of work value orientation, 3 items per type. The types were (1) extrinsic (importance of salary and regular hours, job security, and prestige); (2) intrinsic (importance of utilizing knowledge, science based career, and freedom from close supervision); (3) people-oriented (a career that is beneficial to people and society, association with colleagues with similar interests, and opportunity to meet the public) and (4) a realistic or test characteristic (involving merchandising, competition, and both a profession and a commercial business). He found that Canadian pharmacists clustered, into two primary groups, people–intrinsic—50 percent; realistic–extrinsic—41 percent, and a minority group of other combinations—9 percent. Harvey demonstrated that pharmacy is composed of diverse groups matching the diverse nature of pharmacy with potential role conflict for certain groups in certain work settings.

Quinney found evidence of role conflict among the pharmacists he studied.[11] *Role Conflict* is defined as a subjective, uncomfortable feeling an individual experiences when faced with the performance of two, or more, divergent roles simultaneously. The uncomfortable feeling may be experienced on a scale of none, very little, some/moderate, or very much/extreme. People can and do learn to adapt to or cope with role conflict. He developed two scales, one which measured professional orientation and the second which measured business orientation. He found that pharmacists may be classified into four groups: (1) high professional; (2) high business, (3) high professional and business (a dual group) and (4) low business and professional (an indifferent group). He also found that role conflict was most prevalent among the professional group and least prevalent among the business oriented group.

RECENT RESEARCH OF PHARMACY ROLES

More recent research on pharmacy roles focused more on challenging accepted models and theory of the professional role, providing data to either validate or alter the accepted theory and models in the case of pharmacy.[16–19] Kronus, who built on both Quinney[11] and Harvey's[14] research, examined the validity of the traditional model which posited business and profession in two distinct social institutions with very different and opposing attributes. Kronus found the model to be invalid and that "pharmacists regardless of role orientation were similarly motivated by service and income values."[16] Ironically, pharmacists in business settings expressed more altruism, whereas those in hospitals and clinic settings put more importance on income and prestige.

Kronus also studied the differential influence of professional/occupational characteristics (role orientation and professional activity) and organizational characteristics (work setting with its attending political hierarchy/power structure) on pharmacists' preference of significant others to evaluate their work performance.[17] Kronus found the work setting to be the better predictor of pharmacists' choice. Hospital pharmacists chose physicians; neighborhood (independent) pharmacists chose colleagues, and chain pharmacists chose clients. Again, the professional model was not validated in the case of pharmacy; the situational model (work setting and its characteristics) explained pharmacists' preference for the respective reference group—colleagues, physicians or clients.

Chappell and Barnes continued in the fashion of Kronus in their search for an "understanding of the factors which affect (the) co-existence" of the two roles in pharmacy.[18] Specifically, the focus was on the relationship of role orientation and work setting, and on role orientation and practice behaviors. The authors stated: "The findings point to their lack of correlation (i.e., the two roles) and therefore their possible but not necessary co-existence." The lack of correlation indicated an independence between the two role orientations and thus the absence of a negative interrelationship between the two. They also found that work setting and position were good predictors of role orientation even after controlling for various demographic and work characteristics other than setting. Also owners and managers were more likely to score high on both role orientation scales compared to employees. High professional orientation scores correlated with professional practice indicators.

Another more recent research on role orientation, conflict and career satisfaction among pharmacists and students by Smith, et al.[19] confirmed much of the results of Quinney,[11] Kronus,[16] and Chappell and Barnes.[18] Role typologies from the four studies were summarized in Table 2–1.

SUMMARY OF RECENT STUDIES

The data in Table 2–1 portray a consistent pattern of responses with only two significant differences among the six comparisons of role typologies among the four pharmacist groups: Quinney study versus Smith et al. study and Quinney study versus Chappell and Barnes study. Both comparisons involve the study by Quinney whose sample was skewed toward dual orientation and away from professional orientation because of a special require-

Table 2–1.   Comparison of Role Typlogies in Four Studies

		PERCENTAGE DISTRIBUTION			
Study	*N*	*Business*[a] *Orientation*	*Dual*[b] *Orientation*	*Professional*[c] *Orientation*	*Indifferent*[d] *Orientation*
Quinney	80	20	45	16	19
Kronus	53	23	36	21	21
Chappell & Barnes	299	16	30	36	18
Smith et al.					
Pharmacists	105	14	37	37	12
Students	169	11	54	25	10

[a]High business and low professional score.
[b]High business and high professional score.
[c]Low business and high professional score.
[d]Low business and low professional score.

ment of the research design. The typologies of the students and pharmacists in the Smith study are also significantly different.

Role conflict and career satisfaction data from Quinney and Smith et al. studies were tabulated in Table 2–2. Role conflict and career satisfaction responses were tabulated for each class of role orientation typologies of the two pharmacist groups and one student group.

The career satisfaction responses of pharmacists in the two studies are similar except those pharmacists with indifferent role orientation, who are significantly different. The difference in the overall distribution of responses is not significant. However, more students expressed satisfaction with pharmacy than pharmacists in either study.

Role conflict responses for the two groups of pharmacists again are remarkably similar except for those pharmacists with dual role orientation, who are significantly different. Pharmacists in the two studies with other role orientations do not differ significantly in their role conflict responses. Pharmacists and students who are oriented toward either the professional or the indifferent posture and are more likely to express role conflict with pharmacists being more prone to do so. Role orientation influences the pattern of role conflict response for both pharmacists and students, and role orientation affects pharmacists' career satisfaction responses, but not students to any significant degree.

IMPLICATIONS OF DUAL ROLES

The scores on the business and professional scales are not correlated either positively or negatively. This means that the sentiments behind the scores are compatible in the case of pharmacists. That is why there are many pharmacists and students in the dual orientation group in Table 2–1. It is the largest group for three of the five groups, and equally as large in a fourth group.

Table 2–2. Role Conflict and Career Satisfaction by Role Typology for Three Groups

PERCENTAGE DISTRIBUTION

Group	N	Business Orientation[a]		Dual Orientation[b]		Professional Orientation[c]		Indifferent Orientation[d]	
		Satisfaction	*Conflict*	*Satisfaction*	*Conflict*	*Satisfaction*	*Conflict*	*Satisfaction*	*Conflict*
Quinney[11]									
Pharmacists	80	30	25	70	64	76	77	40	60
Smith[19]									
Pharmacists	105	31	26	68	29	64	84	18	66
Students	169	94	26	87	38	92	65	86	53

[a]High business and low professional score.
[b]High business and high professional score.
[c]Low business and high professional score.
[d]Low business and low professional score.

Pharmacists in all types of practice settings—independent and chain community pharmacies, hospitals and other types of pharmacy related work settings—are highly oriented toward professional practice and, except for pharmacists in nonpractice work settings, there is no significant difference among the groups. This is not true in the case of business orientation. All of the above groups have significantly different business orientation scores except independent versus chain pharmacists. The rank order for the groups is as follows: independent, chain, other, and hospital pharmacists with the lowest mean business score.

Career satisfaction is more prevalent for those pharmacists with either a dual or professional orientation; however, 30 percent or more pharmacists with a business orientation express satisfaction with their careers. Presently, we do not know whether the students in the study have maintained their high level of career satisfaction. We do know that a significantly greater percentage of BS students expressed satisfaction with pharmacy than PharmD students in one study.[19]

Career satisfaction among pharmacists appears to vary according to the setting where they work, but the evidence is not conclusive. The rank order of groups of pharmacists expressing satisfaction with their career is as follows: other, hospital, independent and chain in the Smith et al. study.[19] Other studies have provided similar results although not always in the same order. Career satisfaction and role conflict are not strongly associated; thus role conflict does not generally lead to dissatisfaction with one's career.

Both pharmacists and students with either a business or dual role orientation are less likely to express subjective role conflict. Students are less likely to express role conflict compared to pharmacists, which may reflect the fact they have been less exposed to the real world and thus have not developed the sentiment. PharmD students are more prone to express role conflict than BS students, and this tendency holds for pharmacists. Also, more hospital pharmacists are likely to express role conflict than either independent or chain pharmacists.

The available data indicate that pharmacists are a diverse group of people with varying role orientations and work values, but they are an adaptable group. The data also indicate that pharmacists should not be classified as *either* professional *or* business, but rather they are more likely to accommodate to a dual orientation or a professional orientation with smaller numbers oriented to business or be indifferent. Since either a business or dual orientation is less likely to be associated with role conflict and a dual or professional orientation is more likely to be associated with career satisfaction, it follows that the socializing of students during college should focus on a dual orientation. Professionalism should be emphasized also to maximize satisfaction and to elevate the profession. However, a business orientation and skills are necessary to be successful as an autonomous professional and to minimize role conflict as well.

THE "CLINICAL ROLE"

During the past two decades, the concept of clinical pharmacy has developed to the point that a Section of Clinical Instruction has been recognized within the American Association of Colleges of Pharmacy. The origin and development of clinical pharmacy has been traced by Smith[20] and Gloria Francke.[21] Although the movement is fairly recent, the famous pharmacy educator John C. Krantz alluded to it in 1921.[22]

Clinical pharmacy has become a vigorous force in pharmacy education and practice, but it is not a panacea. It is ubiquitous but ill defined. Although considerable effort has been exerted, especially by members of the American College of Clinical Pharmacy, to make clinical pharmacy a practice speciality, other pharmacy organizations have resisted these efforts successfully so far. Clinical pharmacy does not meet all of the criteria of a practice speciality set forth by the APhA Board of Specialties primarily because of its general and ubiquitous nature.

Although pharmacists frequently refer to the clinical role, it does not at this time meet the criteria of a social role. It has not been firmly institutionalized into society as a separate social role. Perhaps it is best characterized as an enrichment of the professional role.

The primary problem that clinical pharmacy, and its proponents, face is the establishment of a system or method by which pharmacists may be compensated directly for their clinical services. There are only two examples of direct payment for clinical pharmacy services that are generally applicable, viz., pharmacokinetic dosing with consultation and general clinical consultation to extended care facilities. In all other cases, the pharmacist is paid a salary by an organization, usually a hospital, that can justify the salary as a part of its operating costs (as a teaching or service function), or the pharmacist is paid indirectly through the concomitant sale of a product, a drug or a device. This latter practice should not be a deterrance to the delivery of clinical services since this mode of payment is consistent with the tradition of pharmacy.

However, the practice of concomitant sale of product and service does require the pursuit of that tradition, an activity that many "clinical" pharmacists seem reluctant to pursue. Why this reluctance persists is indeed puzzling to many pharmacists, but apparently it reflects a perplexity for "clinical" pharmacists. If pharmacists fully understood social roles as these are structured within pharmacy as an occupation, they probably would have less difficulty seeing the function of clinical pharmacy as an enrichment of the professional role which, in turn, is fully compatible with the business role. Furthermore, they would be able to see that as an entrepreneur, or quasi-entrepreneur, the "clinical" pharmacist will be compensated proportionally and almost directly for the clinical services he renders. It would be beneficial to society, pharmacy in general, and individual pharmacists specifically, if pharmacists would pursue combined clinically enriched professional and entrepreneur-business roles.

The public has indicated through several surveys their desire for more information and services of a clinical nature, and also their willingness to pay for these services. There simply is not any mechanism currently available that will facilitate such transactions without the transfer of a product and only then through continuing patronage. However, there have been few cases reported of pharmacists' charging the patient for substantial consultation on a fee-for-service basis. One pharmacist, Paul Cesarz, reported that he charged $4.50 to $5.00 for a consultation in his pharmacy and $25.00 for a home visit consultation.[23] The consultations took five to ten minutes, and Mr. Cesarz reported he has two or three consultations a day.

THE ENTREPRENEURIAL ROLE

The entrepreneurial role does not exist external to the business role. An entrepreneur is a person who organizes, operates and assumes the risk of a business enterprise. The emphasis is on the risk-taking function when one thinks of the entrepreneur. The manager or administrator performs business functions without necessarily assuming risk of capital. They, especially the manager, assume risk of a different nature, i.e., assume responsibilities for which his reputation and future are at stake.

The entrepreneur is one of the primary reasons the free enterprise systems of the Western economies are different and prosper in comparison to other centrally controlled economies. It is the free enterprise system that nourishes pharmacy as an ancillary (to medicine) yet essentially autonomous (independent of medicine) profession. The amount of required capital and the attending risk may seem to be unsurmountable, but this need not be the case. There are means by which innovative and enterprising pharmacists may finance their own practice. These are dealt with in considerable detail in the chapter on capital planning.

Traits and Model of an Entrepreneur. The greatest challenge facing pharmacists today is the proper blending of diverse talents into a professional-business role. These talents include professional and scientific knowledge, human relations and communication skills, and entrepreneural-managerial knowledge and skills. Lack of any one of these three basic sets of skills is a severe handicap for the aspiring pharmacist-entrepreneur.

The pharmaceutical education should have provided the necessary professional and scientific knowledge. The human relations and communication component is a new addition to the pharmacy curriculum. These should be vigorously pursued; however, these skills can be cultivated and improved through diligent application. Entrepreneural-managerial knowledge and skills may be attained, beginning with appropriate courses in pharmacy management and extending the training through the externship or internship, including a few years of practice with a good mentor.

arch has provided us with a model for a successful small business eneurship. Although the five basic traits of the model may not be the

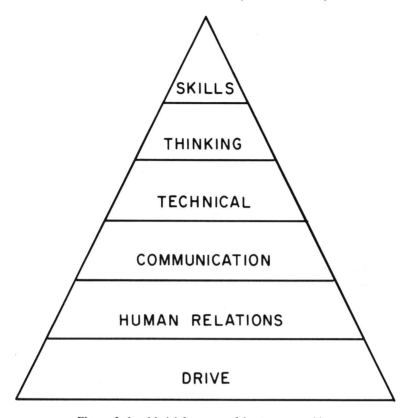

Figure 2–1.   Model for successful entrepreneurship.

only traits involved in a successful enterprise, they are essential. These traits, drive, thinking ability, human relations ability, communication ability, and technical ability, may be organized into a hierarchy from the most innate to those most subject to development through education. This scheme is shown in Figure 2.1

Drive is an inherent trait that cannot be readily acquired. It may be further characterized by initiative, persistence, vigor, and willingness to accept responsibility. One should not rely on himself alone to evaluate himself on this trait or on any of the other four traits of the success model.

Human relations ability can be cultivated, but again the innate personality of the individual plays an important role. Good human relations ability is composed of several elements including ascendency, without being overbearing, emotional stability, cooperation, consideration, cheerfulness, and tactfulness.

Communication ability is a trait that definitely can be cultivated and improved. A college education should provide both written and verbal skills to all graduates; however, this facet of education, along with problem-solving, is one of the greatest weaknesses in pharmaceutical education.

Technical ability can be acquired and is the one characteristic that all recent pharmacy graduates should have in abundance. Indeed, it has been stated that pharmacists are overtrained or overeducated, especially in the sciences. Of course, this point is subject to debate. However, it is doubtful whether pharmaceutical curricula provide *all* the necessary educational tools for the managerial or administrative challenges of managing a successful pharmacy in the highly competitive market of today.

Thinking ability can be developed, but of course it is limited by the person's innate capacity. Thinking ability can take several forms—creative, original, critical, and analytical—all of which are important. Perhaps the most important in pharmacy management is analytical thinking. That is why problem-solving and case study should be incorporated into the pharmaceutical curriculum.

According to authorities in the field of management and administration there is not a unique set of characteristics that will identify a successful executive in a large firm. However, this fact does not negate the success model concept for small business entrepreneurs.

The Small Business Administration has developed a "Check-list for Going into Business" under the general title of *Small Marketers Aids No. 71.* It is available free from any of the field offices or the headquarters in Washington, D.C.

Summary

Social roles are useful in understanding the nature of a profession, especially one such as pharmacy. Recent research has demonstrated that, in the case of pharmacy, professional and business roles are compatible. It follows that the "clinical role" and the "entrepreneurial" role are also compatible since the former is an extension of the professional role and the latter an extension of the business role. Since it is not only possible but expedient to have a dual orientation, this posture will serve the student well and provide him or her with a wider range of practice options, which will maximize the ability to deliver clinical services and secure satisfaction, self-fulfillment and high income.

REFERENCES

1. Banton, M.: *Roles: an Introduction to the Study of Social Forces.* New York: Basic Books, Inc., 1965.
2. Linton, R.: *The Study of Man.* New York: Appleton-Century, 1936.
3. Goode, W.J.: A theory of role strain. *Am. Soc. Rev., 25*:483–96, 1960.
4. Parsons, T.: *The Social System.* Glencoe, ILL: The Free Press, 1951, pp. 168, 180.
5. Hughes, E.C.: Personality types and the division of labor. *Am. J. Soc., 33*:754–68, 1928, and *Men and their Work.* Glencoe, ILL: The Free Press, 1953.
6. Greenwood, E.: Attributes of a profession. *Social Work, 2*:45–55, 1957.
7. Thorner, I.: Pharmacy: The functional significance of an institutional pattern. *Social Forces, 20*:231–38, 1942.

8. Weinlein, A.: Pharmacy as a profession with reference to the State of Wisconsin. Master's Thesis, University of Chicago, 1943.
9. McCormack, T.H.: The druggist's dilemma: problems of a marginal occupation. *Am. J. Soc., 61*:308–15, 1956.
10. Slettin, C.A.: The social structure and idealogy of organized pharmacy. Ph.D. Dissertation, Harvard University, 1959.
11. Quinney, E.R.: Adjustments to occupational role strain: the case of retail pharmacy. *Southwestern Soc. Sci., 44*:367–76, 1964.
12. Quinney, E.R.: Occupational structure and criminal behavior: prescription violation by retail pharmacists. *Soc. Prob., 2*:179–85, 1963.
13. Denzin, N.K., and Mettlin, C.: Incomplete professionalizations: the case of pharmacy. *Soc. Forces, 46*:375–81, 1968.
14. Harvey, E.: Some implications of value differentiation in pharmacy. *Can. Review Soc. Anthrop., 3*:23–37, 1966.
15. Rosenberg, M.: *Occupations and Values.* Glencoe, ILL: The Free Press, 1957, pp. 6, 16–20.
16. Kronus, C.L.: Occupational values, role orientation, and work settings: the case of pharmacy. *Soc. Quart., 16*:171–83, 1975.
17. Kronus, C.L.: Occupational versus organizational influences on reference group identification. *Soc. Work & Occup., 3*:303–30, 1976.
18. Chappell, N.L., and Barnes, G.E.: Professional and business role orientations among practicing pharmacists. *Soc. Sci. Med., 18*:103–110, 1984.
19. Smith, H.A., Branecker, J. and Pence, B.S.: Role orientation, conflict and satisfaction among pharmacists and students. *J. Soc. Adm. Pharm., 3*:18–29, 1985.
20. Smith, H.A., and Swintosky, J.V.: The origin, goals and development of a clinical pharmacy emphasis in pharmacy education and practice. *Am. J. Pharm. Educ., 47*:204–210, 1983.
21. Francke, G.N.: Evolvement of "clinical" pharmacy. *Drug Intell. Clin. Pharm., 3*:348–54, 1969.
22. Griffenhagen, G.B.: Clinical pharmacy = patient involvement, an editorial. *J. Amer. Pharm. Assoc., NS11*:45, 1971.
23. Anon.: Customers at Wisconsin pharmacy pay for R. Ph's counseling service. *Amer. Druggist, 150,* No. 6: 100, June, 1984.

REVIEW

1. What are social roles?

2. Define social role.

3. What are role cognition, expectations, norms and rights?

4. Classify roles and give several examples of each.

5. Describe role strain in the terms Goode used.

6. What is meant by homogeneity of professional groups?

7. Discuss the results of early and more recent research of pharmacy roles. What were the major findings of this research?

8. What is role conflict and how can individuals deal with it?

9. Describe role typology in the case of pharmacy and how do pharmacists classify themselves in respect to role typology?

10. Discuss the implications of dual roles in pharmacy in terms of career satisfaction, role conflict and productivity.

11. Discuss clinical services in terms of social roles and a practice specialty.

12. Discuss entrepreneurship in terms of social roles, especially the business role, the delivery of clinical services and as a means of autonomy.

3

Practice Perspective: Profiles and Opportunities

When speaking of pharmacy practice, traditionally we have meant working in either a community pharmacy (independent or chain) or a hospital pharmacy. This perspective is changing. Before we explore other practice and work options, we should define what we mean by practice. By *practice* we mean pharmacy related work that has a direct impact on the well-being of a patron, patient, client or customer. By direct we mean the impact will be mediated by a direct face to face interaction with the recipient, or through his personal agent, or through a collaborative effort with other persons who are working for the direct benefit of the recipient. By well-being we mean a state of being healthy, happy and prosperous with emphasis on being healthy, but not exclusive of the other characteristics.

Pharmacists' Work Settings

Thus *pharmacy practice* encompasses employment in independent, chain and institutional pharmacies. Institutional practice includes hospitals, extended care facilities (ECFs) with either skilled nursing care or intermediate skill nursing care status, HMOs and other facilities where the expertise of the pharmacist is utilized for the safe and effective use of drugs and health care appliances. See Table 3–1 for a complete summary of work settings.

Approximately 70 percent of working pharmacists practice in community pharmacies—36 percent in independent, another 4 percent in pharmacies located in clinics and medical buildings, and 28 percent in chain pharmacies. Pharmacies located in the clinics and medical buildings are small prescription-oriented pharmacies (sometimes referred to as apothecaries, professional or clinic pharmacies) that are most often owned and operated by independent

34

Table 3–1. Distribution of Pharmacists by Work Setting, 1983

Work Setting	No.	Percentage
Independent Community Pharmacy	62,200	36.4
Chain Community Pharmacy	48,400	28.3
Clinic or Medical Building Pharmacy	6,500	3.8
Other Ambulatory Settings	2,600	1.5
Subtotal	119,700	70.1
Private Hospitals	20,400	11.9
Government Hospitals	9,800	5.7
Nursing Homes	2,200	1.3
Subtotal	32,400	19.0
Total Pharmacists in Practice	152,100	89.1
Pharmaceutical Manufacturing	6,650	3.9
Government Agencies	2,260	1.3
Academic Institutions	2,300	1.3
All Other Employed Pharmacists	7,490	4.4
Subtotal	18,700	10.9
All Employed Pharmacists	170,800	100.0
Estimated Inactive Pharmacists	15,200	NA

Source: Primary—Rucker, T.D., Personal Communication, University of Illinois College of Pharmacy, Chicago, IL, May 8, 1985; Secondary—Teaching Information for Management (TIME), The Upjohn Company, Kalamazoo, MI, 1985, NABP Census of Pharmacy for 1983, and Kapantais, G., National Center for Health Statistics, ADVANCEDATA, No. 85, 1982.

pharmacists. Another 19 percent of working pharmacists practice in institutions, mostly in hospitals. This leaves about 11 percent who work in the pharmaceutical industry, academic institutions, government agencies, and various other organizations. Among community pharmacists, approximately 20 percent are sole proprietors, 12 percent are partners, and 68 percent are managers or staff pharmacists.

Pharmacists' Work Activities

In recent years, emphasis has been given to a new orientation and expanded roles as discussed in Chapter 2. However, pharmacy remains very much the same in many respects as it was 20 years ago. Although the modern watchwords for pharmacy are people orientation, clinical services and patient counseling, other functions have to be performed, many of which are managerial in nature. Good management skills are needed for the efficient application of clinical skills.

From two national studies,[1,2] with over 1,500 pharmacists in each, we now know a great deal about pharmacists' work activities. The data were collected by two open-end questions in one study—one for routine activity and one for critical activity.[1] In the second study, the respondents were asked to estimate the percentage of time spent in each of seven categories or dimensions of work.[2] The data from the former study were compiled in Tables 3–2 and 3–3.

MANAGERIAL ACTIVITY

Managerial functions accounted for more than 50 percent of the total routine and critical activity for all three managerial positions. Among pharmacists in staff position, routine managerial activities accounted for 13 to 45 percent of total routine activity, and critical managerial activities accounted for 25 to 41 percent of total critical activity.

Within the routine managerial category of work, community pharmacists were involved more frequently with inventory and financial matters; hospital directors were occupied most frequently with personnel administration, and hospital staff pharmacists were involved more frequently with inventory and purchasing activity.

Within the critical managerial category of work, proprietors were occupied most frequently by sales and promotion activities (which included important public relations activities) followed closely by general management functions. Both chain managers and hospital pharmacy directors were engaged most frequently in personnel administration followed by general managerial functions. Staff pharmacists were less involved with critical management activities although a significant level of effort was exerted in several of these areas, notably general management, personnel, inventory and sales—excluding inventory in the case of hospital staff pharmacists.

PROFESSIONAL ACTIVITY

Among routine professional and technical work, traditional services occupied pharmacists the most in all positions and settings—with staff pharmacists reporting a higher percentage than their management counterparts. Patient care activities were second in frequency for each position and setting.

Turning now to critical professional and technical functions, patient care activities were most frequently reported by community pharmacists by a margin of approximately 2 to 1 compared to traditional services. For hospital pharmacists, the inverse relationship existed. It should be indicated at this point that those pharmacists who labeled themselves as clinical pharmacists were not tabulated as hospital pharmacists but as clinical pharmacists. Most of these pharmacists indicated their primary employer and affiliation were academic institutions. Personal and professional development, and miscellaneous activities made up the remainder of professional and technical activity classification.

Table 3–2. Distribution of Percentages of Routine Activity of Pharmacists by Setting and Position*

	Independents		Chains		Hospitals	
Activities	*Prop.*	*Staff*	*Manager*	*Staff*	*Director*	*Staff*
ADMINISTRATIVE						
General Management[a]	6	2	8	1	12	2
Personnel[b]	7	4	12	4	23	2
Finance[c]	20	12	14	11	5	2
Inventory[d]	18	18	15	20	10	6
Sales/Promotion[e]	8	7	7	5	NA	NA
Miscellaneous[f]	1	2	*	2	8[k]	*
SUBTOTAL	60	45	56	43	57	13
PROFESSIONAL/TECHNICAL						
Patient Care[g]	16	22	16	18	6	10
Traditional[h]	21	27	23	31	28	71
Professional/Personal Development[i]	1	1	1	1	4	4
Miscellaneous[j]	2	5	4	7	5	3
SUBTOTAL	40	55	44	57	43	87
GRAND TOTAL	100	100	100	100	100	100

Source: Smith, H.A., Reference 1, pp. 210–22

*Percentages were rounded to nearest 1%; subtotals were calculated individually by division and may not be equal to the corresponding sum of percentages. Also * in Table denotes less than 0.5%. Percentages represent the frequency an activity was listed. Data were collected by two open-end questions.

[a]General management includes management, unspecified, planning, organizing, coordinating, directing, decision making, problem solving, reviewing and evaluating, writing reports, writing or revising policies and procedures.

[b]Personnel administration includes recruiting, interviewing, selecting and hiring personnel; orienting and training; scheduling, supervising, motivating and developing, and evaluating and paying personnel.

[c]Finance includes making and managing budgets, monitoring cash flow and expenses, record keeping and third-party billing, managing accounts receivable, calculating and making payrolls, monitoring and changing prices and developing pricing strategies.

[d]Inventory includes all activities associated with purchasing, stock management, and inventory control.

[e]Sales and promotion include advertising design and implementation, displaying, merchandising generally, handling complaints, serving patron/customers and public relations.

[f]Miscellaneous includes the other unclassified managerial activities.

[g]Patient care includes counseling with patients and patrons, consulting with prescribers, recommending O-T-C drugs and Rx accessories, and consulting with nursing home personnel/patients.

[h]Traditional services include dispensing prescriptions, compounding prescriptions, calling prescriber re: refills, answering routine questions, and maintaining patient medication profiles.

[i]Professional/Personal development includes "keeping up," reading journals, continuing education, precepting externs/interns, providing health information, and participating in screening programs.

[j]Miscellaneous includes other unclassified professional or technical activity.

[k]The 8 percent represents administration of clinical programs, both service and teaching, with the specific functions and activities paralleling general administration.

Table 3–3.   Distribution of Percentages of Critical Activity of Pharmacists by Setting and Position*

Activities	Independents		Chains		Hospitals	
	Prop.	*Staff*	*Manager*	*Staff*	*Director*	*Staff*
ADMINISTRATIVE						
General Management[a]	14	8	11	5	15	9
Personnel[b]	11	8	20	8	19	5
Finance[c]	10	3	2	2	6	1
Inventory[d]	8	7	8	8	7	2
Sales/Promotion[e]	16	7	8	11	NA	NA
Miscellaneous[f]	7	5	7	8	5	8
SUBTOTAL	68	38	56	41	52	25
PROFESSIONAL/TECHNICAL						
Patient Care[g]	20	42	24	32	10	26
Traditional[h]	11	13	13	15	31	40
Professional/Personal Development[i]	*	8	6	12	6	10
Miscellaneous[j]	*	*	*	*	1	*
SUBTOTAL	32	62	44	59	48	75
GRAND TOTAL	100	100	100	100	100	100

Source: Smith, H.A., Reference 1, pp. 244–59.

*Percentages were rounded to nearest 1%; subtotals were calculated individually by division and may not be equal to the corresponding sum of percentages. Also * in Table denotes less than 0.5%. Percentages represent the frequency an activity was listed. Data were collected by two open-end questions.

For Footnotes a–j see footnotes a–j to Table 3–2.

COMPARISON OF TWO STUDIES

The studies are not directly comparable because the categories of activity do not match very well. The categories in the Smith study[1] were derived from responses to open-end questions, whereas the categories in the other study[2] were structured within the questionnaire. To have some idea of the correlation between frequency of performance and estimated time spent in the performance of broad categories of work, the data were collapsed into four functional categories: managerial activity of all types, patient care, traditional services (assuming this roughly matched prescription procedures), and all other activity. The percentages of activities were averaged across all practice groups for the Smith study. The data were compared in Table 3–4.

Table 3–4. Comparison of Percentages of Activity[a] in Broad Work Categories in Two National Studies

	Study	
Category of Activity	*Smith*	*APhA—AACP*
Managerial	45	33
Patient Care	15	12
Traditional/Rx Processing	34	47
All Other	6	8
TOTAL	100	100

Source: Smith study, Reference 1; APhA—AACP study, Reference 2.

[a]Percent of frequency of performance of routine activity in the Smith study; estimated percent of time spent in the APhA—AACP study.

Institutional Characteristics of Practice Settings

The characteristics of various types of practice settings will be discussed in terms of general characteristics, advantages and disadvantages.

TRADITIONAL INDEPENDENT PHARMACIES

These pharmacies are the ones that most often come to mind when community pharmacy is mentioned. By convention independent means that no more than three pharmacies are owned and operated by one person or company. By traditional is meant the pharmacy occupies 1,000 sq. ft. or more up to about 7,500 sq. ft., and stock, in addition to prescription drugs, nonprescription (O-T-C) drugs, prescription accessories, health care aids and appliances, toiletries and cosmetics, magazines, cards, writing materials, candy and confections, tobacco and smoking accessories, and other small convenient goods. The propriety of pharmacists' selling tobacco, a health hazard, is one of the current issues pharmacists must deal with.

Some pharmacies specialize in one or more of the following: gifts and party accessories, pet and veterinary drugs and supplies, hypoallergenic cosmetics, a wide variety of health care aids and appliances including the fitting and other special services, and other speciality goods, for example paintings by a local artist. Some pharmacists in this type of setting provide a range of clinical services such as monitoring blood pressure, blood glucose levels in addition to monitoring drug utilization and interactions.

The typical traditional community will occupy 2,500 to 3,500 sq. ft., have $500,000 annual sales of which 50 to 70 percent is prescription sales, dispense 25,000 to 30,000 prescriptions annually, maintain $70,000 to $80,000 of inventory, stay open 60 hours per week, employ two pharmacists including the proprietor or manager, and net $15,000 in profit on a $100,000 investment, if the proprietor is a reasonably good manager.[3] A $20,000 net profit on such an investment exemplifies a high level of management expertise. The total income of the proprietor-pharmacist could be expected to be in the $45,000

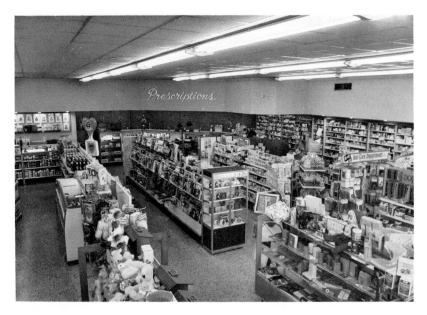

Figure 3–1. Traditional pharmacy: Gardenside Pharmacy, Gardenside Plaza, Lexington, Kentucky.

to $50,000 range before deducting income and social security taxes. See Figure 3–1.

Advantages. If the typical independent pharmacy proprietor were asked why he elected to undertake the ownership of a pharmacy, he would probably give the following typical answers: "to be independent," "to be my own boss," or "to make more money." Clearly, the desire to be one's own boss is a striving for independence, which is one of America's greatest heritages. Whether or not the typical independent pharmacy owner has a true insight into his basic motivations, it is a fact that he elected the course of action as a way of life because of the perceived advantages that appealed to him, such as: (1) being your own boss; (2) doing things the way you like to do them; (3) being secure and independent of the dictates of others; (4) being recognized in the community and playing an important role in its life; and (5) achieving the ego reinforcement motivations of personal pride, status, and self-fulfillment. It is noteworthy that these appeals are primarily emotional in nature, reflecting a basic attitude acquired from the cultural and social background and personal experiences.

The young pharmacist or potential pharmacy owner should be aware of the true nature of these five advantages. Being one's own boss is not absolute freedom. In fact, each patron or patient is "boss" in a real sense. The pharmacist must satisfy the patient's needs and desires, first to attract his patronage, and second to merit continuing patronage. Also "to be the boss" requires a great deal of responsibility and concern, not only with respect to the public, but especially for employees.

If, in fact, a young pharmacist, as a potential pharmacy proprietor, is properly motivated in his desire to "do things the way he thinks they should be done," this is one of the most laudable reasons for undertaking the independent proprietorship of a pharmacy. Certainly, pharmacists should not be encumbered by overpowering commercial interest in making professional decisions. This is one of the fundamental ways pharmacy, with its professional considerations, differs from ordinary small businesses. Similarly, the same thing applies to being independent from the dictates of others. Security in the professional context is a combination of independent discretion and economic and psychologic security. A professional pharmacist feels the need for all three.

The fourth advantage is not restricted to independent pharmacy proprietors, but can be attained by a manager of a chain pharmacy, provided he remains in one community for a sufficient length of time. Also, he must be motivated to seek a significant role in the community. This advantage accrues to an independent pharmacist more readily because of his greater visibility usually, and because the community benefits from the local retention of the profits.

The fifth advantage or appeal is probably the most powerful for most pharmacists. Historically, status and prestige are inherent characteristics reserved primarily for the pharmacist-proprietor in the American pharmacy tradition. This is particularly true in the smaller cities and rural towns. Also, the profit and salary of the independent pharmacy proprietor are considerably more, on the average, than the salary and the bonus of the manager of a chain drugstore, approximately 50 percent more based on *Lilly Digest* data.

Disadvantages. The first disadvantage encountered by the independent pharmacy proprietor is that he is not so independent after all. In fact, he will discover that everyone, in a sense, is his "boss." In other words, some of his ideas may have to be subordinated to those of others. This extends not only to patrons, but also to the banker, the suppliers, the physicians, and others. For example, if a note is due at the bank, the banker may well offer some suggestions, or even make demands, before the renewal of the note, which may affect the manner in which the owner operates the pharmacy. This could also apply to suppliers who may have sold him the opening inventory on credit. It is obvious that the pharmacist and the physician must have professional working relations to function for the maximum benefit to society and each other, and this need not require a simple "yes man" attitude by the pharmacist.

The second disadvantage of ownership is the inherent responsibility and liability. The pharmacist-proprietor must be willing to assume full financial, professional, and legal responsibilities for the entire operation of the pharmacy. This particularly is true of the sole proprietorship. In this regard, the new pharmacy proprietor may have to deprive himself, and his family, during the formative years of the practice until he can develop the practice into a profitable one. This may require several years, depending on the location, type of pharmacy, and managerial ability of the pharmacist-proprietor.

Another obvious disadvantage consists in the long hours and work week during the formative years of the practice. This can be avoided in two basic ways. First, if the pharmacist selects an excellent location and has sufficient capital to begin a going practice, he may be able to employ the second pharmacist soon after beginning his practice. Second, he may form a group practice with other pharmacist(s) with the understanding that each may supplement his income by part-time practice in another pharmacy in another market.

Another disadvantage of independent ownership, and one about which pharmacists frequently complain, is the amount of paper work required. This complaint is exaggerated in the opinion of some. The reasons for the seemingly great burden of paper work are the failure to formalize business and professional procedures, develop good routines, and delegate as much as is feasible and consistent with good professional practice. Adequate records are required to chart the course of an enterprise and analyze its progress, and executed properly, the paperwork is an advantage, not a disadvantage.

In addition to traditional community pharmacies, there is a type of pharmacy that is known by several names—apothecaries, professional pharmacies, prescription pharmacies, clinical or medical building pharmacies. We have chosen prescription pharmacies as the name because it is general in its connotation and does not imply other pharmacies are not professional.

PRESCRIPTION PHARMACIES

This group of pharmacies is generally understood to be a part of the family of independent pharmacy although chain pharmacy firms do own and operate this type of pharmacies. Indeed, there are chain drug firms that operate only this type of pharmacies. These pharmacies generally occupy less than 1,000 sq. ft., stock mostly drugs and health related products, with hypoallergenic cosmetics and toiletries and a few convenient goods frequently stocked as a part of the inventory. Prescription sales constitute 75 percent or more of total sales. These pharmacies often are located in medical clinics or buildings and thus the term ''clinic pharmacy'' is often applied to this subgroup of pharmacies. However, this type of pharmacy may be found in all types of locations, but the pharmacy should be located where it will be convenient and attractive for patrons with prescriptions to patronize. Pharmacists practicing in these pharmacies are in a favorable position to offer a high level of clinical services.

The typical professional pharmacy will have $300,000 to $400,000 in annual sales, of which 75 percent or more will be prescription sales; dispense 25,000 to 35,000 prescriptions annually; stay open 50 hours per week; employ two pharmacists including the proprietor-pharmacist, and net $10,000 to $20,000 in profit on an investment of $45,000 to $50,000. The total income

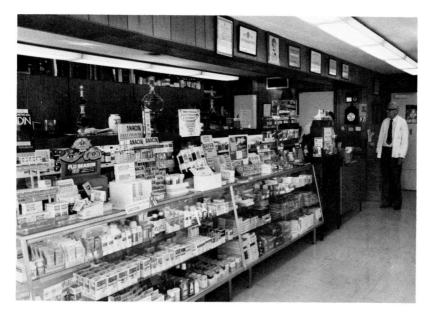

Figure 3–2. Prescription-oriented pharmacy: Hubbard & Curry Pharmacy, Doctors Park, Lexington, Kentucky.

of the proprietor-pharmacist may be in the range of $30,000 to $50,000 before income and social security taxes.[3] See Figure 3–2.

Advantages. The advantages are fairly obvious and include (1) a "professional atmosphere;" (2) lower investment generally; and (3) potentially very profitable for the level of investment.

Disadvantages. The disadvantages are less obvious and include the following: (1) there is a limited number of locations where this type of pharmacy can succeed. Sometimes locations which appear to be well suited for this type of practice turn out not to be so; (2) good locations for this type of practice often require high rent, as much as 10 percent of sales or $20.00 per sq. ft., in some instances; (3) developing a successful practice in these situations often require a longer period of time than in other types of locations and pharmacies; (4) the level of sales and profits is generally limited vis-a-vis other types of locations and practices; and (5) success will require patience and a professional posture with the prescribers while maintaining a "friendly atmosphere" within the pharmacy.

Within the prescription pharmacy group, two fairly recent developments of specialized practices have been developed.

OFFICE PRACTICE/PHARMACEUTICAL CENTER

Some pharmacists, especially younger pharmacists, consider the pharmaceutical center, which was first introduced in 1960, to provide the ideal

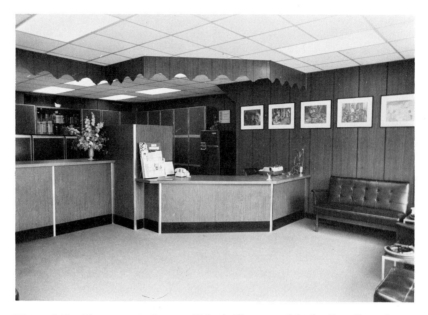

Figure 3–3.   Pharmaceutical center: Baker's Pharmacy, Mt. Sterling, Kentucky.

environment for a highly professional practice. It is estimated that there are now approximately 1,000 pharmaceutical centers, or office practices, in the United States.[4] To be designated as such, the pharmaceutical centers must meet high standards, including the following criteria: (1) no drugs or other products on open display; (2) ample reception area for patients; (3) a patient medication profile system; and (4) the use of a professional fee, either fixed or variable, with appropriate exceptions permissible. The decor of the center is a basic feature also, which causes the center to look more like an office than a traditional pharmacy. See Figure 3–3.

FRANCHISE SYSTEMS

The newest development in pharmaceutical practice is the franchise system involving the entire pharmacy. The idea of a franchise merchandise line, such as Rexall, is old, but the concept of a franchise system has developed within the past two or three decades. It has some of the characteristics of cooperatives, but requires much more stringent controls by the system. There are several organizations offering these systems throughout the country. These franchise systems usually concentrate on prescription services, convalescent/home health care aids, orthopedic appliances, and physicians' supplies.

A typical franchise agreement would include an exclusive use of the franchise name, logo, and trademark within a specified area. The franchisee cannot use any other signs or advertisements except those developed by the franchiser. The total package investment may range from $50,000 to $100,000 and includes approximately 10 percent for launching a promotional program and 20 percent for the franchise license and service fee. The investment is usually financed by the franchiser.

The franchise license and service fee includes assistance in a location evaluation, lease arrangement, setting up the fixtures, equipment and merchandise, and the initial promotional cost. The fee usually includes a management training program to instruct the pharmacist in the management and operating procedures of the system. It may include training in the fitting, servicing, and promotion of the health care equipment and devices.

In some cases, all designated merchandise must be purchased through the system. Usually a computerized accounting system and management assistance are provided routinely. The franchisee-pharmacist usually pays a monthly service fee of 2 to 4 percent of sales for the computerized and managerial assistance. Also, regular promotional and advertising campaigns are furnished, and the franchisee must agree to use a designated percentage of sales for advertising. The pharmacist must participate in a specified percentage of the regional promotional programs. This type of system obviously has inherent strengths, but the question to be answered by a pharmacist contemplating such a venture is whether the cost of the franchise is worth the service received. Additionally, the pharmacist must be willing to forego a considerable degree of independence.

CHAIN PHARMACIES

Whenever chain pharmacies or drugstores are mentioned, a large, highly merchandised enterprise is generally envisioned. This, of course, is not always the case, as indicated in the discussion of prescription pharmacies. Some chain drug firms have developed the strategy of medium size pharmacies with a fairly standardized layout, product mix and promotional strategy in order to maintain a high level of control and operational efficiency. Others have gone to only super drugstores in the 12,000 sq. ft. or more class for all new units. In general, chain pharmacies are much larger with many more departments and variety of merchandise compared to independents. They are highly promoted with advertisements and mass displays, and tend to have lower prices but is not always the case. There are some independent pharmacies that are as large as chain pharmacies, and usually these are vigorously promoted and competitive. See Figure 3–4.

The typical chain pharmacy will occupy 8,000 to 10,000 sq. ft., have annual sales of approximately $2,000,000, of which nearly 25 percent is prescriptions; stay open 80 hours per week; employ three pharmacists, if the manager is a pharmacist; net $100,000 profit on an investment of nearly $300,000 in inventory.[5]

Chain drugstores are classified into four types. The 1983 *NACDS Lilly Digest* sample[5] included the following percentage distribution by type of pharmacies: bantam—25; traditional—45; super—20; supermarket and oth-

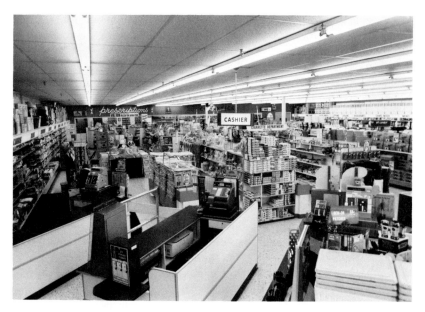

Figure 3–4. Super drugstore: Begley Drug Co., Crossroads Shopping Center, Lexington, Kentucky.

ers—10. The typical *bantam* pharmacy occupies about 5,000 sq. ft.; has annual sales of about $1,250,000, of which prescriptions account for 35 percent; stays open 77 hours per week; employs 2.75 pharmacists including the manager, and nets $54,000 profit on $185,000 inventory investment.[5]

The typical *traditional* chain drugstore occupies 8,500 sq. ft.; has nearly $2,000,000 annual sales, of which about 25 percent is prescriptions; stays open 82 hours per week; employs three pharmacists including the manager, and nets over $90,000 on $275,000 inventory investment.[5]

The typical *super* drugstore occupies 13,000 sq. ft; has annual sales of nearly $3,500,000, of which about 17 percent is prescriptions; stays open 83 hours per week; employs 3.5 pharmacists including the manager, and nets over $200,000 profit on an inventory investment of about $435,000.[5]

The typical *supermarket* with a prescription or pharmacy department occupies about 10,000 sq. ft.; has over $3,000,000 annual sales, of which about 14 percent is prescription sales; the pharmacy stays open 80 hours per week; employs two pharmacists including the pharmacy manager, and nets approximately $225,000 on an inventory investment of approximately $400,000.[5] In all cases, the net profit figure is before income tax is deducted.

Advantages. Some advantages associated with employment in a large organization are: (1) stability of employment and less susceptibility to economic change; (2) fixed hours, paid vacations, insurance, and other fringe benefits; (3) financial strength to carry out the organization's plans; (4) the opportunity to identify and associate with a group; (5) opportunity for advancement in the company with the accompanying status and titles; and (6) opportunity to have anonymity and avoidance of social responsibility to a degree within the community.

Some of these advantages may be partially realized in an independent pharmacy. One of the more recent organizational advancements among independent pharmacists is the establishment of a package of fringe benefits for their employees through an association. These benefits are transferable as long as the employee remains employed by a member of the group. The philosophy has also been extended to group buying, cooperative promotion, preferred provider organization (PPO) and other collective programs. These cooperative efforts provide economic strength to the members of the group along with a measure of the large chain type of security, both psychologic and economic, to the proprietors and their employees.

Disadvantages. The primary disadvantages of employment in a large chain organization are: (1) job insecurity in the sense of frequent transfer, and the resulting lack of sense of permanent local associations and job commitment; (2) receiving blame for certain uncontrollable events; (3) less flexibility in scheduling regular hours and ''time off'' when necessary or desirable; (4) the policies and politics associated with any large organization; and (5) the highly competitive nature of the operation with emphasis on prices.

A brief comment on the first disadvantage is necessary because it may appear to be contradictory. Job security per se should be contrasted with the economic stability of the overall organization. Although the organization can withstand economic changes, even crises, the individual may not feel secure in his job. During an economic recession, a new employee is expendable, but this is not the primary point. The basic point is that the employee must adapt himself to the organization's goals and be productive. Failure to perform as expected may be sufficient reason for dismissal. This should be true in small organizations, but more leniency is practiced in the smaller organizations. Management-by-objectives is the technique designed to avoid this hazard for the benefit of both employee and employer.

Uncontrollable events for which an employee, or especially an employee-manager, may be held accountable are numerous. One example is pilferage by both customers and other employees. This can be controlled to a degree, but complete eradication of this costly crime is not possible with today's methods of merchandise displays and controls. The automatic shipment of goods that will not sell in certain markets is another example. Transfer and re-assignment of personnel are further examples.

Frequency of transfer of personnel, especially management, within a chain organization is a real weakness in establishing loyal patronage on a professional and lasting personal basis. This can, and often does, distract from a complete commitment to the community by pharmacists in a large chain organization; this is not always the case, however. The feeling of anonymity, one among so many others, is a common complaint of our modern-day society. If pharmacists have this feeling themselves, they can hardly transfer a warm, personal, and helpful feeling to the patients and patrons with whom they come in contact. That along with a high volume of prescriptions to dispense may be why there is so little patient consultation provided by some chain pharmacists. However, this fault is found much too frequently among traditional independent pharmacists as well.

Scheduling flexibility need not be a major problem in chain pharmacies, and often it is not. Pharmacists should be aware of company policies and operations in chain pharmacies before accepting a position with a company. Individual needs can be accommodated in most instances with a little effort and ample patience.

It is axiomatic that whenever a sizable group is involved in any activity you will have politics. Conventionally, the term is applied to the activities of government. However, the term is derived from the same root word as "policies" and "polite." Thus, politics will evolve any time a group is formed in which policies are developed and a hierarchy is present. As a general rule, the larger the group, the more likely it is that politics will become a part of the group's activities.

A business firm with a well-defined structure and set of policies has a formal method of controlling activities, making decisions, and achieving goals, which presumably minimizes politics. When efforts are expended to influence decisions, activities, or goals for the benefit of a special group or persons, these efforts are labeled as "politics" in business. Seldom is a business organization of any size free of political activities. This is probably best described by the cliché, "It is not what you know, but who you know." One of the reasons for adopting management-by-objectives is to minimize undesirable politics in business.

The highly competitive posture of most chain pharmacies is well known. The degree of competition varies among chains. Some of the newcomers in the chain drug business have advertised prescriptions at extremely low prices in order to break into a market. Older and established chain drugstores are forced to engage in competitive pricing in order to maintain their market position.

PROFILE OF COMMUNITY PHARMACY

In order to provide a profile or general picture of community pharmacy, three tables were compiled. The first, Table 3–5, is a historic comparison of the number and average sales of independent and chain pharmacies. The second, Table 3–6, shows the distribution of pharmacies by size, i.e., in terms of the number of employees per pharmacy. The third, Table 3–7, shows the distribution of chain pharmacies by size of the firm, i.e., in terms of the number of units per firm.

These tables require little explanation. The growth of chain pharmacies at the expense of independent pharmacies is apparent in Table 3–5. From Table 3–6 it appears that pharmacy is predominantly small businesses with an

Table 3–5. Comparison of Chain and Independent Pharmacies, 1935–1983: Number and Average Sales

	Independents		Chains[a]	
Year	Number	Mean Sales[b]	Number	Mean Sales[b]
1935	52,899	$ 17,285	3,798	$ 83,800
1939	53,723	27,600	4,180	96,200
1948	53,553	53,145	3,402	244,700
1954	44,551	109,000	NA[c]	NA
1958	47,697	106,800	3,751	382,900
1963	45,853	131,700	4,465	477,400
1967	40,902	166,800	5,342	648,600
1972	42,891	204,800	8,651	787,900
1983	33,892	494,600	16,203	1,722,100

Source: Census of Business, several editions, 1940–1972, for years 1940 to 1972; for 1983, *American Druggist, 189* (No. 5): 20; May, 1984.

[a]Chain drugstores of four or more units under same ownership and management.

[b]Mean sales are mean annual sales.

[c]NA denotes data not available.

average of 10 employees per firm. However, independent pharmacies make up practically all of the first two brackets and about 25 percent of the third bracket. About one-half of chain pharmacies are owned by seven firms. The other half is owned by the other 140 firms. There is a considerable amount of concentration in the chain drug industry, which could be exaccerbated by mergers, a growing trend in recent years.

Table 3–6. Distribution of Pharmacies by Number of Employees

Number of Employees	Number of Pharmacies[a]	Percentage[b]
1–4	15,146	30.6
5–9	14,987	30.3
10–19	13,520	27.3
20–49	4,976	10.0
50–99	370	0.7
100–249	52	0.1
250–499	NR	1.0
500–999	NR	
>1000	1	0.0
TOTAL 504,689	49,052	100.0
MEAN 10	NA	NA

Source: *County Business Patterns, U.S. Summary,* U.S. Dept. of Commerce, Bureau of Census, 1982, p. 69.

[a]The total number includes both proprietary stores and drugstores; however, the 49,052 number is less than the 49,527 total for proprietary and drugstores with payroll in 1982 because not all data for two brackets were reported.

[b]The percentages are based on 49,527 pharmacies.

Table 3–7.   Distribution of Chain Drugstores by Size of Firm, 1984

Size of Firms Number of Units	Number of Firms	Total Number of Units
Over 1,000	3	4,305
500–999	4	2,608
100–499	18	3,936
50–99	11	766
25–49	22	776
10–24	39	589
4–9	50	297
TOTALS	147	13,277

Source: *NACDS Membership Directory, 1984 ed.*, National Association of Chain Drugstores, Inc., Alexandria, VA. Not all chain drugstores are listed in the directory.

INSTITUTIONAL PRACTICE

A pharmacist may elect to practice in one of the several types of institutions. See Table 3–1. The hospital is the primary employer of pharmacists in institutions; however, skilled and other nursing homes, and penal institutions employ pharmacists, either full-time, part-time, or as consultants. Although the duties of the pharmacist vary considerably with the type of institutions, the basic duties are common to all. There are as many differences between hospital pharmacy practice in an acute short-term general hospital and a long-term mental or tuberculosis hospital as there are between hospital practice and other various types of institutional practice. See Tables 3–2 and 3–3. The following characteristics, advantages and disadvantages apply primarily to hospital practitioners.

Characteristics. There are certain basic distinctions between the institutional pharmacist and the general, community pharmacist:

1. The institutional pharmacist primarily serves patients confined to the institution, with the exception of those outpatients having prescriptions dispensed at the institutional pharmacy.
2. The institutional pharmacist's professional relationship involves primarily the physician and the nurse, his involvement with the patient often is an indirect one through the nurse. Again, the exceptions are the outpatients and certain large teaching hospitals in which "clinical" pharmacists serve patients directly on the floor, taking drug histories, providing information in certain instances, and monitoring the drug regimen.
3. Most institutional pharmacists operate on a nonprofit basis, but in a revenue/expenditure budget context, but the trend is toward for-profit proprietary hospitals. The distinction between profit and nonprofit should not be overemphasized because hosptial administrators often expect the director of pharmaceutical services to generate revenues in excess of expenditures to offset deficits in other departments. Thus the

director of pharmaceutical services, or chief pharmacist, is expected to produce a profit or a surplus.

4. A final distinction is that an institutional pharmacist must be knowledgeable and feel comfortable in a bureaucratic organizational structure, especially in larger institutions. He must understand the interrelationships in the organization, the lines of authority, responsibility, and communication, and be able to function efficiently within the organization.

Advantages and Disadvantages. The *advantages* of institutional practice include: (1) insulation from severe economic, competitive pressures, but this is changing; (2) opportunity to relate to and consult more frequently with other health professionals; (3) opportunity to influence prescribing patterns through the Pharmacy and Therapeutics Committee; (4) opportunity to teach other health professionals and assist in research, especially in the large, teaching hospitals; (5) opportunity to engage in limited manufacturing of pharmaceuticals in larger institutions; and (6) opportunity for advancement in the larger institutions.

The *disadvantages* include: (1) limited direct contact with the patient and the resulting absence of patient consultation concerning prescriptions (with the exception noted above); (2) almost complete absence of direct contact with patrons and the opportunity to assist in the primary care of patients except in ambulatory clinics; (3) less opportunity to function independently in several facets of practice common to community practitioner; and (4) absence of the opportunity to be self-employed and the advantages inherent in proprietorship.

HOSPITAL PHARMACY

The first U.S. hospital pharmacy was established in the eighteenth century; however, the practice of pharmacy in hospitals grew slowly until World War II. Following WWII, hospital pharmacy began to flourish under the influence of the American Society of Hospital Pharmacy (ASHP), which was established in 1942 under the aegis of the APhA. One barometer of the growth of hospital pharmacy is the membership in the ASHP. By 1960, the active membership had reached 2,700. By 1970, the active membership had more than doubled, reaching almost 5,600. In the next five years, the membership had increased another 40 percent, and by 1980, the active membership was 9,973, almost 80 percent above the 1970 figure. In 1983, active members numbered 14,429, a 45 percent increase over the 1980 figure.[6]

Obviously the growth of hospital pharmacy was fueled by the increased use and significance of drugs in hospitals. This growth paralleled the development of new and powerful drugs by the pharmaceutical industry, and paralleled the growth of prescription sales in community pharmacies. The importance of and market for acute care hospitals has grown astronomically since 1940.

The Eli Lilly Company publishes the *Lilly Hospital Pharmacy Survey*[7] annually beginning in 1976. Their survey covers over 2,000 hospitals and includes pertinent data on hospitals in addition to information on hospital pharmacy. The typical hospital in the survey for 1983 had a mean bed capacity of 246, 69 percent occupancy rate and a mean hospital stay of 7.1 days. The typical hospital inpatient pharmacy is open 96 hours per week; employs 7 full-time equivalent (FTE) pharmacists, 6.6 FTE technicians, 2.9 FTE other support personnel; maintains a $121,550 inventory with a turnover rate of 7.2, and occupies 1,629 sq. ft. work area.[7] On an average, hospitals employ a pharmacist 1.1 hour per week for each bed in the hospital.

Approximately 40 percent of the sample provided outpatient prescription services. For nearly every bracket of bed capacity, hospital pharmacies with outpatient prescription services had greater values for the following statistics: purchases, inventory, hours per week pharmacies were open, and hours per week worked by all personnel.[7]

The number of hours per week pharmacist(s) devote to pharmacy management ranged from 10 for small hospitals with less than 50 beds to 99 for hospitals with 500 or more beds. The figure for 100 to 199 bed range was 29, and for 200 to 299 bed range, 59. Drug distribution occupied pharmacists the most, followed by management, and then clinical services.[7]

NURSING HOME PHARMACY

The term nursing home is used in a generic sense and encompasses skilled nursing facilities (SNFs) intermediate care facilities (ICFs) and other related facilities. Related facilities include personal care facilities, homes or centers for mentally retarded persons and other disabled persons requiring care other than intensive or extensive nursing care. One other generic term, long-term care facilities (L-TCF's), has become "fashionable" in recent years.

Every SNF and ICF is required, under medicare and medicaid standards, to employ a pharmacist either full-time, part-time, or as a consultant. The latter arrangement is most often used. The consultant pharmacist may or may not provide drugs to the patients in the facility. The consultant may practice in an independent community pharmacy, a chain community pharmacy, a hospital pharmacy, a pharmacy that specializes in providing drugs and services to L-TCF's, or devote full-time services to L-TCFs working out of an office or his/her home. Some 800 pharmacists practice full-time in pharmacies located within the facility.[8] The number of full-time consultants providing information-based services, but not drugs, is increasing.

There is one apparent discrepancy in the data in Table 3–1, and that is, not all of the 2,200 nursing home pharmacists are necessarily stationed in the nursing home. Of the 2,200 nursing home pharmacists, 800 were stationed and practiced full-time in L-TCFs, the other 1,400 devoted full-time or a majority of their time to nursing home services. In addition, another 11,100 pharmacists were reported in 1977 as working part-time or as a consultant in L-TCFs.[8]

Economic Characteristics of Practice Settings

COMMUNITY PHARMACY

Of the approximately 120,000 pharmacists practicing in community pharmacy in 1983, 40 percent practiced in approximately 16,200 chain pharmacies.

Growth of Chains. There was a steady increase in the numbers of chain pharmacies in the 1950s and 1960s. Beginning in 1970, the rate of increase took a tremendous jump, nearly doubling between 1972 and 1983. This increase in the number of chain pharmacies over the years was primarily at the expense of independent pharmacies. The number of chain pharmacies increased by 12,450 between 1958 and 1983, while the number of independent pharmacies decreased by 13,800. More significantly, the average annual sales of chain pharmacies increased by over $1,300,000 during the same period, while average annual sales in independent pharmacies increased by only $388,000. However, the percentage change in the average annual sales during that period was approximately the same for independent and chain pharmacies. See Table 3–5 for additional data and trends.

All independent pharmacies did not fare equally in their competitive struggle with chain drugstores and other mass merchandising stores. For example, in 1982 small independent pharmacies (sales under $250,000) had 9.2 percent of the total retail drug market, medium size independents (sales of $250,000–$500,000) had 15.2 percent of the market, and large independents (sales over $500,000) had 18.8 percent of the market. Both small and medium size independent pharmacies had a lesser share of the market in 1982 compared to 1981, whereas large independent pharmacies increased their share of the market, but at a lower rate compared to chains.

Strength of Independents. The above picture of the economic plight of independents is not quite as dismal as it appears on first analysis. The increase in the number of chain pharmacies is real and substantial, and this fact cannot be extenuated by any rationalization or explanation. However, the much greater growth in total sales by the chains is due in large measure to the increase in the average size of the total store and the wider assortment and variety of goods offered for sale.

There is good reason to believe that the independent pharmacies could have maintained a greater share of the total retail drug market, especially for those products normally sold in independent pharmacies, had they utilized better management and marketing skills. Even the superior financial leverage enjoyed by chains could have been more nearly matched by independents had they practiced some form of capital aggregation as explained in Chapter 8.

In the prescription department, which is the area of greatest economic and professional interest, independent pharmacies have performed about as well as chain pharmacies in recent years as shown in Table 3–8. There is ample opportunity for success for those independent pharmacists who know and practice good management and professional skills along with a good marketing

Table 3–8. **Comparison of Chain and Independent Pharmacies, 1981–1983: Prescription Sales**

Item	1981	Percent[a] Change	1982	Percent[a] Change	1983
Mean Annual Sales					
Independents	$ 417,422	8.2	$ 451,828	9.5	$ 494,572
Chains	1,416,482	6.8	1,512,979	13.8	1,722,102
Mean Rx Sales					
Independents	213,498	17.0	249,695	14.7	286,524
Chains	190,901	15.5	220,534	18.4	261,110
% Rx/Total Sales					
Independents	51.1	—	55.3	—	57.9
Chains	13.5	—	14.6	—	15.1
Mean No. of Rx's					
Independents	28,773	5.6	30,394	1.5	30,841
Chains	26,085	2.6	26,767	4.1	27,862
Mean Rx Charge					
Independents	7.42	10.8	8.22	13.0	9.29
Chains	7.32	13.3	8.29	14.2	9.37
Mean No. of 3rd Party Rx's					
Independents	7,788	10.6	8,613	2.9	8,863
Chains	5,997	6.0	6,355	5.1	6,679
% 3rd Party/Total Rx's					
Independents	27.1	—	28.3	—	28.8
Chains	23.0	—	23.7	—	24.0

Source: *Amer. Druggist, 189* (No. 5): 20, 1984.

[a]Percent Change denotes percent changes during years between 1981–1982 and 1982–1983, respectively.

strategy. Of course these opportunities exist for chain pharmacists who do likewise. The independent pharmacist has the advantages of being a more permanent constituent of the community and has greater flexibility of decision making and action.

Economics and Competition. To provide a broader perspective of the economics of community pharmacy, data on disposable income, total drugstore sales and market share of chain and independents were compiled in Table 3–9. These data indicate that drugstore sales increased faster than disposable income in three of the six years, and overall for all six years. Chain drugstore sales increased more each year than independent pharmacy sales. Independent pharmacy sales growth was well below disposable income growth each year except 1982. The consumer price index (CPI) for the same years was included as a guide for interpreting the data in terms of constant dollars.

For years pharmacists have been concerned about losing sales of health and beauty aids (HBAs) to food stores and mass merchandising. Table 3–10

Table 3–9. Summary of Selected Economic and Market Indicators, 1977–1983

			Total Drugstore		Chains		Independents		
Year	D I[a]	D I%[b]	$ Sales[c]	% C[d]	% M[e]	% C	% M	% C	CPI[f]
1977	$5,545	NA	$22.2	8	47.1	14	52.9	4	100
1978	6,155	11.0	24.3	10	49.8	16	50.2	4	108
1979	6,820	10.8	27.2	12	52.3	17	47.7	6	120
1980	7,430	8.9	30.3	12	54.8	16	45.2	7	136
1981	8,318	12.0	33.4	10	55.3	12	44.7	8	150
1982	8,706	4.7	36.2	8	56.8	11	43.2	5	159
1983	9,806	12.6	39.7	10	57.4	11	42.6	8	164

Source: Nielsen Review of Retail Drugstore Trends. Chicago, IL, 1983, 1984

[a]DI denotes per capita disposable income, which is per capita personal income less taxes and social security.

[b]DI % denotes annual increase in per capital disposable income.

[c]Sales denote the total annual sales in $ billion in all drugstores, pharmacies and proprietary stores.

[d]% C denotes the percent annual change compared to previous year.

[e]% M denotes the percentage share of the total market.

[f]CPI denotes consumer price index with the base of 1977 = 100.

was constructed to demonstrate that this concern was well founded. Beginning in 1981, grocery stores have maintained a majority share of HBAs sales.

Some pharmacists may not be concerned about these trends because they perceive little health implications in the use of these products. This perception is incorrect; much benefit may be realized by the proper use of O-T-C drugs, and toiletries as well. As a corollary, much harm may result from the misuse of HBAs not to mention the waste. Pharmacists have an economic and profes-

Table 3–10. Summary of HBAs Sales, 1977–1982

	Total HBAs		Drugstores		Grocery		Mass Merchandisers	
Year	$ Sales[a]	% C[b]	% M[c]	% C	% M	% C	% M	% C
1977	6,766	10	37.7	7	48.1	11	14.3	14
1978	7,619	13	36.6	9	48.3	13	15.1	19
1979	8,487	11	36.0	10	49.2	13	14.8	9
1980	9,802	15	36.0	14	49.7	17	14.3	17
1981	11,327	14	35.7	11	50.2	17	14.1	17
1982	12,480	10	34.7	7	51.0	12	14.3	12
1983[d]	19,312	10	37.8	6	47.1	12	15.1	15

Source: Nielsen Review of Retail Drugstore Trends, A.C. Nielsen, Chicago, IL, 1983, 1984.

[a]Annual Sales in Millions $.

[b]% C denotes percent annual change compared to previous year's sales.

[c]% M denotes percentage share of total market.

[d]1983 data are for 49 HBA product categories compared to 25 *major* product categories for the other years.

sional stake in the HBAs market, but they have neglected the opportunity to vigorously pursue this market with tasteful and effective merchandising, and with strategically placed signs of caveats and signs that say: "Consult the pharmacist for proper use of these products." Pharmacy educators share the blame by neglecting to teach pharmacy students the significance of these products and how to counsel patients effectively in their proper use.

The *Lilly Digest*[3] and the *NACDS Lilly Digest*[5] provide a wealth of economic data on the operations of community pharmacies. Data from these sources will be used in later chapters to illustrate financial problems and managerial solutions to them.

HOSPITAL PHARMACY

As stated previously, the hospital market generally and hospital pharmacy market specifically have increased immensely since 1940. This increase was the result of the invention and utilization of high technology including drugs in hospitals, and escalating the cost of acute hospital care. The cost of hospital rooms with the attending services has far outpaced all other components of the CPI. Because of these trends, the federal government issued the diagnosis related groups (DRGs) guidelines for reimbursement for hospital care under Medicare and Medicaid. This prospective approach (as opposed to the retrospective approach) was similar to the method of paying community pharmacists for drugs and prescription services from the inception of Medicaid. The DRGs and other market constraints, such as private investment based on profit motive and thus cost reduction, have brought acute hospital care into the realm of the "real world" market. These economic influences have simply accelerated the already noticeable trends in the number, size and potential efficiency of hospitals as illustrated in Table 3–11.

Among general hospitals, the size of hospitals has increased along with the gross number of beds, while the number of hospitals decreased. The mean daily census per hospital increased, while the occupancy rate and daily census have decreased in relation to population trends. Occupancy rate has begun to increase again in recent years. The objective should be to increase occupancy rate while holding daily census per 1,000 population constant or decreasing it, thus making more efficient use of available resources. The length of stay is also declining, another sign of efficiency. The pharmacist and efficacious drugs have played a strategic role in these trends.

The trends have been more dramatic in the case of special hospitals, which resulted from the closure of many large tuberculosis hospitals—from 107 to 11 in 10 years. The number of beds in tuberculosis hospitals declined by 92 percent. Although the number of psychiatric hospitals increased by 2 percent, the number of beds decreased by 56 percent. Overall there were decreases in every statistic associated with speciality hospitals except occupancy rate, with no change, and full-time equivalent employees per 100 beds, an increase of 15 percent.

Table 3–11. Number of Hospitals and Related Statistics by Selected Years

Item	1970	1976	1978	1980	% Change 1970–80
General Hospitals					
Number	6,553	6,361	6,270	6,176	− 5.8
Mean Bed Capacity	153	168	171	175	14.4
% Increase in Beds	NA	7.0	0.5	0.6	8.1
Mean Daily Census/					
Hospital	118	125	126	132	12.0
Occupancy Rate[a]	77.4	74.6	73.6	75.6	− 2.3
Length of Stay in					
Days	9.0	8.1	7.94	7.86	− 12.7
Daily Census/1,000					
Population	3.8	3.7	3.6	3.6	− 5.3
FTE/100 Beds[b]	223	262	275	293	31.4
Special Hospitals					
Number	1,064	910	889	875	− 17.8
Mean Bed Capacity	498	342	310	288	− 42.2
% Decrease in Beds	NA	41.2	11.6	8.5	52.4
Mean Daily Census/					
Hospital	425	281	254	245	− 42.4
Occupancy Rate[a]	85.0	82.1	82.0	85.0	0.0
Length of Stay in					
Days	143	81	70	68	− 52.4
Daily Census/1,000					
Population	2.2	1.2	1.0	0.9	− 59.1
FTE/100 Beds[b]	371	412	426	428	15.4

Source: Straham, G.W., Reference 9.

[a]Occupancy Rate $= \dfrac{\text{Average Daily Census}}{\text{Number of Beds}} \times 100$

[b]FTE denotes full-time equivalent of employees per 100 beds.

The proprietary or "for profit" hospitals have gained a substantial share of the hospital market within the past decade. This trend, together with the emerging management enterprises that manage the entire hospital for a fee, will very likely sweep the entire hospital industry into the free enterprise system before the end of the century. These trends will provide a different environment within which hospital pharmacists will practice. As these conditions become more prevalent, prescription drug marketing will have to change to avoid violations of the Robinson and Patman Act and other antitrust laws. These trends towards large organization and increased economic power will favor the concept of preferred provider organizations (PPOs). Small hospitals, as well as independent pharmacies, will have to devise a framework that will enable them to form PPOs and aggregate capital in order to compete with the large firms. This will be addressed in more detail in Chapter 8.

Table 3–12.   Population Statistics and Nursing Home Beds[a] for Selected Years

	Population in Millions			% Change Per Year 65 +[c]	Beds per 1,000 65 +[b]
Year	Total	65 +[b]	% of Total		
1983	236.60[d]	27.38[d]	11.6	2.4	NA[e]
1980	226.55	25.54	11.3	2.8	57.2
1976	218.33[d]	22.94[d]	10.5	2.3	56.3
1970	203.30	20.13	9.9	NA	43.4[f]

Source: Census Data, U.S. Bureau of Census; Nursing Home Beds; Straham, G.W., Reference 9.

[a]Nursing homes with 25 beds or more.
[b]Age 65 and over.
[c]The % Change per year over the total period of 1970–83 was 2.77.
[d]Estimated.
[e]NA denotes not available or not calculated.
[f]The year was 1969 for this particular statistic.

The institutional differences between community pharmacy and hospital pharmacy will fade into the remote background, as their common interest of sustaining an autonomous profession gradually replaces previous animosity. The practice of medicine will continue toward the corporate structure type of organization. Status for occupational groups—pharmacists, physicians, nurses, dentists, and others—will in the future depend to a large degree on their ability as a group to practice economic and managerial skills as well as clinical skills.

NURSING HOME PHARMACY

Nursing home pharmacy is the fastest growing segment of pharmacy. This is the result of changing demographics, as shown in Table 3–12, and the enactment of Medicare and Medicaid. Between 1970 and 1983, there was an annual 2.8 percent increase in the population age 65 and over, which was twice the 1.25 percent growth rate for the total population. The increase in the population age 75 and over was greater than that of the 65 and over group. The amount of drugs, sickroom supplies and health appliances used by the older population is several times that of the rest of the population, and this pattern increases with each passing year.

The number of nursing homes increased rapidly during the 1960s after the enactment of the Medicare and Medicaid programs. The growth has been less dramatic since the passage of the amendments in 1972 that increased the standards for SNFs and ICFs. The rate of growth in nursing homes and related statistics between 1969 and 1980 are shown in Table 3–13. The leveling of the growth trend after 1973 is apparent.[9]

A 1977 survey of nursing homes and related facilities was more comprehensive in terms of types of homes and residents and employee characteristics.[8]

Table 3–13. **Number of Nursing Homes[a] and Related Statistics for Selected Years**

Item	1969	1973	1976	1980
No. of Nursing Homes[a]	11,465	14,089	14,133	14,567
Mean Bed Capacity	73.6	86.0	91.4	100.2
Beds/1,000 Population				
Age 65 and over	43.4	56.8	56.3	57.2
Occupancy Rate[b]	90.0	90.6	91.7	91.0
Residents in Millions	0.759	1.099	1.184	1.329
Residents/Home	66.2	78.0	83.8	91.2
FTE Employees/100 beds	55.0	57.2	57.1	62.9
% by Type of Ownership:				
Government	6.0	6.8	7.1	6.1
Proprietary	72.4	72.7	72.9	73.4
Nonprofit	21.6	20.5	20.0	20.5

Source: Straham, G.W., Reference 9.

[a]Number of nursing homes with 25 beds or more.

$$^{b}\text{Occupancy Rate} = \frac{\text{Average Daily Census}}{\text{Number of Beds}} \times 100$$

That survey covered 18,900 facilities of which 19.05 percent was SNFs only, 24.34 percent was a combination of SNFs and ICFs (i.e., with beds certified for each category), 31.75 percent was ICFs only, and 24.87 percent was not certified in either category.

It has been estimated that there were 15,000 certified nursing homes in 1985 with about 25 percent SNFs only, 35 percent combination of SNFs and ICFs, and 40 percent ICFs only. The estimated gross revenues for all nursing homes in 1985 was $39 billion. The per diem cost per resident was less than $40.[10]

Summary

Young pharmacists today have many practice opportunities. Pharmacy, as every other social institution, is constantly changing ever so slowly but at an increasing pace. With changes come new challenges and opportunities. The pharmacist who has developed his perspective will be able to discern those opportunities that best match his personality and utilize his skills.

Many of the good opportunities in the future will depend on the ability to adjust to a changing environment and the ability to blend clinical and managerial skills. Those pharmacists who depend on narrowly defined skills will discover that his opportunities will be narrowly defined as well. Advancement will be slow and the opportunity to become a fully independent, autonomous practitioner will elude the pharmacist with narrowly based skills. Specialization is one avenue for advancement, but pharmacy has few genuine specialities. This may change; however, those with broadly based skills will be in a better position to discern and select from a wide variety of opportunities.

REFERENCES

1. Smith, H.A.: *Innovative Career Counseling Manual for Pharmacists,* Bethseda, MD: A.A.C.P., 1985.
2. Rosenfeld, M., Thornton, R.F., and Glazer, R.: *A National Study of the Practice of Pharmacy,* Washington, DC: A.Ph.A.—A.A.C.P., 1978.
3. Deiner, C.H. (editor): *The Lilly Digest,* Indianapolis, IN: Eli Lilly and Company, 1984.
4. Personal Communications: Huffman (Jr.), D.C.: Executive Vice President, American College of Apothecaries (ACA), Memphis, TN, May 1985.
5. Deiner, C.H. (editor): *NACDS—Lilly Digest,* Indianapolis, IN: Eli Lilly Company, 1984.
6. *Amer. J. Hosp. Pharm.,* various issues, 1960–1984.
7. Deiner, C.H. (editor): *Lilly Hospital Pharmacy Survey,* Indianapolis, IN, 1984, plus other editions.
8. Sirrocco, A.: Employees in nursing homes in the United States: 1977 national nursing home survey. *Vital and Health Statistics,* Series 14, No. 25, Feb 1981.
9. Straham, G.W.: Trends in nursing and related care homes and hospitals. *Vital and Health Statistics,* Series 14, No. 30, 1984.
10. Personal Communications: Webster, T., Executive Director, American Society of Consulting Pharmacists (ASCP), Arlington, VA, May 1985.

REVIEW

1. Define pharmacy practice and differentiate it from other pharmacy related work.

2. Describe the various settings where pharmacists practice.

3. What percent of pharmacists practice in each of the practice settings in question 2?

4. What are the other types of pharmacist employment and the percentage of pharmacists working in each?

5. Discuss the work of pharmacists in independent, chain and hospital pharmacies in terms of various administrative and professional functions, both routine and critical.

6. Discuss the growth of chain pharmacy over the past 50 years and contrast this to the economic status of independent pharmacy. Why has this trend developed? Could this have been avoided?

7. Discuss the institutional characteristics of traditional independent, professional, chain, hospital and nursing home practice. What are the distinguishing features of each? What are the advantages and disadvantages of each?

8. Discuss the office type of practice in terms of unique features, appeal and future. Explain in your own words why this type of practice has not grown as some had projected.

9. Discuss the franchise system. What are the advantages and disadvantages of this type of practice.

10. What are the special strengths of independent pharmacy?

4 | Managerial Perspective: Nature of the Management Process

What is Management?

The *classic definition of management* is the art and science of planning, organizing, directing, and controlling human effort and resources for the general good within the organizational framework and economic environment of the firm. The essence of management is *decision-making*. Its unique function is choosing between alternative means of moving toward an objective. The decision-making process involves the following *factors:* (1) identifying and defining the problem; (2) analyzing it; (3) developing alternate solutions; (4) deciding upon the best solution; and (5) converting the decision into effective action. In carrying out this mandate, the manager has to weigh the risks of every course of action against the expected gains. Then, having decided, he must clearly communicate the orders and provide the necessary leadership to get results. Many people shun this sort of responsibility. Only a few seek it, and they become leaders, knowing that there is a possibility that a decision may be wrong, and also knowing that this chance may be minimized if some basic rules and procedures are followed.

Management and administration are often considered synonymous by many employed in the field. However, with the changing characteristics of business—especially the changing economic environment, the vast size of many businesses, and the evolving bureaucracy in business—authorities now make a distinction between the two. The *administrator* is one who adapts to his environment in order to survive in it and obtain sustenance from it. The *manager* relates to and manages his environment. He is more risk-oriented and relates directly to his resources in order to control, manipulate, and direct them for gain.[1]

Administration or management of a business is a network in which every decision is connected in some way with every other decision that has preceded it and will have a bearing upon decisions to be made in the future. A manager needs the qualities of a statesman to see his organization in all its relationships. He has to know the organization's objectives and policies, what resources he can call upon, and the capabilities of those who will make his decisions effective, and then he must produce plans that take all these into account. This is the leadership function of management. Every employee has a stake in leadership, because the manager is accountable not only for the success of his organization, but also for the continued employment and the satisfaction of all those associated with it. Many business decisions are routine and re-petitive to the experienced manager, but he must patiently keep in mind that particular problems may be new to the staff. Therefore, it is part of a manager's duty to provide the necessary guidance and explanations.

Two cardinal principles of management are: (1) the decision must be ad-equate to solve the problem, and (2) authority must be commensurate with responsibilities. There is no use in attacking a tank with a bow and arrow, and it is wasteful to shoot sparrows with a cannon. Delegation of responsibility without giving the necessary authority to carry out the responsibility is unfair to the subordinate. It leads to frustrations and ineffective administration. However, authority is not the only means of controlling and of influencing the activities of others; indeed, it may not be the best means of controlling the actions of others in many circumstances. A disregard for the latter principle probably is the most common failure among managers and administrators.

In his book entitled *A Philosophy of Administration,*[2] Marshall E. Dimock states that administration ought to be studied according to the scientific method, but that administration ought not to aim at being a science. Yet, any philosophy of administration must be capable of passing the acid test of science, i.e., management must be capable of empiric validation based on the results of past or present experience, and it must be capable of further predictions and planning of future goals.

Practicing pharmacy in an economy such as ours demands *foresight, judg-ment, resourcefulness, knowledge,* and *courage.* Only the person who applies all these qualities in making decisions may expect to advance his practice.

Styles of Management

There are basically five distinct styles of management that have evolved from the days of classic capitalism. They are:

	HARD NOSE ←──────────────────────────→ NO NOSE					
Style	*Autocrat*	*Authoritariancrat*	*Bureaucrat*	*Democrat*	*Particicrat*	*Abdicrat*
Source	Self	Position	Rules, systems, procedures	Majority	Group	Diffused
General mode of com- muni- cation	Directives and order giving		Explainer and explana- tion	Discusser and discus- sion	Joint determiner and determina- tion	Random

Figure 4–1.   Leadership styles continuum. (Adapted from Caskey, C.C.: Developing a leadership style. *Supervision*, April, 1964. By permission of *Supervision* and the National Research Bureau, Inc.)

1. The "Captain-of-Industry" style that pre-dated and later coexisted with the establishment of "scientific" management in 1885.
2. The "Hard-Nose" style of the mid 1910s to the 1930s.
3. The "Human-Relations" style of the 1940s and the early 1950s.
4. The "Management-by-Pressure" style of the early 1950s to mid 1960s.
5. The "Management-by-Objectives" style beginning in the mid 1960s.

The various management or leadership styles are depicted as a continuum in Figure 4–1.

CAPTAIN-OF-INDUSTRY STYLE

This style is represented by the strong individualistic person who amassed a fortune through drive, hard work, ingenuity, and good luck. Well-known examples of this type of entrepreneur of the nineteenth century include Andrew William Mellon, John Davidson Rockefeller, Andrew Carnegie, and Henry Ford, although the last began his industrial career in the early twentieth century. These people represent only a few of the outstanding capitalists of this era. All had different personalities and characteristics, although some type of composite personality profile might be synthesized from their major attributes. Even if a person with this composite personality profile could be found, there is no assurance he would be a successful businessman. There were, of course, common traits among these men. These included a drive, a dream, and definite short-term and long-term goals.

This style of management gradually declined as our industrial society became more mature and institutionalized. That is, large corporations began to adapt to social pressure, largely via legal regulation, and began to operate accordingly. With the adoption of the principles of "scientific" management, introduced by Frederick W. Taylor around 1885, this change in the style of management was accelerated.

"Scientific" management was based on the principles and techniques of analyzing each job down to the smallest elements that could be identified and measured in terms of the time required to perform the task. These elements were then organized into a work cycle for each job, and standards were set for each job by the use of stopwatches and statistical procedures. Thus, the workers were reduced to an almost robot level, and the base pay scale, raises, and bonuses were based on meeting or surpassing the work standards.

HARD-NOSE STYLE

After the enactment of the Sherman Anti-Trust Act in 1890, the Clayton Anti-Trust Act, and the Federal Trade Commission Act in 1914, corporate policies became more restrained in commercial dealing. However, under the increasing competitive influence brought about by these laws, management sought newer ways to compete. Armed with the techniques of "scientific" management, large corporations were in a position to demand high standards of work performance, thus lowering the unit production cost. This economic and political background provided the basis for the hard-nose policy of management from about 1914 through the 1930s.

HUMAN-RELATIONS STYLE

This style of management was ushered in by two major events. First was the growth in size and strength of the unions, especially after the passage of the Wagner Act in 1935. This Act gave the unions the right to assemble, associate together, negotiate, and strike if necessary without anti-trust sanctions. More importantly, World War II brought about a scarcity of workers, and it was necessary to motivate employees through good human relations programs to increase the productivity needed for the war effort. This philosophy was enhanced by two other factors: first, price stabilization, which eased the competitive pressures, and second, the research findings of the social scientists. This also was an era when fringe benefits became important considerations in lieu of frozen pay increases. Human relations served management well, except that it was often used primarily for its "cosmetic" effect, rather than reflecting fundamental change in management philosophy.

MANAGEMENT-BY-PRESSURE STYLE

This style of management originated under the economic conditions following World War II. These conditions were characterized by increasing demand, prices, and costs. Without returning to the old hard-nose policy, except in labor negotiations, management exerted pressure to hold costs down, increase productivity, and obtain a larger share of the growing market. Pressure was exerted to produce more by gearing promotion and other economic incentives to productivity, while maintaining increased fringe benefits, but putting less reliance on the policy of good human relations. This was the era when a good manager was known as someone "who could make things happen."

Meanwhile, "scientific" management had not been ignored by the personnel and industrial engineering departments. On the contrary, the tools of "scientific" management had been refined, and it was augmented by the observations of such famous management authorities as Peter Drucker.[3] "Scientific" management was being enriched and humanized by the appreciation of research findings of the industrial psychologists and social scientists. The works of Joseph Tiffin[4] and Douglas McGregor[5] were good examples.

MANAGEMENT-BY-OBJECTIVES STYLE

The formulation of this style, perhaps better labeled as *a method and a philosophy* of management was based on analysis of the defects of the previous styles or methods of management and a synthesis of some of the better aspects of the previous methods. Since it is goal-oriented, it obviously has some of the better characteristics, philosophy, and concepts of the pressure style. Management by objectives, frequently abbreviated as MBO, accommodates all that is best in the human relations style, and it can also accommodate and use the results of well-designed behavioral science research.

Since its premises are not based on any set of personality traits or a personality cult, it is not incompatible with the "captain-of-industry" type of manager as long as the manager accepts the premises and philosophy set forth. Although it can accommodate the "hard-nose" style, the effectiveness of management by objectives is greatly lessened by this style and philosophy. MBO is designed for managers and professionals; however, the principles are applicable to any work group with some overall goals. Above all, management by objectives, like so many really useful methods, is a very simple, common sense, and logical method. One wonders why it took so long to discover it. Like many discoveries, management by objectives, though simple in content, required extraordinary insight into the various elements of the system. It was described first by Peter Drucker,[6] and later in more detail by Odiorne.[7,8]

Management by Objectives

Odiorne gave a concise *definition* of management by objectives.[9] He stated,

> In brief, the system of management by objectives can be described as a process whereby the superior and subordinate managers of an organization jointly identify its common goals, define each individual's major area of responsibility in terms of results expected of him, and use these measures as guides for operating the unit and assessing the contribution of each of its members.

The key words in the definition are *jointly identify* and *process*. This establishes MBO at participatory management, a term often misunderstood. The subordinate person does indeed participate without management losing ultimate control, and the participation must be meaningful for the subordinate employee. In addition to the employee's participation in identifying his goals and responsibilities, he is often consulted in those decisions that affect him directly.

MAJOR PREMISES

The major premises of management by objectives are as follows:[10]

1. Business management takes place within individual firms, which collectively form a major and integral component of the economic system. The economic system has undergone drastic change over the past 45 years, requiring greater social awareness and responsibility on the part of business management. The premise has a special significance for pharmacy, since health care is continuing to undergo drastic changes as a result of strong social and political pressure for improvement. MBO is directed toward meeting these changes and the new requirements.

2. Management by objectives presumes that the first step in management is to identify the goals of the organization, which are consistent wtih the goals of society. All other management methods and subsystems follow this preliminary step.

3. Once organizational goals have been identified, orderly procedures should be instituted for distributing responsibility among individuals in such a way that their combined efforts are directed toward achieving those goals.

4. Management by objectives assumes that managerial behavior is more important than manager personality, and that this behavior should be defined in terms of results, measured against the manager's goals rather than in terms of overall goals for the entire organization.

5. It also presumes that while participation is highly desirable in goal-setting and decision-making, its principal merit lies in its social and political value rather than its effects on productivity, though even here it usually has a favorable impact.

6. It regards the successful manager as a manager of defined situations, which fall within the overall purpose and scope of the firm or organization. Success is attributed to the managerial behavior best suited to achieve results with respect to defined situations and objectives. This means that there is no best pattern of management, but that management should be discriminatory, relating to specific goals, yet responsive to the larger socioeconomic system within which it operates.

PHILOSOPHY AND CONCEPTUAL FRAMEWORK

Management by objectives is essentially a system of incorporating into a more logical and effective pattern the things many people are already doing, although in a somewhat chaotic manner, or in a manner that obscures personal risk and responsibility. Management by objectives is basic and simple, yet flexible enough to incorporate subsystems such as economic order quantities and personnel development programs. Also, management by objectives does not exclude it from being a part of a larger system, especially the value system of the organization.[11]

The system of management by objectives is *not a "cookbook" approach to management* in which "cut-and-dried" procedures are followed blindly. Such an approach would render management by objectives impotent and useless. When such an approach has been used, experience has shown repeatedly that the people who are supposed to implement it never accept it. Instead they consider it as one more mechanism and an exercise in futility.[12] The system of management by objectives goes beyond a set of rules, a series of procedures, or even a set method of management. It is a *philosophy, a way of thinking,* and a *system* that incorporates objectivity, logic, and scientific management procedures. It also bridges the gap between participatory management and firm organizational control.

Odiorne described the *conceptual framework* for the implementation of the system of management by objectives:[13]

1. The system *utilizes* the basic *organizational structure* or *hierarchy* of the business and *makes it work.* This induces vitality and personal involvement of the people in the firm, and the system can be applied to a small independent pharmacy with a single proprietor, to a large drugstore chain operation, a drug wholesaler, or a pharmaceutical manufacturer.

2. Management by objectives *stimulates the growth and development* of an organization by involving all key employees, causing them to grow and develop. This is accomplished through the mutual development of statements of *expectations* and the necessary *criteria* for measuring the results.

3. The system *assigns risk* via mutual agreement and participation in the whole process. It stresses ability and achievement rather than personality and ties the employee's progress—pay raises, promotion, and even tenure—to the results achieved as measured against the objectives. Both *objectives* and their attainment are *mutually determined* by the employee and his supervisor.

4. Management by objectives is *especially applicable to professional and managerial* employees and may be extended to department supervisors, technical positions, or clerical employees with some modification in the method of setting standards and measuring results. However, at the lower level the employees may not be as capable of identifying viable objectives as are employees at higher levels.

5. Management by objectives *helps to overcome many chronic problems* of managing professionals and store managers by negating many, if not all, of the chronic problems discussed below.

SOLUTION FOR CHRONIC PROBLEMS

The problems of management fall into two major areas: (1) problems of managing professionals and pharmacy managers and (2) problems encountered by the small business proprietor in managing employees. However, these two sets of problems are not necessarily peculiar to either category.

The solution to some of the chronic managerial problems by the application of management by objectives has been described by Odiorne[13] as follows:

1. Management by objectives provides a means of *measuring the true contribution* of managerial and professional personnel.

2. By defining the common goals of people and organizations, and measuring individual contributions toward reaching these goals, the possibility of *obtaining coordinated effort and teamwork* is enhanced without eliminating the personal risk.

3. MBO provides solutions to the key problem of *defining the major areas of responsibility* for each person in the organization, including joint or shared responsibilities.

4. MBO processes are geared to *achieving the results desired, both for the organization as a whole and for the individual contributors*.

5. It *eliminates the need for people to change their personalities*, as well as for appraising people on the basis of their personality traits.

6. It provides a means of *determining the span of control of each manager*.

7. It offers an *answer to the key question of salary administration*— "How should we allocate pay increase from available funds, if we want to pay for the results?"

8. It aids in *identifying potential for advancement and in finding promotable people*.

Steinmetz et al. described the common "pitfalls" of managers of small businesses as follows:[14]

1. *Wasting time* as the most common hazard to good management.

2. *Putting fun things first, not first things first*, resulting from inability to establish appropriate priorities.

3. *Inability to delegate*, resulting from the close personal identification with the entire business enterprise.

This last problem was viewed by Steinmetz and his co-authors as one that is very difficult to overcome. Nine reasons were outlined to relate why managers and small business proprietors fail to delegate work.

1. They are little Napoleons who must satisfy their own ego by keeping all authority.

2. They feel that they can do it better themselves, and they refuse to permit others to do it in a "substandard" manner.

3. They are unable to communicate to their subordinates precisely what it is that they want done, when, where, and how much.

4. They lack confidence in their subordinates' abilities to do the work which should be delegated to them.

5. They feel that they lack feedback or other control mechanisms by which the subordinate can be "checked on."

6. They are afraid that their subordinates will "outshine" them or otherwise prove that they know as much or more about the job than the boss.

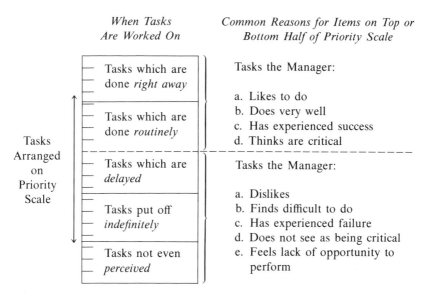

Figure 4–2. Managerial performance priority scale. (Adapted from Caskey, C.C.: Developing a leadership style. *Supervision,* April, 1964. By permission of *Supervision* and the National Research Bureau, Inc.)

7. They are afraid to trust anyone besides themselves.

8. They suffer from a martyr complex—because they desire to have people feel sorry for them, they refuse to delegate work which logically could be done by other people.

9. They are possessed by a "guilt drive"—they feel guilty if they have nothing to do and delegating work to others leaves them in that "awkward" position.[15]

There must be an explanation for these chronic problems, and "pitfalls" of management. The explanation lies in two dimensions: first, the failure to adopt an effective method of management such as management by objectives, and second, the natural tendency to put off less enjoyable tasks and concentrate on tasks that are more to our liking. An arrangement of performance priorities which depicts this dilemma is shown in Figure 4–2.

Management by objectives provides an opportunity for assigning appropriate priorities to tasks and objectives as well as a means of avoiding many of the related problems.

Installing the MBO System

There are some necessary conditions before the system can be installed properly. It must have the endorsement of the principal manager in the organizational unit.[16] This would be the proprietor of an independent pharmacy or the partners of a partnership. In a small chain of drugstores (4 to 25 units), the president and probably the board of directors should endorse the system. In a larger chain of drugstores, the system should be first installed in a district or regional operational unit with the endorsement of the principal manager. The manager of any functional division of a drug wholesale or manufacturing firm could endorse the system. However, it is better if the endorsement comes from top management and the system is implemented from the top down to the lowest level that is practical.

BASIC CHANGES

After obtaining the appropriate endorsement and before the actual installation of the system, the initiator of the system must involve the higher echelon of management in *three phases of changes* within the firm:

1. A *familiarization process* must be implemented, beginning with top management and proceeding down to the others involved, using the appropriate communication channels.

2. *Performance goals for the organization* as a whole must be set by the top echelon of management, but *individual goal-setting methods* must be developed and extended down through the organization to the lower levels.

3. The *necessary changes* must be made in such areas as appraisal system or performance review, salary and bonus procedures, delegation of responsibility and authority, and policy clarification.

IMPLEMENTATION

There are basically *four stages of the actual implementation* of the system:

1. Establishing the goals for the firm, and then for each manager or individual involved. This is done usually at the beginning of the budget year.

2. Determining the means of measuring performance, including the necessary *criteria* for *measuring* the *results* for the firm and each individual involved.

3. Reviewing the results with each individual and assessing the achievement of the goals. This is done usually at the end of the budget year for the firm, but periodically for the individual.

4. Making any necessary modifications in goals or criteria that the reviews indicate. This is done usually at the end of the budget year.

Each of these stages should be broken down into *specific steps and/or elements* for efficient implementation and for good results.

1. *Setting Goals for the Firm.* Those goals should be identified which the principal manager(s) or executive(s) can reasonably expect to achieve. Some of the more common goals are given in Table 4–1.

2. *Clarifying the Organizational Chart.* The organizational chart, or the informal relationship among the employees of a small firm, should be reviewed to determine the best method for assigning responsibilities in order to achieve the goals of the firm.

Table 4–1. Setting Goals for the Firm

Goal	Criteria
Profitability	$\dfrac{NP}{Sales}$; $\dfrac{NP}{Investment}$; NP (in percentages)
Competitive position	Share of the market; Market penetration
Expense control	Functional expense as % of sales; Dispensing cost/Rx
Productivity	Sales increase & Rx's increase
Employee relations	Turnover rate; Average tenure by position; Reported complaints: Suggestions
Inventory control	Turnover rate; Out-of-stock incidences; Economic order quantity, and Sources of purchasing
Public relations	Reported complaints; Returned merchandise; Compliment reports; Survey reports
Professional relations	Pharmacist avg. tenure; Prescriber complaint reports; Survey results of special projects

3. *Setting Goals for Subordinates.* Finally, implementation must be carried out on an individual basis for each employee who will assume a significant responsibility within the organization. Each employee should be asked to write down his objectives for the ensuing year. Then a date should be set to review these with him or her. The employee should be asked to organize his goals into four categories: (1) routine duties, (2) problem-solving goals, (3) creative goals, and (4) personal development goals.

Meanwhile, the immediate supervisor should construct a list of objectives before the meeting with the employee. At this meeting, the two sets of objectives should be reviewed and reconciled into one set by mutual agreement. Two copies of the new set of objectives should be typed, one for the employee and one for the supervisor. Then the supervisor should ask what he can do to help the employee to achieve his objectives, and any suggestions or requests should be documented.

4. *Measuring Results against Goals.* Some of the goals for the firm cannot be measured until the end of the year, whereas others can be reviewed monthly or quarterly. This is also true for some individual goals; however, many of the individual's goals should be reviewed frequently, depending upon the length of employment and scope of responsibility. Weekly reviews should be conducted for new employees, especially if they are not experienced in the

work. Managers should review the progress of their supervisors on a monthly basis. At these meetings, goals may be altered or suggestions given, as indicated by the progress to date. Appropriate criteria are essential to determine whether goals have been attained.

5. *Annual Review of Results*. At the end of the budget year, each employee should have an annual review of the results achieved as measured against his goals. And, the employee should participate in this assessment. Again, criteria are essential. New goals should be set based on the past year's performance, keeping in mind that the employee should be challenged to do even better during the next year. The principal manager should also review the performance of his unit or area of responsibility with his superior. The review of the achievements of the firm should be performed by the proprietor or the chief executive officer, with the assistance of the appropriate staff. New sets of goals are established and the cycle is repeated each year.

MISCONCEPTIONS OF MANAGEMENT-BY-OBJECTIVES

Pharmacy students because of emphasis on biological and physical sciences in their educational background tend to have difficulty in developing an appreciation and understanding of the subtleties and complexities of MBO. Although MBO is comparatively simple vis-a-vis other management systems, it is not as simple as some students tend to make of it. There is the tendency to view MBO as (1) setting goals; (2) achieving goals; and (3) measuring the results in terms of primary effects only. The tendency is to reduce the process to its simplest possible terms—objectives that are easily identified and defined and results that are easily defined and measured. This oversimplification fails to take into account that, in the long-run, achieving primary effects will depend largely on achieving secondary and tertiary effects.

Setting goals or objectives is *not* MBO; almost everyone has goals and objectives. Management by objective msut be *formally* implemented and executed, and it must involve all key employees. Without the full implementation, the process is quasi-MBO at best.

In the evolution of management styles, there have been incremental changes from ''Captain-of-Industry'' to MBO, almost imperceptibly at times, in attitude toward management and employees. MBO is compatible with human relations but less so with other styles. Thus, MBO is compatible with theory Y and the humanistic approach to management to be discussed next. MBO may be compatible with the traditional approach to management but it most likely will not be as practiced by most managers. It follows then that MBO may be, but is less likely to be, compatible with the classical school of organizational theory of behavior. MBO definitely is compatible with both branches of the behavioral school and the management science school of organizational theory of behavior. Organizational theory of behavior will be discussed in a later chapter. See Table 4–2 for a comparison of MBO tenets with other management methods.

Table 4–2. Comparison of the Tenets of MBO with Other Methods

Basic Tenets of MBO	*Status of other Management Methods*
1. Broad goals are established for this firm.	True with other methods.
2. Goals are translated to more specific objectives for a given period.	Yes, in most cases.
3. Goals are translated to specific objectives for various levels and/or departments.	Yes, in some cases.
4. Each person affected by this translation participates formally in this process in meaningful manner.[a]	No, not formally and rarely done in a meaningful manner.
5. Goals and objectives are expressed in measurable terms or criteria.	Often but not in all cases.
6. Evaluation on an established periodical basis utilizing tenet 5 above.[b]	Evaluation usually is performed but often tenet 5 may not be used and may not occur as regularly.
7. MBO is a *philosophy,* a *method,* a *style,* an *approach;* it is *flexible* and *compatible* with certain aspects of other management methods, and certain organizational behavior theories but *not* compatible with others, e.g. theory X; it synthesizes the *best from other methods* and *styles.*[c]	Not true, for the most part, of the other methods, styles or approaches.

[a]This is the singular, most distinguishing mark of MBO; that is why MBO is called PARTICIPATORY MANAGEMENT, not just participatory work.
[b]This is the second most distinguishing mark of MBO.
[c]This is the third most distinguishing mark of MBO.

RESULTS OF MANAGEMENT-BY-OBJECTIVES

The *primary effects* of management by objectives are tangible results in the form of profit, increased sales, growth, and lower costs. The *secondary effects* are less tangible, but very valuable in that management itself becomes more efficient and more responsive to the needs of the firm, its employees, and society. Public and professional relations are enhanced. MBO reduces the stifling effects of bureaucracy. *Tertiary effects* are seen in improved employee morale, improved service, improved delegation, and a happier business family. Employee relations are improved as measured in terms of turnover rate, tardiness and other measures of employee satisfaction.

Traditional versus Humanistic Approach to Management

McGregor[5] provides us with an excellent treatise on the subject of traditional theory versus modern humanistic theory of managerial direction and control.

Humanistic approach to management is not analogous to the humanistic approach to philosophy. He labeled these two approaches to management theory X and theory Y, respectively. To a large extent, theory Y is based on Maslow's "hierarchy of needs" theory of motivation and is consistent with Herzberg's "dual factors of job satisfaction" theory of work motivation.[17,18] Both works will be discussed in more detail in chapters 9, 10 and 12.

THEORY X

McGregor maintains, and rightly so, that every managerial act or decision is based on an underlying theory of human nature, either explicit or implicit—more often the latter. The traditional approach to managerial direction and control relies on authority and is based on the following assumptions, constituting theory X.

1. *"The average human being has an inherent dislike of work and will avoid it if he can."*[19] Like Herzberg, McGregor sees this as an Adamic concept of life—the necessity of work for a livelihood as a punishment for the original sin of eating the forbidden fruit. This enslaved condition of man was drastically modified by the Abrahamic concept of life, a life based on faith and promise, and was modified still further by the Christian approach to life. It is strange that after 4,000 years (the span of time since Abraham) or even 2,000 years (the time since Jesus Christ) that much of modern-day management is based, at least implicitly, on a theory of enslaved mankind. It is even stranger that such a theory would persist in view of enlightened self-interest, which is contrary to such a theory as shown by McGregor.[5] However, this assumption is deep-seated in traditional management.

2. *"Because of this human characteristic of dislike for work, most people must be coerced, controlled, directed, threatened with punishment to get them to put forth adequate effort toward the achievement of organization objectives."*[20] According to McGregor, the rationale for the traditional approach is as follows: "The dislike for work is so strong that even the promise of rewards is not generally enough to overcome it. People will accept the rewards and demand continually higher ones, but these alone will not produce the necessary effort. Only the threat of punishment will do the trick. The current wave of criticism of 'human relations' (beginning in the 1950s, but it still exists in some quarters), the derogatory comments about 'permissiveness' and 'democracy' in industry, the trends in some companies toward recentralization. . .—all these are assertions of the underlying assumption that people will only work under external coercion and control."[20]

3. *"The average human being prefers to be directed, wishes to avoid responsibility, has relatively little ambition, wants security above all."*[20] This assumption is seldom, if ever, actually expressed openly today with our modern-day "social awareness." Political and social opinion would not permit it. However, this assumption still underlies much of modern managerial policies and strategies.

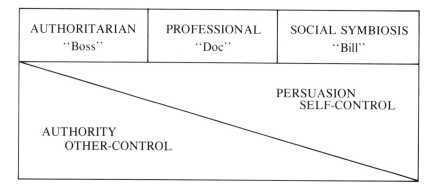

Figure 4–3. The relationship among levels of social control and methods of organizational control.

If the above analysis seems severe and harsh, an independent analysis of the managerial policies and strategies of many firms, especially larger firms, will affirm the accuracy of this analysis. There are, of course, exceptions. Smaller organizations, because of the intimacy among the personnel, are less prone to theory X; nonetheless it exists in the small organization. Theory X is especially stifling in an organization of professionals; therefore, it should be avoided by all means in the management of a pharmacy.

THEORY Y

Theory Y is not based on any soft, permissive, or pampering approach to management. It *is* based on a fundamental departure from the traditional use of *authority,* as exemplified by theory X, in management. It does not abandon authority altogether. There is still a need and a place for the exercise of authority under certain conditions. It certainly is *not* an abdication of authority; it does *reserve* authority for those special circumstances when other methods of control fail or are not appropriate. What are the methods of control other than authority?

Persuasion, in its many forms, is a powerful tool for social control. Persuasion can range from an appeal for assistance of help (entreaty) to an assertion that a certain course of action will be to the advantage of the person receiving the message (argument). Persuasion, to be convincing, must be logical, credible, and of the proper emotional tone for the situation. In the usual sense, persuasion is devoid of threat or fear.

There are at least three general levels of social relationships or control in organizations. One is that of complete *authority.*

A second level of social relationship or control is that of *professional* and *client* such as the relationship between an attorney and his client or a physician and his patient. This is an *unbalanced interdependent* relationship. A higher degree of control is reserved for the professional component of the relationship.

A third level of social relationship or control is *social "symbiosis"* through *mutual social interdependence*. This is best exemplified by the membership on an athletic team. It also exists among colleagues in an organization. To the extent that workers in an organization are colleagues, they naturally form a mutual social interdependence, and self-control replaces, to a large extent, other control.

The relationship among the three levels of social relationships or control, and the methods of exercising that control, authority and persuasion, are depicted in Figure 4–3.

The Assumptions of Theory Y. Based largely on Maslow's hierarchy of need theory of motivation, McGregor formulated six assumptions underlying theory Y.

1. *"The expenditure of physical and mental effort in work is as natural as play or rest.* The average human being does not inherently dislike work. Depending upon controllable conditions, work may be a source of satisfaction (and will be voluntarily performed) or a source of punishment (and will be avoided if possible).

2. *"External control and the threat of punishment are not the only means for bringing about effort toward organizational objectives. Man will exercise self-direction and self-control in the service of objectives to which he is committed.*

3. *"Commitment to objectives is a function of the rewards associated with their achievement.* The most significant of such rewards, e.g., the satisfaction of ego and self-actualization needs, can be direct products of effort directed toward organizational objectives.

4. *"The average human being learns, under proper conditions, not only to accept but to seek responsibility.* Avoidance of responsibility, lack of ambition, and emphasis on security are generally consequences of experience, not inherent human characteristics.

5. *"The capacity to exercise a relatively high degree of imagination, ingenuity, and creativity in the solution of organizational problems is widely, not narrowly, distributed in the population.*

6. *"Under the conditions of modern industrial life, the intellectual potentialities of the average human being are only partially utilized."* *

These assumptions call for a drastically different managerial strategy from those of theory X. Such a strategy requires the *selective adaptation* of the methods of control rather than a single absolute form of control. By selective adaptation, McGregor has in mind the unique combination of control, reward, and organizational environment that will motivate the worker to accomplish both the organization's *and* his own goals, which are completely compatible.

---

*From McGregor, O.: *The Human Side of Enterprise.* New York: McGraw-Hill Book Co., 1960.

The principle by which the organization's goals and the individual worker's goals are made compatible is *organizational integration*. This principle is profoundly different from the "scalar principle" of traditional organizational theory, which is manifested by authority that has been derived and "scaled" (delegated) throughout the organization, as illustrated by the organizational chart. Organizational integration simply means developing goals for both the organization and the individual that are compatible and mutually supportive. The student should realize by now that this integration principle of McGregor is the "heart and soul" of management by objectives. Whereas MBO is a *method* and a *philosophy*, theory Y is a *theory* and *philosophy*, and the two approaches to management are similar. Indeed, MBO is not effective unless the integration principle is freely applied to the end that participatory management is achieved, i.e., each individual participates in management to the extent that he is involved and is affected by the outcome.

Improving Decision-Making

As indicated previously, decision-making is the essence of management, although it doesn't represent all that is management. The process of decision-making follows closely the scientific method of investigation. The major difference is that, in using the scientific method in research, most of the facts are known and most of the variables are controlled, whereas in making decisions, many factors and variables are unknown. This is known as making decisions under the condition of uncertainty.

This handicap is reduced considerably when the decision-maker can ascertain more of the facts through surveys of samples. New data being derived from a sample of the universe of data can be relied upon only with a degree of probability. By following a procedure of revising probabilities based on Bayes' Theorem, the degree of uncertainty can be reduced. Although discussion of this technique is beyond the scope of this text, additional information on its use can be found in *Statistical Analysis for Business Decisions*.[21] Let us now consider some of the basic principles of decision-making that every manager can use.

PRINCIPLES OF DECISION-MAKING

It is necessary in the convulsive scene of business life to assign values to our problems and to set priorities. Clearing up simple mechanical difficulties is different from reaching a decision on a course of action which involves people, budget, and markets. It would be helpful if we had some general principles to guide us in this effort.

The *first principle* is that one needs to give *patience,* time, and thought to decision-making, especially when one is on unfamiliar ground. Decisions come easily to the sales manager who has been on the job twenty years, as long as they involve only the factors to which he is accustomed. When a new factor is introduced, or the manager moves into an area where he is a stranger, he must take time for orientation.

The *second principle* is weighing the *gain versus risk* principle. The power of deciding involves the danger of going astray, and that is the essence of deciding. Going astray involves some kind of penalty, and that is the essence of error. The consequences of a decision are part of the total problem, and should be considered as factors in it. We must balance risk against gain, and be neither deterred by the one nor dazzled by the other.

The *third principle* of decision-making involves *anticipation* in terms of results and problems arising from the decision. The manager is subject to one trial not common to the worker: he has the continual feeling of incompletion. His job is never done. His energy drives him to the consideration of the next job while the present job is still in the works, and he needs to keep his balance in both.

The *fourth principle* is that decisions are best made when there is a *master plan* to guide the manager. There is no necessary virtue in ''planning'' itself. Its value depends upon what the plan is for, what ends it will serve, what difficulties it is designed to overcome—difficulties arising from the caprices of fate, the actions of competitors, and the quirks of human nature. Without a plan, fluid though it may be, decisions cannot be reached intelligently. Management by objectives is a method that provides the necessary stability for solid decision-making.

The *fifth principle* is to *balance* the *urgency* of the decision against *deliberation*. Mere speed in coming to decisions may have small relevance at the top business management level where a person's contributions to the enterprise may be the making of two or three significant decisions a month. This is not to say that we should debate or stew over every problem. We are probably too much given to sending someone out with a red flag in front of every new idea. On the whole, it is wiser, after giving the matter adequate thought, to make a decision promptly and crisply than to linger over it and lose momentum and drive.

These five principles may be viewed simultaneously in respect to interrelationships. The first and fifth principles are related in that each has a time dimension. However, the first principle includes a personality dimension, patience, which constrains the time dimension while introducing a mental element, thought. The fifth principle emphasizes balance which constrains time to a degree but avoids procrastination, and thus promotes expeditious action. The second principle is like the fifth in that it involves balancing, but risk, not time, is the primary dimension. The third and fourth principles are interrelated in that the third principle directs the decision maker to view the future in terms of results and new problems, whereas the fifth principle directs the decision maker to utilize his master plan in making the correct choice.

To make a sound decision, it is not necessary to have all the facts, but it is necessary to know what facts are missing so that we may make allowances for same and decide the degree of rigidity to give to our decision. Some managers, in trying to avoid off-the-cuff masterminding, make it a practice to take time to sleep on a problem. This can be useful if a tentative decision has been reached or workable alternatives outlined so that the subconscious has something tangible to push around.

Little good can be said about procrastinating. Any business will become paralyzed if there are persistently long delays in the making of managerial decisions. They cause waste of time among personnel, loss of teamwork, and forfeiture of faith in management.

There are, of course, times for postponement, when a resolute determination to take no action until more facts are available is a constructive contribution to a wise decision. The warning is against unwise or frivolous procrastination. We must keep in mind that to make no decision is itself a decision, and as such must be justified.

PREPARATION FOR DECISIONS

Decisions appropriate to the situation cannot be made unless there is adequate knowledge of facts and the forces acting upon them. There must be available a large store of memories of previous experiences and things learned which can be linked with the current problem.

The reasoning process requires frames of references or units of comparison gathered through experience and study. When we have sufficient data in our minds, our recall mechanism ranges over them, assesses them, takes a little of this and a little of that, relates them significantly, and produces a decision. What we call "good judgment" is the ability to bring together new facts and relate them to the archives of our memory to arrive at a decision.

The pharmacist must never stop adding to his stock of knowledge and understanding, but this need not be a burdensome task. If pressure is inherent in his daily routine, he will find it relaxing as well as useful to spend his leisure hours deliberately engaged with new ideas and new theories which will enlarge his horizons.

It is not profitable to think of the capable decision-maker in terms of a cartoon stereotype—as a table pounder, a window gazer, a pacer of the office, an aspirin user, or a man with a wet towel around his head. One general belief may be given credence in some measure: the person who makes important decisions may not always be sweet-tempered. He is under pressure, he takes risks, he wrestles with the task of getting his ideas carried out, he has little patience with incompetency.

Some firms make no provision for the stress of management. Their managers are loaded with detail instead of being relieved of all trivia, so that they may devote their special talents to important things.

STEPS IN MAKING A DECISION

The manager who wishes to develop the habit of making decisions with wisdom and effectiveness might do well to consider the following *steps:*
1. Have an objective in mind before attempting a decision.
2. Look at the situation generally, and from it extract the problem.
3. Put the problem into words.
4. Remove all of the irrelevant substance from the problem and separate it into its component parts; in other words, "tidy up" the problem.
5. Do the preparatory research thoroughly, and brush aside preconceived ideas.
6. Consider all the facts and develop alternate solutions or options and predict the effects of each option.
7. Think through to a solution and set up some controls to ensure that the decision works.

The first job is to find the real problem, divesting the situation of all irrelevant details. Masses of data may look impressive, but only those facts that apply to the problem are worth considering. It is quite right to see the pattern of the total situation and how the parts fit together, but successful managers have the capacity to reduce the whole picture to simple terms.

A problem only becomes intelligible when it is put into words. There simply is no magic formula for decision-making, but the manager who approaches the point of decision by setting out his problem in an orderly way stands a better chance of reaching the right outcome than one who relies on snap judgments.

A problem can be solved if the person responsible grasps its nature, gauges its true dimension, decides what to do about it, and takes immediate steps to cope with it. He breaks a big problem down into small, easily tackled units, changing a vague difficulty into a specific concrete form. He may go so far as to answer one "yes or no" question and then ask others until the major problem is solved. One method advocated by some experts is "take it apart." The problem is first put in writing. Beneath this, in two columns, are written the arguments "for" and "against." When this is done seriously and honestly, the "pros" and "cons" can be counted and weighed.

Managers may smooth their way by having all proposals and problems in order before moving toward decisions. Almost every problem needs to be explored through such questions as these: (1) Why is this necessary or desirable? (2) What can it be expected to accomplish? (3) How can it be worked out? (4) Who will do it? (5) Who will be affected by it? (6) What harmful situations might result?

Superiority in decision-making rests on a solid basis of preparation, with a grasp of all the possibilities. When you reach a tentative conclusion, try to knock it down with dispassionate energy. Ask: "What will happen if . . . ? Does this decision take care of A, B, and C possibilities?" By proceeding in this way, the business executive borrows a bit of the value of the scientific method and spirit, the resolute asking of the questions: "What else?" "What if?"

You need to pay attention to detail in the preliminary stages, while keeping in mind the end purpose. Toscanini, the great conductor, is quoted as having said "In rehearsing a musical work, the important passages can frequently take care of themselves; it is the supposedly unimportant phrase or line that demands careful consideration."

The manager needs suppleness of mind. He shoulld display enthusiasm, but not the sort of zeal that blinds him to facts. He should recognize that his opinion on a matter is only something that falls between ignorance and understanding. It is knowledge in the making. To change an opinion in the face of new facts is a sign of vitality, progress, and intelligence.

In the course of deliberation, he will have taken advantage of subconscious thought. All creative thinking, including scientific research, emerges from the subconscious. The "passed to you for action" memo which consciousness receives may be couched in vague terms, and may have to be worked into shape. But this is no mystical process; it goes on hour after hour throughout our lives. It is, however, an advantage to recognize it so that fullest use may be made of it.

Last in this group of seven suggestions is the "thinking through" of the proposed decision to its conclusion. This involves testing every step leading to the decision as well as anticipating what may follow from it.

When you have reached the point where you have gathered the facts and tested them, thought about them, and weighed the consequences, then make your decision. Here are two illustrations on the folly of hesitating. Buridan, a French philosopher of the twelfth century, told us about the ass which was placed midway between two equally attractive bales of hay, and died of starvation because he couldn't choose which one to eat. Robert Browning's poem reminds us that Saul, crowned king at a time when one swift blow would have scattered his foes and united his friends, stood midway between his duty and his task, and indecision slew him.

"FOLLOW-THROUGH"

We have located and defined our problems, collected facts, and weighed the favorable against the unfavorable; we have listened to what can be said by experts, friends, and enemies; we have checked the accuracy of our information and of our thinking; we have various solutions; and we have arrived at a decision. What do we do next?

The fatal thing to do is to put the decision in a "pigeon-hole." The only place to put a good decision is into action. An idea has been born, it has evolved, and has been transformed into a decision. Now the manager must direct and participate in the execution of the decision.

It would be a mistake at this point to spend time looking back to see if you are too far from shore. You are obligated, having made the decision, to develop a certain amount of blindness to the possibility of failure. By that act you give confidence to those who must do the work of implementing the decision. However, it would be wrong to cling to a course if some vital new facts in its disfavor become known, but don't change your mind merely because you are running into obstacles. The road may be strewn with rocks, but that merely means that it is a rough road, not that it is going in the wrong direction.

Be sure that your decision is promulgated clearly. Unless you organize and clarify for your people the unrelated ideas and facts with which you have wrestled, they cannot be expected to respond with effective action. They must know what change in behavior is expected of them, what change to expect in the behavior of others with whom they work, and what change will be made in the working conditions. This is the manager's directional guidance. Together the manager and the employees establish the goals and determine the methods to achieve them.

Mechanical problems associated with your decision are relatively simple compared with the human problems. For example, your decision may change the apparent status of workers, and it is astonishing how surely someone will be annoyed and deeply pained by any wrong done to this feeling of self-importance. This is one reason for careful consultation of all those who are to be affected by the decision. It will give you the benefit of their experience and their ideas, and make them participants in whatever comes to pass.

Being a decisive manager doesn't mean being truculent, or living apart. To be part of the working force was emphasized as a necessity of management by speakers at the Duke of Edinburgh's Study Conference in Oxford. The manager must make the time to keep in touch with subordinates. Only thus can he appraise the spirit of his people, tap their interest, and ensure their cooperation in carrying out plans upon which he decides. Human motivations and human emotions are involved as factors in the solution of every problem.

Of this one can be sure: no decision can be better than the people who are assigned to implement it. Their enthusiasm, competence, and understanding determine what they can and will do.

Summary

The student may be wondering why he should bother with these various styles and methods of management and the brief background surrounding each. The answer is that all of these styles or methods of management, except management by objectives, and possibly theory Y, can be found in the various pharmacy practices—independent proprietorships, chain drugstores, or institutional pharmacies. If we include the pharmaceutical industry, we probably could find some fairly good examples of all these methods and theories. The young pharmacist will encounter one or more of these management styles, or perhaps some combination of them. An understanding of the nature of the various management styles and the boss's personality will aid a pharmacist to develop a better rapport and working relationship with his supervisor and to be a better manager.

The various theories, principles, techniques, procedures, and methods of management have been presented. Major emphasis was given to management by objectives and the importance of good decision-making. Management by objectives improves all aspects of management, but its greatest impact is on performance and performance evaluation. It enables the manager to communicate with a subordinate without causing the subordinate to become defensive. Although every technique and procedure may not be applicable to every small independent pharmacy, most of the procedures and *all the theories and principles,* especially those related to management by objectives and decision-making, *apply* to any type of pharmacy or pharmaceutical enterprise. Indeed most of the principles and techniques can be applied to an individual in managing his time and personal affairs.

Most young pharmacists intend either to own their own pharmacy or to become a manager of a chain drugstore or a chief pharmacist in a hospital. A word of caution is in order. Neither management by objectives nor theory Y is a panacea, and there still is room for improvement, which is reflected by the title of the book *Beyond Management by Objectives.*[22] For a more comprehensive comparison of the classical, behavioral, and management science schools of thought on management, see *Fundamentals of Management* by Donnelly, Gibson, and Ivancevich.[23]

REFERENCES

1. Odiorne, G.S.: *Management by Objectives—A System of Managerial Leadership.* New York: Pitman Publishing Corp., 1965, p. 39.
2. Dimock, M.E.: *A Philosophy of Administration.* New York: Harper and Row, 1958.
3. Drucker, P.F.: *The Practice of Management.* New York: Harper and Brothers, 1954, p. 280.
4. Tiffin, J.: *Industrial Psychology.* 3rd ed. New York: Prentice-Hall, Inc., 1952.
5. McGregor, D.: *The Human Side of Enterprise.* New York: McGraw-Hill Book Co., 1960.
6. Drucker, P.F.: *op cit.,* Chapter 11, pp. 121–136.
7. Odiorne, G.S.: *op cit.,* (the entire book).
8. Odiorne, G.S.: *Management Decisions by Objectives.* New York: Prentice-Hall, Inc., 1969.
9. Odiorne, G.S.: *Management by Objectives, op cit.,* p. 55.
10. Adapted from Odiorne, *ibid.,* pp. vii and viii of Preface.
11. *Ibid.,* p. 66.
12. *Ibid.,* p. 67.
13. *Ibid.,* pp. 54, 55.
14. Steinmetz, L.L., Kline, J.B., and Stegall, D.P.: *Managing the Small Business.* Homewood, Ill.: Richard D. Irwin, Inc., 1968, pp. 146–148.
15. *Ibid.,* p. 148.
16. Odiorne, G.S.: *Management by Objectives, op. cit.,* p. 68.
17. Maslow, H.: *Motivation and Personality,* 1st ed. New York: Harper and Brothers, 1954.
18. Herzberg, F.: *The Motivation to Work.* New York: John Wiley & Sons, Inc., 1959.
19. McGregor, D.: *op cit.,* p. 33.
20. *Ibid.,* p. 34.
21. Spurr, W.A., and Bonini, C.P.: *Statistical Analysis for Business Decisions.* Homewood, Ill.: Richard D. Irwin, Inc., 1967, Chapters 15–17.

22. Batten, J.D.: *Beyond Management by Objectives*. New York: American Management Association, 1966.
23. Donnelly, J.H., Jr., Gibson, J.L., and Ivancevich, J.M.: *Fundamentals of Management: Functions, Behavior and Models*, 3rd ed. Dallas: Business Publications, Inc., 1978.

REVIEW

1. Define management in classical terms.

2. What is the essence of management?

3. What are the two cardinal principles of management and the consequences of the failure to follow these two principles?

4. Discuss in philosophic and practical terms the differences between managers and administrators.

5. Name and describe the five historic management styles or methods, including the approximate time frame and the socioeconomic changes taking place during each era.

6. Associate the source of power and the general mode of communication with the six "styles" of management that can be identified today.

7. Define management by objectives, and discuss its six major premises, its basic philosophy and conceptual framework.

8. Explain the proper manner and sequence of implementing management by objectives and the consequence of poor implementation.

9. Explain how management by objectives accommodates the value systems of society and the special techniques and subsystems of management.

10. Discuss how management by objectives can be used in overcoming chronic problems of both professional managers and small business entrepreneurs.

11. What are nine reasons given for failing to delegate work?

12. Explain the priority scale for arranging tasks used by some managers.

13. Discuss the entire process of setting objectives for the firm, managers, supervisors, and individual employees, including the criteria for measuring the achievement of the objectives.

14. What are the four categories of individual objectives?

15. Explain the purpose and procedure of the annual review.

16. Briefly describe the primary, secondary and tertiary effects of management by objectives.

17. Contrast the traditional approach to management with the modern humanistic approach to management.

18. Discuss theory X as it applies to management.

19. What are the assumptions underlying theory X?

20. Discuss theory Y as it applies to management.

21. What are the assumptions underlying theory Y?

22. Contrast authority versus persuasion as basic methods of management and the three levels of organizational control.

23. Discuss the five factors and principles of decision-making, including implications of each.

24. Discuss the preparation and the follow-through of decision-making.

25. Outline the seven steps in decision-making and briefly explain the purpose of each.

26. Explain how management by objectives relates to the statement: "Of this be sure: no decision can be better than the people you have to carry it out."

PLANNING

This section includes four chapters. Chapter 5 deals with planning in general as guidelines for other functions. It also includes factors, such as risk, to be considered in choosing a practice. The sixth chapter treats the subject of location evaluation in terms of its viability for the type of practice one is planning. Although the process of this chapter fits within the rubric of marketing research, it is also a major component of the overall practice plan. The seventh chapter discusses the planning and designing of the layout of the pharmacy. Chapter 8 deals with capital planning including sources, available credit, interest, capital or financial leverage, and an innovative capital structure plan. Also, Chapter 8 includes reasons for having a private practice; the advantages and disadvantages of purchasing an established pharmacy, establishing a new pharmacy or entering practice as a junior partner; estimating the price of an established pharmacy and the capital required for establishing a new pharmacy.

5 | The Planning Process

Planning is more than simply making a list of wishes. This is what is sometimes meant when young people say they are planning their future. Of course, this simplistic approach is not utilized by the serious student. Recently, I was asked to read and evaluate over 100 scholarship applications including essays. This experience taught me that college freshmen are mature and serious about planning for their future. Many have the ability to assess their strengths and weaknesses, likes and dislikes, financial resources, and potential of a particular vocation to provide the needs and desires they envision. Yes, likes, dislikes and wishes are a part of planning, but they are subordinate to the more difficult elements of planning.

Planning is one of two general types, strategic and tactical. Strategy is the overall plan for moving to a major goal. It is usually of a long-term nature. In contrast, tactics is the securing an objective designated by the strategy. Thus, tactics tend to be short-term in nature and focused on a specific objective in contrast to strategy which focuses on broader goals.

Planning is the setting of goals, assessing the resources that will be needed and the availability of those resources, developing alternative approaches to obtaining the goals, assessing the risks inherent in each approach, and then deciding on the best approach. Even this definition is somewhat of an over-simplification of the process.

Developing the Plan

SETTING GOALS

Goals may be broad and general or they may be specific; they may be long-term or short-term; they may have a high or low priority, and goals may have a high or low probability of being achieved. Thus, the first order of business is to sort out the goals, and then focus on those goals that are relevant, have high priority, and are achievable.

Next, goals should be classified as short-term or long-term and general or specific. Often a set of specific, short-term goals, which should be labeled objectives, must first be achieved in order to accomplish a broader, long-term goal. Thus identifying, sorting and arranging goals and objectives is a necessary first step of planning.

Goals, of course, must be consistent with life's purposes. Goals must be purposefully set in harmony with social, economic and legal boundaries. This principle is one of the premises of MBO discussed in the previous chapter. Thus planning is an essential aspect of the MBO style of management.

As we saw in the previous chapter, goals often require criteria in order to determine when a goal has been accomplished and to what degree. Some goals are accomplished completely or not at all, whereas other goals may be accomplished in degrees. Avoiding business failure is an example of the former; making a satisfactory net profit is an example of the latter. Criteria are obviously required for the second goal. For example, we might specify a net profit of less than 2 percent of sales as unsatisfactory, 2 to 4 percent as acceptable, and over 4 percent, very desirable. Criteria as well as goals must be reasonable; for example, a net profit of 15 percent of sales generally would not be reasonable.

ASSESSING RESOURCES

Resources are usually thought of as being one of two kinds, *natural* and *human*. There is a third kind, *spiritual,* which is included, either implicitly or explicitly, within the human category. This is quite acceptable because a spiritual resource is activated in an individual human or mediated through an individual person. All three kinds of resources are necessary in achieving most worthwile goals.

It is helpful to think in terms of concrete goals in order to better understand needed resources. For example, establishing a new pharmacy practice will require a finite set of resources. First and foremost is the pharmacist-proprietor and his or her abilities and drive. These should be assessed as objectively and precisely as possible. In addition, other personnel will be required; some on a temporary basis in the initial phase of organizing the practice and others in the future as the practice progresses. Some of the initial human resources include a banker, an attorney, an accountant (unless the pharmacist is sufficiently proficient), a drug wholesaler, fixtures supplier, and possibly other suppliers.

Implicit in the above list of human resources is a series of other resources. These include capital or money, a building and lease arrangement (else purchase the building which would require much more capital and place a strain on limited capital and/or credit), fixtures and equipment, and a stock of drugs and other goods. There are other resources that are not implicit in the list of human resources. These include a desirable location, an efficient layout design, physicians and other prescribers near the site of the pharmacy, and amicable business relations with a long list of other people and firms.

Planning requires more than just identifying these resources. Each must be assessed as to adequacy, cost, functional capacity, and affordability. The assessment of each major category of assets usually constitutes a major project. It will require much effort and time. Each presents a challenge and the utilization of all the professional and managerial skills of the pharmacist.

DEVELOPING ALTERNATIVE APPROACHES

Not every plan will be subject to a series of realistic alternative approaches. However, many goals within a plan are achievable by more than one approach. Each approach may have advantages and disadvantages associated with it. It is this aspect of planning along with the risk inherent in each approach that is most challenging.

Again, a concrete example is useful in discussing this topic. Therefore, the establishment of a pharmacy will be our frame of reference. Our alternatives are several and far reaching in their characteristics. First, the desired type practice will dictate many variables and thus limit many of the factors for considerations. However, because of the self-limitations associated with this step, it may not be practical to use this step as the chief criterion for selecting alternatives. In other words, it probably would be wise to have several options at this point.

Second, with two or more types of practices in mind, the location should be considered next. Again, several options are desirable perhaps two or more for each type of practice. It is best to start with the broad issues and progress toward more specific ones. The part of the country in which to locate should be considered. The changing economic climate makes some areas of the country more attractive than others. The weather climate is another consideration along with social and cultural match between the people in the area and the pharmacist. Following this is the consideration of which part of a state—large, medium, small cities or rural towns. The process is the same as above. The identification and selection of a general location is relatively easy, but the evaluation and selection of specific locations is not so easy. (Types of locations and their analysis and evaluation are discussed in the next chapter.) Of course, the type of location will have to be compatible with the type of practice. At this stage the alternative approaches are beginning to take form in terms of type of practice *and* location as well as different areas of the country and state.

The third step will be the assessment of the kinds of fixtures and equipment needed for each alternative and these will have to be selected. The same is true for the inventory of goods to be stocked. The best source of supply is also a consideration.

The fourth step will be the assessment of the finances—the amount of capital required, the amount the pharmacist has, and the amount that will have to be borrowed. Again, the sources and cost of the capital (interest) are important considerations. This will have to be done for each practice alternative that remains viable.

The fifth step is the most difficult of all—assessing the risk and potential payoff of each alternative. This is *the task* of the *entrepreneur.*

ASSESSING THE RISK[1]

There are two kinds of risk, endogenous and exogenous. Exogenous risk exists outside the market or economic system in the form of a disaster such as storms, lightning, fires, winds and the like. It is nearly, if not entirely, impossible to factor these risks into a business or marketing plan except in the form of insurance. This kind of risk is discussed in a later chapter.

The type of risk under present discussion is endogenous or market risk which exists as an integral part of our free enterprise, economic system. Thus, *risk* is a basic managerial concept with definite implications for planning because there is always some degree of risk or uncertainty in planning. Risk is involved from the time a pharmacist decides to purchase or establish a pharmacy. However, the scope of interest at this juncture is large, and any attempt to define and assess the assumed risk would have to be based on a simple success or failure criterion. Such a criterion would be indicative of the amount and manner of organizing and deploying the accompanying resources, including systems and controls for their deployment. Thus, we would not be assessing risk per se, but evaluating the entire enterprise.

Although the pharmacist is not expected to conduct research on the nature of risk or to perform complicated statistical calculations, a review of some aspects of the research on market risk will enable the pharmacist to better understand and deal with risk. There is a large body of literature on the nature of risk and the best construct to be used for operationalizing and measuring risk for experimental purposes. (A construct is a concept that has been defined in a manner that permits its measurement or quantification.) Many of these studies are found in the psychological literature and deal with risk in decision making in simple situations involving relatively small amounts of money. There has been a substantial number of studies involving large amounts of money in risky decisions in both simulated and real business situations. These have been reported in the accountancy, management science and marketing literature.

The computations in most of these studies generally involve estimations of two or more parameters: (1) the *expected return* or payoff as measured by the mean or median of dollar amounts, the percentage representation of these, or the expected value or utility, and (2) the *uncertainty* of the return as measured by the variance, standard deviation, the below-mean-semivariance, or some other probability expression of uncertainty. Choices among various opportunities are represented by probability distribution functions (F).

The variables involved in risk may be combined in various ways as models or equations. A general expression might be F (μ, σ^2) where μ represents the mean expected return and σ^2 represents uncertainty in the form of variance over a range of outcomes. The probability distribution has three regions of interest. Let x represent the return on opportunity A, then $F(x)$ is the probability A's return *will not* exceed x; $1 - F(x)$ is the probability that A's return *will* exceed x, and $F(x-)$ is the limiting value of $F(y)$ as y approaches x from below and is the probability that A's return *will be less* than x. Thus, the three regions of interest are: (1) a return equal to x; (2) less than x; and (3) more than x.

Before discussing the risk construct and the more useful models of assessing risk behavior, some general guidelines are necessary. (1) Investment opportunities must be treated as mutually exclusive so that implementation of one necessarily precludes the implementation of all others. (2) The returns or outcomes of all choices are assumed to be measured on a common monetary or percentage scale over a single or common time period. This includes present value of future earnings and all other time related values of money. (3) Investment opportunities from which a choice is made are always represented by either a probability distribution or a utility function. (4) It is assumed that distributions have finite means, variances as well as all other such estimations, and that decision makers perceive these to be accurately and reliably measured and presented. (5) All other things being equal, return (μ) is good, more is preferred to less, and uncertainty (σ^2) is bad, less is preferred to more.

There are two basic types of behavioral models used to describe risk, but this is of little interest to pharmacists. There is one classification criterion that should be stated, and that is the compensatory or noncompensatory criterion. There are no trade-offs with the latter type. Noncompensatory models require that the decision maker assign an importance order to the parameters under consideration. In the compensatory models, the decision maker may trade off a certain degree of risk for a reduced amount of return, or some other trade-off combination. The trade-off rule is necessary to account for individual differences among decision makers. The compensatory models are normally represented by a utility function, $U(\mu, \sigma^2)$, in which μ again represents the payoff or return and σ^2 represents the risk.

The Risk Construct. From a statistical perspective, variance (σ^2) is an attractive construct to represent and measure risk, but it is not so attractive intuitively or from the decision maker's perspective. The weight of empirical studies strongly supports those models which conceptualize risk as the *failure to obtain a level of return,* a contingent-process model based on the probability of loss. Loss may be perceived within the range of a return less than a target return (which may be defined by convention within an industry or by prime interest rate) to a ruinous loss. The data make it quite clear that risk is not perceived by decision makers simply as variance; they weigh "negative" returns, however defined, more heavily than "positive" returns in evaluating an outcome distribution.

The Combination Rule. How do decision makers combine risk and return, whether in a compensatory or noncompensatory fashion? Although the data are not conclusive, the studies so far suggest that decision makers utilize a hybrid model that combines both a compensatory and a noncompensatory rule. First, a noncompensatory rule is followed in which risk of ruinous loss places a constraint on the range of choices. Ruinous loss is avoided at all costs it seems. Then risk in the form of a target semivariance, probability of below-target return or some other below-target parameter interacts with the mean (expected) return in a trade-off, compensatory fashion. Note that, in the second stage of the process, risk is still perceived to be more on the negative, below target side of the probability outcome distribution. People simply do not want to lose, not even entrepreneurs.

Individual Differences and Group Behavior. People do differ in their decision-making behavior as would be expected. However, there are patterns of decision behavior based on background and, to a lesser degree, on personal preference for risk. Research has shown that the personal risk preference characteristic plays a lesser role than two other factors: training and experience, and the risk-taking situation, i.e., the type of business, company policy and financial circumstances.

Decision-making behavior within a given company tends to converge. This is the result of a common selection process, similar training, and a common environment of decision feedback, company policy and industry norms. Thus, group decisions, a common mode of decision making in industry, generally are arrived at by group consensus, which, in turn, is a result of a combination of central tendency of normative behavior, influence of leaders and group process. This pattern of behavior is consistent with the conservative decision-making behavior described above as being most common in the business environment and reflected by the hybrid noncompensatory: compensatory-trade-off model.

Summary. Risk is viewed as the failure to obtain a certain level of return which is seen first as possibly ruinous loss, and then anchored by a target return. Risk taking may be represented by a probability distribution function or a utility function. Either expression will normally, in the real world business decision context, have two or more parameters (μ, below-target semivariance, or similar risk representation). A noncompensatory contingency constraint rule operates to avoid ruinous loss, then the compensatory trade-off between return and risk (μ,r) is exercised. The utility function is an appropriate one where trade-offs are operative. The general form, R: $U(\mu,s_t^2)$ is an appropriate representation, where R is ruinous loss risk and is avoided, if possible, μ is the mean return, and s_t^2 is below-target semivariance and represents risk in the trade-off region. The expression might take the following operational form: R: $U(\mu,s_t^2) = $ R: $a\mu - bs_t^2$ where a and b are weights and are specified by the decision maker.

Experimentally, the decision makers would choose between pairs of risky and known or target investment alternatives. In practice, the decision maker would choose between two or more risky options and weigh each against the other. Thus, for four alternatives A, B, C and D, the decision maker would have to make six comparisons—A:B, A:C, A:D, B:C, B:D and C:D. Then he would probably weigh his most promising alternative against the return from a low-risk investment of the same amount in the money market.

DECIDING ON THE BEST APPROACH

Deciding on the best approach to take is no different than the decision-making process discussed in Chapter 4. The principles of decision making which are most likely to be emphasized will depend to a large degree on the nature of the perceived risk and the amount of capital involved. The larger the investment in relation to the net worth of the firm the more likely the entrepreneur will deliberate and use patience. Also, the noncompensatory constraint of avoiding ruinous loss will be more likely to be operative under these conditions. Also, a similar posture will be taken when the perceived risk is great. The reader should not be led to believe that potential loss in the form of high stakes and/or high probability of failure is the all controlling factor. If that were true, little economic progress would be made. Returning to the case of establishing a pharmacy practice, the pharmacist would at this point have the following elements of his plan. Type of practice—traditional independent pharmacy; location—home state, city with a population of 10,000 and county with 10,000 additional people, economic indicators just below national norms, seven physicians, three existing pharmacies employing two pharmacists each, two of which are located in the "downtown" area and one in small shopping center at the edge of the town; and a new site at a shopping center about twice the size of the other shopping center. The site building occupies 4,500 sq. ft. (45′ × 100′) next to the supermarket which is located at the end of the "strip" toward the town. The shopping center is scheduled to be completed and ready for occupancy in six months. Also, the location has been evaluated as a part of the risk assessment and general strategy, and the potential of the location and site was not only adequate but superior to all other alternatives investigated.

Implementing the Plan

DEVELOPING A TIME TABLE

Each approach may require a different time table because each may involve different resources, expertise, impediments and time. First and foremost, he would have to estimate the capital needed, at least an approximation. Next he would determine the amount of capital of his own that he could invest, and based on these data, determine the amount of capital he would have to borrow. Needless to say, these and the foregoing steps would have to be accomplished as rapidly as possible in order to secure the building and thus this opportunity before some other enterprising pharmacist did. This is to be done by day five.

The next step, and a crucial one, is to secure a lease for the building on reasonable terms that are consistent with the value of the location. This is to be accomplished by day 10. Preliminary inquiries have been made already and the pharmacist is on the list of preferred tenants. There is evidence based on research that chain pharmacies have gained ground on the independents not so much because of superior day-to-day operational competitiveness but because of securing the leases of the better sites. On the average, chain pharmacies pay higher rent than independent pharmacies, but they have more productive sites. Whereas chain pays about $6.35 per sq. ft. for rent (2.5 percent of sales), independents pay about $5.05 per sq. ft (2.4 percent of sales). However, the chains will realize sales about four times that of independents with about three times the space. Obviously the independent needs to be more aggressive in seeking good location sites and be prepared to pay the going rate for the lease to be in position to be fundamentally competitive.

The third step is to make arrangements to purchase the necessary fixtures and equipment. Catalogues and other information have already been assembled. This step is scheduled to be completed by day 30. The actual installation is scheduled for month five.

Fourth, arrangements for the purchase of the opening inventory are already underway with the delivery of the goods scheduled for month five plus two weeks. The only exceptions are the perishables. One week is allowed for stocking and displaying the merchandise with assistance from the prime wholesaler.

The fifth step is to arrange for the utilities to be connected one week prior to the grand opening.

The sixth step is to secure the pharmacy permit, the DEA license, the local business permit effective on the opening date.

The seventh and last step is the details of the grand opening promotion. The pharmacist will begin this phase one month prior to the opening date. He will work with local newspaper, radio station and his prime wholesaler.

Checking Progress. The time table is developed in detail along with progress dates as well as completion dates for each major step and aspect of each step. Progress is monitored and checked off on the planning schedule. If any part of the plan has to be abandoned, contingency plans will have to be put in operation.

CONTROL SYSTEMS AND RISK

Whatever the scope of a plan, whether it is establishing a practice or adding a new line of products, appropriate system(s) for control is/are needed. For a practice, all of the major systems and controls should be planned and ready to be implemented on opening day. For a smaller project such as a new line of products, perhaps the only system required is to integrate these products into the inventory system. However, the pharmacist should track the sales and estimated profit of the new line of products for several months to determine the profitability and whether to continue the line.

Although systems and controls are discussed in detail in later chapters, an overview of the utility of systems in relation to risk is useful at this point. It is quite obvious that appropriate control systems can, under certain conditions, minimize the loss that may result from inherent risk of a new venture. Risk and control should not be viewed as opposite ends of a continuum however. These are two very different concepts. For example, all of the control systems available to the Ford Motor Company did not reduce the risk of marketing the Edsel in the mid 1950s. Better marketing research may have prevented this marketing disaster, but marketing research is not a control in the usual sense. The role of control systems is more prominent and critical as the scope of a planned venture increases. The more complicated a venture is, the more elements there are that can go awry, and thus a greater need for systems.

In addition to the inherent value of control systems, they provide a powerful psychologic force for the entrepreneur, especially the timid or bureaucratic type. Appropriate control systems not only reduce the danger inherent in a risky venture, systems in place can boost the propensity of entrepreneurs to assume greater risks. Thus, we have two psychological constructs, the propensity to assume risk and the propensity to utilize systems. An entrepreneur may have either a high or low propensity for the one and either a high or low propensity of the other. Based on these two principles, five basic types of entrepreneurs are identified in Figure 5–1 in a grid format.

Actually, the grid approach to this two-factor representation allows the portrayal of various degrees of either factor. Since systems do cost, more and more systems are not the solution. There needs to be a balance between the use of systems and the degree of risk one is willing to assume.

BUSINESS FAILURE: A MAJOR RISK

Business failures have increased in recent years, especially during periods of recessions of the business cycle. The recessionary pressures have been exacerbated by high interest rates during the past decade. Business failures were at an especially high rate during the 1981–82 recession. Fortunately, pharmacies are among the less failure-prone retail trade. In a survey of 255 Illinois towns and cities, Converse found that during 1925 to 1930, 24 percent of drugstores failed compared to 46 percent for all types of retail stores.[2] Recent data support this finding. The data, although not conclusive, indicate that a high percentage of failures occur with businesses that have been in existence for only a few years, and probably small firms are more susceptible to failure than larger firms; however, the data again are far from conclusive. The problem of uncertainty arises from different definitions of business failure used by the various reporting agencies and some gaps in the reported data, especially among smaller firms.

Extent of the Problem. In 1983, Dun and Bradstreet, one of the largest business analysis and credit rating firms in the country, reported 145 drugstore failures with total current liabilities of $23,380,000 for an average of $161,240

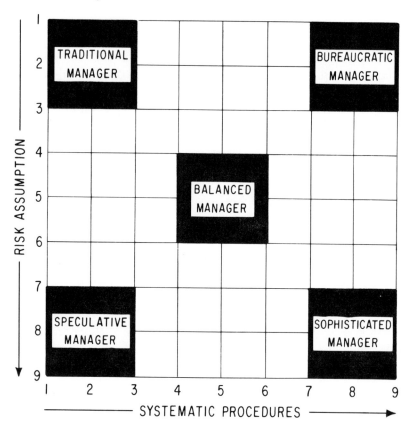

Figure 5–1. Grid representation of the propensity to assume market risk and control systems.

per drugstore.[3] Although these figures are consistent with the concept of a small business in the context of business generally, that average current liabilities figure is nearly five times the 1983 average for the *Lilly Digest* sample that reported balance sheet data. In fact, the $161,240 figure is about three times the average current liabilities figure for pharmacies with sales over $600,000 and less than five years old. One may readily conclude that there were ample reasons for these pharmacies to have failed.

Causes of Failure. Why do pharmacies fail? Two early studies—one by Baer[4] in Pittsburgh during the 1924–34 period and one by the Department of Commerce[5] in St. Louis during the early 1930s—provided data that for the most part agree with later research. It is especially noteworthy that in the St. Louis study only a few failures could be attributed to the economic conditions of the Great Depression to a significant degree. For example, one-third (10 of the 30 failures) were located on site where previous pharmacies had failed. Only two of the pharmacist-proprietors maintained adequate financial records.

Rent and other operating expenses were high in relations to sales. Overextension of credit was another symptom of inadequate financial acumen. And 20 of the 30 supplied less than 30 percent of the initial capital.

Smith, in a study of failures and changes of ownership among Indiana pharmacies (1946–54), found similar results.[6] The former owners indicated poor location was the most frequent cause of failure followed by inadequate sales, excessive operating expenses and inadequate capital. None of the pharmacists who closed their pharmacies checked lack of experience as a cause of failure, whereas 50 percent of those who sold their pharmacies did.

Dun and Bradstreet publishes in their house publications[7] a review of business failures in two ways: (A) the underlying or root causes and (B) the related apparent or visible causes. These causes, along with the historic percentages of occurrence, are for A followed by B in brackets: disaster [burglary, fire, flood, strikes]—3; fraud [falsification of records, facts, etc.]—2; neglect [bad habits, family difficulties, poor health]—10; lack of training and experience—45 and incompetence—40. These latter two root causes were reflected by inadequate sales—50, inventory problems—20, excessive expenses—15, excessive fixed assets—10, poor location—20, problems with accounts receivable—5, and lack of competitive practices—20. The latter series reflects multiple causes and thus, exceed 100 percent.

Kelly and Campbell reported that there was a definite relationship between population shifts and pharmacy closings.[8] More recently, Thomas and Evanson conducted a comparative study of 90 pharmacies that had closed, 117 pharmacies that had changed ownerships, and 191 ongoing pharmacies.[9] They found that significantly more of the closures had been in business five years or less, and that closed pharmacies had significantly lower sales, fewer prescriptions, lower total earnings (net profit plus proprietor salary), and lower percentage of total earnings on sales. There was not a significant difference in the physical size of the pharmacies in the three groups, the size of the city where located, the type of location (in respect to closed and ongoing pharmacies), and the use of 12 financial ratios in making operational decisions.

One of the most significant findings is the fact that only 25 percent of the entire sample utilized the return on equity (percent net profit of net worth) in making financial decisions, whereas approximately two-thirds utilized the inventory turnover rate and percentage cost of goods of sales. This is indicative of a rather low order of appreciation of the utility of the more significant financial ratios. This conclusion was reinforced by the lack of correlation between sales or profits and the use of financial ratios.

Relationship Between Failure and Planning. The data definitely indicate that most business failures are the result of poor planning or essentially no plan at all. There are indications of poor site location, inadequate capital and insufficient understanding of capital requirements, no integrated operational plans, and generally inadequate business skills and thus a poor plan.

Policies and Procedures

An appropriately constructed policies and procedures document will serve as the master plan for a pharmacy practice. A policies and procedures document should not address every conceivable problem that may be encountered in the future. The document should include the following components. First, it should present the pharmacist's philosophy of practice in rather general but definitive terms. This statement should include what the pharmacist believes is *not* the practice of pharmacy.

Second, the document should outline the goals of the pharmacy. Again, these should be in general but not vague terms. Goals, not objectives, should be stated at this point.

Third, appropriate professional behavior should be outlined for each major category of personnel: pharmacists, technicians and clerks.

Fourth, personnel policies and procedures should be thoroughly but concisely described. These should include employment procedures, qualification for each permanent position, salary and work schedules, sick days, vacation, and other fringe benefits policies, safety and security rules, basis for dismissal, and any other area that is important to the pharmacist.

Fifth, the policies on meeting, greeting, serving and thanking the patron or patient should be made clear.

Sixth, the policy of handling transactions, cash, cashiering, charges and other similar conduct should be made explicit.

Seventh, the policy and procedure of handling prescription orders, the finished prescription, exempted preparations and poisons are critical considerations and should be emphasized in the policy and procedures document. The steps and requirements for dispensing prescriptions and counseling patients should be detailed for the pharmacist.

In addition to the general policy and procedure document, special statements may be constructed for various functions and areas of practice. Some examples include purchasing policies including receiving, marking and stocking goods, maintenance of certain areas in the pharmacy including cleanliness; handling returns and complaints; pricing, charging, procedures for opening and closing the pharmacy, and other items of a specific nature.

All of the above policy and procedural matters are for the benefit of all personnel and each new employee should receive a copy of the document. In addition to this document, the pharmacist-manager may want to formulate policies for various functions that only he or his assistant manager would be concerned with. This category of policies might include some directives on purchasing, pricing or prescription fees, financial ratios and guidelines, and control mechanisms. For example, at what inventory turnover rate would be set for discontinuance of a product or product line?

There are various policies and procedures manuals available from the professional societies of various types of practices. American College of Apothecaries (ACA) has their Standards of Practice and a Comprehensive Policies and Procedures Manual for professional pharmacies. The American Society of Consultant Pharmacists (ASCP) has a code of ethics and a Policies and Procedures Manual for Consultant Pharmacists. The American Society of Hospital Pharmacists (ASHP) has not only a general Policies and Procedures

Manual but also a set of guidelines on nearly every major phase of institutional practice. The American Pharmaceutical Association (APhA) has a code of ethics and Standards of Practice but these are guidelines for individual pharmacists and not managerial or operational policies and procedures.

One final point on policies and procedures manuals—they are not documents you can write and then forget about them. No policies and procedures manual will ever be written perfectly the first time, and they need to be reviewed and updated periodically.

REFERENCES

1. Much of this section was adapted from review articles by Libb, R. and Fishburn, P.C.: Behavioral models of risk taking in business decisions: A survey and evaluation. *J. Account. Research, 15*:272–92, 1977.
2. The study was reviewed in Hooke, G.B.: Retail mortality and pharmacy. *J. Amer. Assoc. Pract. Ed., 12*:701–02, 1951.
3. "The Dun and Bradstreet Business Failure Quarterly Report," Economic Analysis Dept. Dun and Bradstreet Corp., New York, 1983.
4. Hooke, G.B., *op. cit.*
5. Feiker, F.M.: *Causes of Failure Among Drug Stores*, Washington D.C.: Bureau of Domestic and Foreign Commerce, Domestic Series No. 59, U.S. Dept. of Commerce, 1932.
6. Smith, H.A.: An evaluation of the causes of drug store failures from 1946 through 1954. Master's Thesis, Purdue University, 1956.
7. Ref. 3 and Dun's Business Month: see for example, Duncan, J.W.: Falloff in business. *Dun's Business Month, 125*:69, April, 1985.
8. Kelly, E.T. and Campbell, N.A.: Study of extrinsic factors involved in community pharmacy closing in Massachusetts, paper presented to the Econ. and Adm. Sci. Section of the APhA Acad. of Pharm. Sci., Washington, D.C., April 16, 1970.
9. Thomas (III), J. and Evanson, R.V.: A comparative study of pharmacy closures and changes of ownership with a group of ongoing pharmacies, paper presented to the Econ. and Adm. Sci. Section of the APhA Acad. of Pharm. Sci., Montreal, Can., May 9, 1984.

REVIEW

1. Outline the planning process step by step.

2. Discuss each step in the planning process.

3. Name the two kinds of risk, describe and define each.

4. What is a construct? Define risk as a construct.

5. How is risk measured?

6. Explain the combination rule.

7. Discuss individual differences and group behavior in respect to decision making.

8. What are control systems? Differentiate between propensity to take risk and to use control systems.

9. Discuss business failures. What are the apparent causes of business failures? What are the underlying causes of business failures? How can one prevent business failures?

10. Discuss policies and procedures. What should these include? Compose a policies and procedures document for "your pharmacy practice."

6 | Planning and Evaluating a Location

The importance of a good location to the success of a pharmacy practice can hardly be overemphasized. This point is readily understood if one considers the extreme case, for example, of the so-called "ghost town." Many small rural communities that once thrived and supported a physician and pharmacy can no longer do so because of the *migration* from rural to urban and then to the suburban areas. This migration has been brought about by technologic and sociologic changes, the mechanization of farming, the deterioration of the quality of life in the inner core of the cities, and the appeal of suburbia to the more affluent taxpayers. Migration has reduced the market value of some locations while increasing the value of others. These changes have been enhanced by the increasing reliance on the automobile and the development of planned shopping centers.

Another way to view the importance of the location is to recognize the *frequency that locations are* or *should be, evaluated* and reevaluated. At first, one might think that the typical pharmacist will evaluate one location once in his entire practice. This is a myopic and static view of the subject. A more dynamic and practical view of location evaluation is to consider that a pharmacist reevaluates his location implicitly each time he renews his lease, and although more subtly, he reevaluates the location each morning when he turns the key to unlock the door. The pharmacy proprietor should formally evaluate his pharmacy when he renegotiates his lease, every five years, or when he detects a protracted decrease in sales, whichever comes first. Mobility of the population and shopping patterns dictate it. Even the newly graduated pharmacist evaluates a location when he accepts his first position and each new position. After all, it could be the pharmacy where he will practice the remainder of his lifetime.

One should also consider location analysis in the light of the *relationship of a poor location with business failures*. Although the selection of a poor location is considered by experts, such as Dunn and Bradstreet, as a symptom

102

of the underlying deficiencies of inexperience or incompetence, it is one of the major apparent causes of business failures. Good management and aggressive promotions cannot overcome a weak location. The data accumulated during a thorough location analysis will provide the basis for the *marketing* and *promotional strategy* that the pharmacist-manager can use later, in promoting the pharmacy.

The basic principle, therefore, is simple. Locate in or near high population density, and where competition is not too severe. This does not mean that one should avoid all rural towns and the inner core of the cities. There are people in these places who need health care services, including pharmaceutical services. Several government programs, such as urban renewal, Medicaid, and others are available to assist the people in these areas. Also, it has been shown that people in these areas relate favorably to the community pharmacist. For these, the pharmacist is often their first medical care contact and resource. The pharmacist can function effectively as a medium of entry into the medical care system for the underprivileged people in these locations.

Classification and Definitions

Locations may be classified in two general ways—*geographic* and *functional*. The geographic classification is further classified broadly into either *rural* or *urban* areas. Urban areas constitute a much smaller proportion of the geographic area, but a much larger proportion of the population. According to the definitions used by the United States Census Bureau and other government agencies, ''urban places'' comprise all incorporated and unincorporated places having 2,500 inhabitants or more, and certain other towns, townships, and counties classified as urban in the *1970 Census of Population*.[1] A complete definition of urban places may be found in the *1970 Census of Population*.[1] All other areas, of course, are designated as rural areas.

GEOGRAPHIC AND DEMOGRAPHIC CLASSES

Market Size. The term urban places is used for all the urban classifications including the smallest classification unit, towns with a population of 2,500 or density of 1,000 persons per square mile, and the largest classification unit, the standard metropolitan statistical area. Urban places are further classified as follows: (1) standard metropolitan statistical areas (SMSA), (2) urbanized areas (UA), (3) cities (C), and (4) other urban places (OUP).

A definition of each of the above classifications will provide the basis for understanding the nature of the various types of urban locations. The definition of an individual SMSA involves two components: (1) the central city and the corresponding central county, and (2) a social and economic relationship and integration of contiguous counties which are metropolitan in character. A standard metropolitan statistical area must include a city with 50,000 inhabitants or more, or two cities with contiguous boundaries and a combined population of 50,000, the smaller of which must have a population of at least 15,000.

The population of the contiguous counties must be primarily nonagricultural in nature as indicated by 75 percent of the labor force. This criterion may be met if a minimum of 10 percent of the nonagricultural population in the central county or counties either work or live in the contiguous counties, or a minimum of 10,000 nonagricultural people either work or live in each contiguous county. In addition, 50 percent of the population in the contiguous counties must have a population density of 150 persons per square mile in an unbroken pattern radiating from the central city.

The criteria of economic integration are fundamental to the concept of SMSA. Either 15 percent of the workers living in each of the contiguous counties must work in the central county (or counties), or 25 percent of the people working in a contiguous county must live in the central county or counties. If the above criteria are not met, other information may be used to demonstrate social and economic integration. These include newspaper circulation, telephone listings, analysis of charge accounts of retail stores in the central cities, the extent of delivery service, official traffic counts, public transportation, and local planning, which demonstrate a social and economic interrelationship of the central city (or cities) with the outlying contiguous counties.

An *urbanized area* is similar to the SMSA, but the emphasis is placed on population density in a defined geographic area rather than social and economic integration. An urbanized area is defined as a city of 50,000 inhabitants or more, or twin cities of 50,000 people or more, the smaller of which must have a population of at least 15,000. In addition it includes the surrounding area that meets the following criteria: (1) contiguous incorporated places with 2,500 inhabitants or more, (2) contiguous incorporated or unincorporated places with less than 2,500 inhabitants, but having 100 housing units or more in a closely settled area, (3) contiguous unincorporated census districts with a population density of 1,000 inhabitants or more per square mile, and (4) any other census district within one and a half miles of the main city of the urbanized area meeting the population density criterion to eliminate enclaves or indentation of one mile or less in the circumference of the total urbanized area.

The designation "city," in general, refers to a political subdivision of a state which is incorporated and has a population of 25,000 inhabitants or more. The Bureau of Census recognizes unincorporated cities with 25,000 population or greater, but since this classification has the same general characteristics as incorporated cities, we have chosen not to differentiate between the two. Finally, there are all of the other urban places that do not fall into one or the other classifications. The above classifications have been tabulated and given common names in Table 6–1.

Type of Location. In addition to the above general geographic classifica-

Table 6–1. Modified Classification of Geographic Locations

Bureau of Census Designation	Approx. Population	Common Name
Standard metropolitan statistical areas	100,000 or more	Metropolitan area
Urbanized areas	50,000 or more	Large cities
Cities	25,000–49,999	Small cities
Other urban places	2,500–24,999	Large towns
Towns in rural areas	less than 2,500	Rural towns

tions, locations may be classified more precisely according to their characteristics and scope of commercial services and functions provided. These locations may be classified as (1) central business district (CBD); (2) major outlying retail districts (MORD); (3) neighborhood or suburban residential locations (NSR); and (4) shopping centers (SC).

The first two classifications are recognized by the Census Bureau and defined in the *County and City Data Book, 1967*. The *central business district* is described as an area of high concentration of retail businesses, offices, theaters, hotels, and other services, and an area of high traffic flow. Central business districts have been delineated officially only in cities with a population of 100,000 or more; however, a central downtown shopping district can be presumed to exist in all cities of 25,000 population or greater. Although business has declined drastically in the central business district over the past several decades, the refurbishing of these areas, especially the development of downtown malls, halted the business decline in some of these locations.

The *major outlying retail center* has been defined by the Bureau of Census as a concentration of retail stores located inside a standard metropolitan statistical area in which the central business district is located, but outside the central business district itself, which includes, among other stores, a major general merchandise store, usually a department store. Major outlying retail centers normally do not include the larger planned suburban shopping centers, but rather the older neighborhood developments which meet the above requisites. There is a major distinction between shopping centers and other major retail centers. Shopping centers are planned and well designed for efficient shopping and off-street parking, while the older type of major retail centers grew in a haphazard and unplanned manner.

The *residential neighborhood* or *suburban location* is just what is implied by the words. The term "neighborhood" is used most frequently to denote a location in the older residential part of a city, whereas the term "suburban" is used to denote a similar location in the newer, sprawling residential developments in the cities. This type of location is characterized by a few convenience stores and service establishments without a particular design. Generally, they have been established to serve the residents within an immediate area of approximately a mile radius. A pharmacy located in an older neighborhood section traditionally has been referred to as the "neighborhood pharmacy." The term "corner pharmacy" is sometimes used to refer to the same type of pharmacy located on the corner; however, the term "corner pharmacy" (or drugstore) is more frequently used to designate a traditional pharmacy in the smaller cities and rural towns.

The neighborhood or convenience shopping center differs from the older neighborhood or suburban location in that the shopping center must have been planned and designed in such a way that each establishment complements the others and attracts patrons to the center. Accessibility to the center is a prime requisite. Also, the neighborhood or convenience shopping center normally will have a greater variety of stores and services than the older neighborhood location.

A new type of pharmacy location found in the newer suburban section of our cities has been described as an "island" location in the *American Druggist*. The *island location* may be described as a single, free-standing building in a residential area. It houses the pharmacy and is surrounded by a parking area— thus the label, "island" location. Infrequently, a second commercial or service establishment will be located in the building. The island location was born of economic necessity. It provides the independent pharmacist a location with adequate off-street parking at a cost he can afford. Rental charges in the better shopping centers are prohibitive for some independent pharmacists. In addition, the independent pharmacist has difficulty obtaining a lease in the larger centers because the developers prefer lessees with greater assets and a high credit rating, the reason being that the developer will use the credit strength of the larger lessee as leverage in obtaining funds from financial institutions for developing the center. One usually will find a modern conventional pharmacy in the island location; on occasion, a prescription speciality shop may be located in an island location. It is apparent that the island location is a special case of the neighborhood or suburban residential location. Figure 6–1 shows a view of a typical island location.

SHOPPING CENTERS

Shopping centers are further classified and defined according to the size of the trading area and the classes of goods that are prevalent in the center. These are summarized in Table 6–2.

Neighborhood Centers. This type of shopping center is frequently designated as a *convenience* center. It consists of a few stores that purvey primarily convenience goods such as food, drugs, some hardware goods, liquor, and variety store items. It serves a district approximately the size of a grade school district, normally a radius of two to three miles. These centers are usually of the "strip design" along one side of a street.

Community Centers. Community centers are sometimes referred to as *suburban* centers. They are larger than the neighborhood centers, consisting of a dozen or more stores that carry convenience goods, some shopping goods, and limited specialty goods. These centers approximate the size of a city high school district with the usual radius being three to five miles. They sometimes

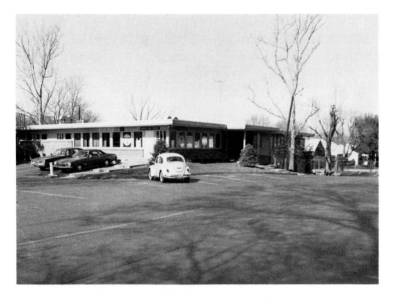

Figure 6–1. View of a typical island location.

draw patrons from distances up to ten miles. Nearly all types of stores and goods may be found in these centers including a junior-size department store, frequently a branch super-variety store, or a full-size department store. These centers are usually of the ''strip'' or ''mall'' design.

Regional Shopping Centers. This type of center is the largest of shopping centers, characterized by a large department store—more frequently, two department stores— and one or more general line stores such as pharmacies, groceries, hardware stores, and variety stores. These centers draw trade for shopping goods such as clothing and appliances, from as far as 50 miles away and occasionally farther. Several designs may be found among these centers. The regional center designation is often misused. Few shopping centers are actually regional in their characteristics.

Table 6–2. Classification of Shopping Centers

Common Name	Radius of Drawing Area	Dominant Class of Goods
Neighborhood	Up to 2–3 miles	Convenience goods
Community	Up to 3–5 miles	Convenience and shopping goods
Regional	Up to 50 miles or more	Convenience, shopping & specialty goods

FUNCTIONAL CLASSES OF LOCATIONS

So far we have discussed five general classes and four specific geographic types of location that are generally familiar to most students and pharmacists. In addition, locations may be classified functionally as suscipient, interceptive, or generative. These terms are less familiar. This classification is distinct and any of the geographic classes of location may be further classified in this manner.

A *suscipient* location is one to which patrons are coincidentally or impulsively attracted while away from their place of residence for any primary purpose other than shopping. Thus, a pharmacy located in a hotel, an airport, a resort area, and similar places is a suscipient location. Pharmacies located in clinics and hospitals are special cases of this class of location. Although these latter examples must be considered prime locations, care should be exercised not to overestimate their value. This is especially true of the pharmacies located in clinics with a large number of low prescribing specialists.

The *interceptive* location receives its label from the fact that the strategy of such a location is to intercept patrons on their way to a shopping district, a major outlying retailing center, or a shopping center. This strategy is most effective among convenience and speciality shops located, for example, between a large office building and the central downtown business district. A pharmacy located near but not within a clinic is an example of this type of location.

The *generative* location is the most common among this classification. It derives its name from the fact that patrons are attracted to it for the purpose of shopping—thus it generates business. Obviously, the central downtown business districts, the major outlying retail centers, and the shopping centers are examples of the generative class. Most pharmacies in the small cities, rural towns, and neighborhood locations fall within this class. In many instances, one would have to investigate the particular situation surrounding the pharmacy to classify its functional location accurately.

In summary, a location may be one of the general geographic locations (SMSA, urbanized city, smaller city, other urban place or large town, or a rural town). Additionally, a location site may be in a central downtown business district, a major outlying retail center, a shopping center, a neighborhood or suburban area, or an island location. Any of these locations may be classified further as suscipient, interceptive, or generative. Each particular type of location has its advantages and disadvantages, but in the final analysis each individual location must be analyzed and evaluated for its market potential.

Variables Affecting Choice of Location

DEMOGRAPHIC

Demographic factors are the primary variables in the selecting of a location. These factors are important because they determine to a large degree the need of, if not the demand for, health care services. The aged and infants use more medication than other age groups. Ethnic groups sometimes require special consideration in their specific needs and demands. Other variables include the *economic activity,* the *social and cultural institutions of the community,* the *type of pharmacy,* and the *pharmacist's inclinations and desires.*

ECONOMIC

The primary measures of economic activity are the *per capita income* and the *median family income.* The underlying factors of economic activity include *economic input factors* and *economic organization.* To investigate these, the following questions should be raised. Is the economy of the community primarily agricultural or industrial, or does it include both? If it is primarily agricultural, does the community rely mostly on one or two crops, or is the agriculture diversified? If it is an industrial community, does it rely primarily on one or two basic (heavy) industries such as steel, or is the industry of the community diversified? The implications of the questions should be obvious. Reliance on one major crop involves heavy risk from drought, floods, and other disasters. The same is true with a single industry since risks inherent from strikes, riots, or failure of the company to obtain a government contract are real.

INSTITUTIONAL

Supportive social and cultural institutions are important to the growth and development of a community. These institutions include the economic institutions, such as banks, and the proper number and types of shops and stores. Adequate transportation, utilities, professionals, services, good educational and health institutions, and religious and cultural institutions are also important parts of the social and cultural institutional milieu. Of course, natural resources are vital, but human resources are the most important of all. Often a community has a dearth of skilled artisans and professionals, and these people are essential to the growth of a community. Physicians within the general area are essential for a successful pharmacy.

PHARMACY TYPE

Another variable to be considered is the type of pharmacy practice to be established. For example, a large super drugstore is hardly feasible in a rural town with a population of a thousand or less. At one time it was thought that the strictly prescription shop was not feasible in a small community with less than 10,000 population. This theory has proved to be erroneous, since several pharmacists have successfully established this type of practice in some of our smaller communities. *Pharmaceutical centers* have also been successful in smaller communities. The pharmacist's inclinations and desires are important considerations in the selecting of a location and constitutes yet another variable.

Variables Significantly Related to Sales

Obviously all four categories of variables discussed above are important and they probably are statistically significant. However, little research has been conducted in respect to the importance or significance of these variables to the success of pharmacy sites. Kottas in a study in 1980 attempted to identify statistically important determinants of sales volume of pharmacies.[2] He focused on pharmacy size, traffic count, number of physicians in the trading area, value of houses in the area, and population within the trading area. His sample of 44 pharmacies included 37 independents and seven chain units located in Austin, Texas.

Not surprisingly, multiple stepwise regression analysis revealed that size in sq. ft. and type of pharmacy were the two most significant variables, explaining about 74 percent of the variation in sales. Focusing on independent pharmacies only, the three most significant variables were hours the pharmacy was open in a week, number of physicians within one mile, and number of years the pharmacy had been in operation. These factors explained 46 percent of sales variations.

Kottas utilized a statistical technique (factor analysis, both principal component and orthogonal rotation) to identify the primary factors among 17 independent variables. Then using the lead or most prominent variable in each of the six factors, multiple stepwise regression analyses were applied to (1) all 44 pharmacies, (2) 42 pharmacies after eliminating the highest and lowest sales volume, and (3) standardized data for the 44 pharmacies. None of these analyses provided much additional insight into the relationship between sales and the various independent variables. Size was the only consistent variable that explained variation in sales when all 44 cases, including the one large chain pharmacy, were analyzed. When the 42 cases, excluding the large pharmacy, or the 37 independents were analyzed, hours per week the pharmacy was open and type of pharmacy usually were the significant variables.

Although population within one mile, physicians within one-half mile, hours per week pharmacy was open, size of the pharmacy, number of pharmacies within one-fourth mile and traffic count were consistently the lead variable in the six primary factors (with one or two exceptions), these were submerged in the regression analyses except as noted above. The seven chain pharmacies were an insufficient number for a balanced analysis, but they exerted overwhelming influence on the regression when included. Only the independent pharmacies should have been included for the full series of analyses. Cluster analysis was not helpful either. In general, it may be stated that the results supported conventional wisdom on this subject to a fairly high degree.

In 1983, Fassett investigated 51 of 54 clinic pharmacies in the greater Seattle area for the purpose of determining operating characteristics and identifying clinic and pharmacy variables that were related to prescription volume.[3] Two variables, third-party index (i.e., number of third-party programs accepted) and size of the pharmacy (sq. ft.) were significantly associated with prescription volume, i.e., new prescriptions, refill prescriptions and total prescriptions, respectively. Clinic size and clinic ownership, rent basis (percentage rent, per month dollar amount or combination), direct telephone lines and discount for physician supplies failed to predict prescription volume in any form.

In terms of new prescription volume, two variables—third-party index and number of prescribers (weighted by specialty and percentage of prescription likely to be dispensed in the clinic pharmacy and calculated from data in Table 6–4)—were significant predictors. Contrary to expectation, neither clinical services nor convenience services explained variation in prescription volume.

Although several measures of the prescriber variable were significant in explaining the volume of new prescriptions, the one described above (based on specialty and percentage dispensed locally) was the best predictor. The lack of significant predictable power for clinical and convenience services does not mean that these services were unimportant. They may have been uniformly provided in either an exceptional manner or an ordinary manner. The same may be true for a number of other independent variables. The sample was composed from a fairly homogeneous type of practice.

A study of geographic patterns of pharmacy patronage among the elderly in Flint, Michigan provides another view of the significant variables related to location of urban pharmacies.[4] This 1982 study, based on interviews of 131 older persons with low income, focused on perceptions and actual behavior in the purchase of prescriptions. Most respondents, whether black or white or residing in either of the three residential areas, felt that a convenient neighborhood pharmacy was either important or very important for their well being. There was a positive correlation between the perceived importance of a nearby pharmacy and actual distance traveled to purchase prescriptions, i.e., those who felt nearness to be very important traveled the shortest distance. Having access to an automobile was not a factor in their perception of the importance of a pharmacy nearby.

However, respondents overall did not patronize the nearest pharmacy, but on the average, "bypassed" seven pharmacies closer to their residence and traveled 1.9 miles to purchase their prescriptions. Whereas 53 percent of white respondents traveled less than one mile and 80 percent traveled less than two miles, only 31 percent of black respondents traveled less than one mile and 54 pecent traveled less than two miles. Although more whites drove (70 to 55 percent), more blacks were driven by family or friend (30 to 12 percent) with approximately equal use of an automobile. Only 12 percent of whites and 3 percent of blacks walked to the pharmacy for a distance less than a mile in all instances. Three percent of whites and 9 percent of blacks utilized a bus, traveling on the average 3.8 miles. Residents in the two areas predominantly populated by blacks traveled to the central business district-hospital "corridor" for prescriptions, probably reflecting the mode of obtaining health care generally.

The reader should be aware that this sample was atypical; however, it probably represented the inner urban population fairly well.

Analysis of the Market Potential

DELINEATING THE TRADE AREA

Once a pharmacist has identified tentatively a location, or perhaps several locations, he must delineate more precisely the trade area of each. There are several methods of accomplishing this task.

Interview Method. The *interview* technique, which is the most accurate and the most costly method, is also time consuming. The primary requisite is that an appropriate sample of the people in the projected trade area be selected. The object is to determine where the people purchase, or would prefer to purchase, the particular goods and/or services in question—in our case drugs and pharmaceutical services. The projected trade area is then divided into smaller units (usually census units), and each unit is sampled and studied individually. This method has the following advantages:

1. The researcher can better analyze the smaller units and more readily perceive and make sounder judgments concerning the various factors requiring judgment.
2. The multiplicity of many discrete judgments tends to prevent accumulative error, since the chances are greater that errors in judgment will cancel eath other.
3. Unusual situations—including demographic, economic, and social variables—can be uncovered through the interviews.

A *modification of the interview technique* may be used to evaluate central business districts, major retailing centers, or large shopping centers. The object is to interview a sample of the foot traffic passing a particular site during appropriate time intervals and identify the addresses of those passing the site. A plot of the addresses on a map will identify the boundary of the trade area. Based on the distribution of the sample, a percentage value can be assigned to each discrete population unit surrounding the site under consideration. These percentages are then multiplied by the population in each population unit to estimate the potential more precisely. Questions pertaining to the reasons the people are in the immediate trade area are included in the interview. Thus, the percent of people making pharmaceutical purchases can be used to estimate the potential for a pharmacy.

Of course, the accuracy of the modified interview technique varies with the type or class of location and pharmacy, as well as the sampling procedure used. For example, this technique is usually successful for drugstores located in central business districts, major retail centers, and the large regional shopping centers of a metropolitan area. However, since pharmacies primarily sell convenience goods and services, they do not attract many patrons from the outer fringes of the metropolitan area to the same degree as stores handling many shopping goods, and this must be taken into consideration in evaluating these locations for a pharmacy. Yet, the entire trading area must be considered as the base when this method is used.

Reilly's Law. The second technique of delineating the potential trade area of a location is *Reilly's Law of Retail Gravitation*. The usefulness of Reilly's Law is restricted primarily to rural towns, small city locations and shopping centers. Reilly's Law is represented by the following formula:

$$D_{a \to b} = \frac{d}{1 + \sqrt{\dfrac{P_b}{P_a}}}$$

where:

$D_{a \to b}$ = Outer limit of the trading area of community A, expressed in miles, along each major paved road between community A and community B.

d = Distance in miles between community A and community B.

P_a = Population of community A.

P_b = Population of community B.

The assumption underlying this equation is that patrons normally travel to the larger and more accessible community. A modification of this equation substitutes, in the case of two shopping centers, the square feet of space in the respective shopping centers for the population of the communities and the driving time for the distance between the communities, respectively. However, the application of the modified formula for estimating the trade area of a shopping center may be in some cases less valid than the original formula for estimating the trade area of rural towns and small cities.

An example, shown in Figure 6–2, illustrates how Reilly's law is applied. The pertinent data are as follows:

Town X—under consideration, population 10,000.
Town A—20 miles north of X, population 20,000.
Town B—30 miles south of X, population 30,000.
Town C—10 miles west of X, population 10,000.
Town D—15 miles east of X, population 15,000.

The calculations of Reilly's formula are as follows:

$$\text{Town A:} \quad D_{x \longrightarrow a} = \frac{20}{1 + \sqrt{\dfrac{20}{10}}} = \frac{20}{1 + 1.41} = \frac{20}{2.41} = 8.3 \; miles$$

$$\text{Town B:} \quad D_{x \longrightarrow b} = \frac{30}{1 + \sqrt{\dfrac{30,000}{10,000}}} = \frac{30}{1 + 1.73} = \frac{30}{2.73} = 11.0 \; miles$$

$$\text{Town C:} \quad D_{x \longrightarrow c} = \frac{10}{1 + \sqrt{\dfrac{10,000}{10,000}}} = \frac{10}{1 + 1} = \frac{10}{2} = 5.0 \; miles$$

$$\text{Town D:} \quad D_{x \longrightarrow d} = \frac{15}{1 + \sqrt{\dfrac{15,000}{10,000}}} = \frac{15}{1 + 1.23} = \frac{15}{2.23} = 6.7 \; miles$$

Since the trade area in this case is a rectangle, the area in square miles is calculated by multiplying the length times the width ($19.3 \times 11.7 = 225.8$). Thus, the area is 225.8 square miles. Sometimes the configuration of the trading area will approximate a circle. In such cases, the formula for the area of a circle is utilized ($A = \pi \gamma^2$).

It is obvious that Reilly's Law can be employed with a minimum expenditure of time, money and effort. It is a reasonably accurate technique for a rural setting, but it must be used with caution in an urban situation. In an urban setting the situation is more complex, and factors other than distance and population must be considered to be equally and sometimes more important.

Record Sampling Method. A technique for estimating the trade area of an existing pharmacy is to *sample the prescription file* and/or *charge accounts* and plot the addresses of the customers on a map. The sample should be sufficiently large, about 400 prescriptions or accounts, and selected randomly. The area represented by the plot of the addresses represents the trade area of the pharmacy. This technique is discussed in more detail in the section of relocating a pharmacy.

Vacuum Method. Another technique, used in the *vacuum method,* is the delineation of the boundaries by applying the *trading criteria* listed in the next paragraph. This technique is best utilized when the geographic boundaries of the trade area can be well defined, such as rural areas, small urban towns, most neighborhood districts in cities, and small convenient shopping centers. The vacuum technique has been applied, however, to nearly all classes and types of locations and pharmacies.

The first step in the vacuum technique is to delineate geographically the

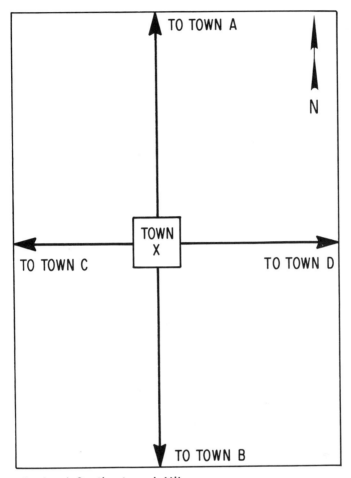

Scale: 1 Centimeter = 1 Mile

Figure 6–2. Diagram showing the application of Reilly's law of retail gravitation.

trade area. The county boundary is most frequently used for rural areas and smaller urban towns when the populations of neighboring towns are approximately equal. For neighborhood or residential locations in cities, the trade area for the site is determined using one or more of the following criteria and applying it to each major street leading to the site: (1) the distance to the nearest pharmacy; (2) two miles or ten minutes driving time from the site; or (3) any natural "traffic barrier" such as rivers, or a busy railroad crossing. The geographic limits of the trade area for central business district, major retail center, and large regional shopping centers cannot be determined by this technique.

Table 6–3. U.S. Expenditures* for Pharmacy Products in 1983

Category	Expenditures in $ Millions	% of Person-al Income†	Per Capita Expenditures	% of Pharmacy Sales
Prescriptions	$16,706	0.791	$ 72.90	35.34
O-T-C Drugs#	4,251	0.201	18.55	8.99
Home Health Care & Sickroom supplies	551	0.026	2.40	1.17
Foot Care Products	172	0.008	0.75	0.36
Baby Care Products	776	0.037	3.40	1.64
Feminine & Personal Hygiene Products	779	0.038	3.50	1.69
Optical Care Products	637	0.030	2.80	1.35
Contraceptives	186	0.009	0.80	0.39
Subtotal	$24,078	1.140	$105.10	50.93
Dental Care Products	661	0.031	2.90	1.40
Shaving Products	366	0.017	1.60	0.77
Fragrances, Cosmetics & Skin Care	3,260	0.154	14.15	6.90
Hair Care Products	1,898	0.090	8.30	4.01
Subtotal	$ 6,185	0.292	$ 26.95	13.08

Gifts	534	0.025	2.35	1.13
Photo Supplies	2,291	0.108	10.00	4.85
Stationary & School Supplies	984	0.047	4.30	2.08
Household Products	1,365	0.065	5.95	2.89
Hosiery	1,481	0.070	6.50	3.13
Subtotal	$ 6,655	0.315	$ 29.00	14.08
Magazines	1,617	0.077	7.05	3.42
Candy & Gum	1,434	0.068	6.25	3.03
Tobacco Products	1,772	0.084	7.75	3.75
Food & Beverages	5,532	0.262	24.15	11.70
Subtotal	$10,355	0.491	$ 45.20	21.90
GRAND TOTAL	$47,273	2.238	$206.25	100.00

*Source: *Drug Topics*, July 2:22, 23, 1984, and represent sales in pharmacies and drugstores only.

†Estimated based on *Drug Topics* (*ibid.*) and various government publications.

#O-T-C Drugs include cough and cold products, analgesics, vitamins, digestive aids, laxatives, diet aids, hemorrhoid remedies, dermatologicals, external analgesics, first aid and miscellaneous products.

ESTIMATING THE MARKET POTENTIAL

When the trade area has been delineated, one can proceed to estimate its sales potential. Two demographic units and economic measures are available for this purpose: (1) the number of families and the median family income, and (2) the population and the per capita income. The latter criteria are preferred since they provide for inclusion of individuals not living in family households.

The *first step* in estimating the market potential is to ascertain the population of the trade area. This may be accomplished in one of two ways: (1) get the information from a reliable source, such as government publications, postal lists, Chambers of Commerce, or tax rolls for adults and school rolls for children, or (2) count the number of households and multiply this by the mean number of persons per household. The United States average was 2.73 persons per family in 1983.

The *second step* is to multiply the population by the per capita income for the area. An alternate method is to multiply the number of families by the median family income for the area. This calculation gives the total personal income for the entire area. If the trade area has many persons, either young or old, living alone, the number of persons and the per capita statistics should then be used. The estimated per capita personal income in the United States was approximately $9,220 in 1983, and the per household median income was approximately $20,885 and the mean household income was $25,400. The disposable income was approximately 84 percent of the personal income. The personal income is then used to estimate the potential for the trade area by applying the appropriate percentages or per capita figure from Table 6–3. The appropriate figure is based on the contemplated departments in the pharmacy, e.g., prescriptions, over-the-counter drugs, home health care, foot care, baby care, personal and feminine hygiene, optical and contraceptive products will produce an expected potential sales volume of 1.14 percent of the personal income. An alternate method to obtain this figure is to multiply the per capita expenditures for various drugstore products by the population of the trade area to determine its potential. This is probably the most accurate and the preferred method in most instances, especially when the population is known or can be determined accurately. This step gives the gross potential pharmacy sales for the trade area.

The *third step* is to estimate the sales volume for the competing pharmacies located in the trade area; the remainder of the expenditures is available to the new pharmacy. The sales volume of each pharmacy within the trade area can be estimated by multiplying the estimated payroll, including the proprietor's salary, by a factor of six for independent pharmacies and 10 for chain pharmacies. An alternate method is to determine the gross square footage of each competing pharmacy and then to apply the appropriate sales per square foot figure from the *Lilly Digest* to each pharmacy. This figure will provide an estimate of the sales volume for each pharmacy. Each procedure is based on the statistics reported in the latest *Lilly Digest*[5] and is valid for most pharmacies with sales volumes over $100,000 a year.

The *fourth step* is to subtract the estimated sales volume of the competition in the trade area from the gross potential sales volume, for that particular trade area. This is the "potential" available for a new pharmacy, which is called the *"vacuum" potential.* Of course, these people currently are obtaining their drugs and pharmaceutical services from some source, but the significance of the vacuum potential is that a new pharmacy, properly located, should have a better chance of attracting and holding these patrons than any other pharmacy. In addition, the pharmacy may attract some patrons from existing pharmacies and nondrug outlets. The ability to do this will be determined by the relative strength of the several location sites and management. Estimating and adjusting for the relative strength of the several pharmacies in the trade area (including the new pharmacy) is the *fifth* and *final step,* and is discussed in detail in the following section.

ESTIMATING RELATIVE STRENGTH

The relative strength of pharmacies should be estimated from several points of view, some of which are more significant than others. For example, proximity to physicians' offices is important for prescription shops, whereas foot traffic may be a determining factor in the location of a conventional pharmacy, especially for a super drugstore in a shopping center or a downtown location. To arrive at these estimates, a weight should be assigned to the following factors:

Size. Size probably is the most significant factor in determining the sales of a traditional pharmacy.[2] However, size alone will not produce sales. The size should be consistent with the type of pharmacy, type and potential of the location, and the promotional plan the pharmacist envisions. Also, the size of a pharmacy is subjected to the law of diminishing returns to scale. For each type of pharmacy, there is a threshold or minimum size. Therefore, the size of a traditional independent pharmacy should range between 1,000 sq. ft. as a bare minimum and some upper limit depending on the number and types of departments—approximately 6,000 sq. ft. The following somewhat arbitrary 1–10 assessment scale was developed to assist in comparing pharmacies on this factor.

Units of 1,000 sq. ft:	0.5	0.75	1	2	3	4	5	6
Scale Values:	-2	-1	1	4	6	8	9	10

> Each factor should be assessed on a 1 to 10 scale. Prescription pharmacies should occupy between 500 to 1,000 sq. ft. Chain drugstores are classified as bantam (4,000 to 6,000 sq. ft.), traditional (6,000 to 12,000 sq. ft.) and super (above 12,000 sq. ft.).

Shape. Traditional pharmacies are most efficient when customers are readily drawn throughout the pharmacy. Thus, the most efficient design is a rectangular shape with the short side facing the street. An ideal ratio between the length and width of the front is 2.5 to 1. The 1 to 10 efficiency scale of the pharmacy should be decreased some for less than an ideal ratio. However, the percent efficiency should be decreased considerably if "L" shapes or hidden alcoves exist within the store. These configurations tend to make it difficult to activate all of the selling area. Super drugstores may be either square or slightly rectangular. Decrease the efficiency scale slightly for a super drugstore as the space departs from the square or near-square configuration. Shape is not as crucial in the prescription pharmacy, but clumsy alcoves make the store difficult to lay out.

Front. Except for a few locations, the entirely or nearly entirely glass front should be considered ideal. As the front departs from this ideal, the 1 to 10 visibility scale should reflect this. In recent years, there has been a trend away from the completely glass front for two reasons. (1) In view of the current energy "crunch," this front may not be the most efficient. Thermal-pane glass and double-pane glass are better than ordinary glass-pane windows in this respect. (2) With the increased cost of real estate, building (rent), fixtures, insurance, and other relevant factors, pharmacy entrepreneurs can ill afford to use much space that is not productive in sales. However, a view of the prescription department from the sidewalk is desirable. A partial "open" glass front is probably the answer. In heavily traveled downtown districts, a display window front may be desirable, but good vision into the pharmacy is also desirable because "people go to people." An entrance above or below street level may reduce volume potential, and an allowance for this should be made in the efficiency rating.

General Appearance. The overall appearance of orderliness and cleanliness is important. The pharmacy should be well lighted and clean, and have pleasing color combinations, attractive displays that are not jumbled, and a professional atmosphere. This factor should be assessed on a 1 to 10 appearance scale for each pharmacy.

Parking. In modern shopping centers, a ratio of three square feet of parking area to one square foot of selling area is considered the *bare minimum*. In the better centers, a ratio of at least four and one-half to one is maintained. If the ratio of parking area to selling area falls below this value in a shopping center, the parking scale is decreased. In older existing shopping districts, where no such ratio can be established, it would be wise to make an observation at peak selling periods. Parking spaces should always be available near enough to the location under consideration so that it will be more convenient to stop and shop there than to go to another pharmacy. In downtown shopping locations, parking is quite a different matter. Most shoppers usually park in some commercial facility and shop several stores on foot. However, if commercial parking facilities in a downtown shopping area are distant from the location, the rating for this factor should be decreased. Finally, if all parking spaces in the shopping district or area are filled during peak periods the rating should be decreased.

Traffic. Passing foot and car traffic are of promotional value and should also be considered. Minimums or ideals depend on whether the site being considered is in a central business district, a major retailing center, or a shopping center. They also depend on the type of pharmacy being considered. Passing traffic is qualitative and traffic going to and from work is much less valuable than shopping traffic. Persons driving home from work are more likely to stop for shopping than are those going to work. Thus a site on the right side of the street when the traffic is moving toward the residential area of a city is preferred over the opposite side of the street. This premise is especially applicable to small, convenient, strip shopping centers and to neighborhood locations, if other factors are equal. A foot and car traffic count, showing the number of passersby in a given period, should be made during several periods selected at random. Surveys should be made both at the proposed location site and at the competing pharmacies in the same trading area. The site with the greatest traffic count is given a rating of 10. Other sites are rated as a ratio of their traffic count to the count of the best site. If the pharmacy is in a shopping center, it should be located in the most active end. Also, it should be easily accessible and visible from the main thruway.

Proximity to Merchants. Pharmacies, particularly those without strong traffic-building departments, need to be located either near the population center or near strong traffic-building stores. A spot adjacent to an aggressive supermarket or department store is considered to be best, and the business proximity rating should be adjusted accordingly for those not adjacent to such stores.

Proximity to Physicians. This factor is important for prescription pharmacies, less essential for traditional pharmacies, and still less essential for super drugstores. One can make estimates of the number of prescriptions written by physicians in the area. Table 6–4 provides data to assist in making these estimates. This table is especially applicable to clinic pharmacies. The prescriber proximity rating should be made on the bases of the *nearness* to prescribers and calculated from the index value in Table 6–4 and the number of each kind of prescriber (specialist) in the same market area.

Proximity to Other Health Facilities. A medical clinic near the pharmacy would constitute a location with a 10 rating for this factor. A hospital with active outpatient clinics should be rated rather high, but less than 10. This factor, as with the one above, is important for prescription pharmacies and less essential for the other types.

Summary. Care should be exercised in attaching too much significance to some of these factors for certain types of pharmacies. On the other hand, these factors should not be ignored. The following weights were given to the respective scales described above in order to have one overall efficiency assessment of a pharmacy for comparison purposes: shape—0.5, front—0.5, general appearance—0.5, parking—1.0, traffic count—0.25, proximity to health facilities—0.25, proximity to businesses—1.0, proximity to prescribing—2.0, and size—4.0 for a total of 10. Even though these weights were

Table 6–4.   Annual New and Renewed Prescriptions Filled by Pharmacies, by Specialty

Specialty	Annual New and Renewed Prescriptions	% Filled Locally	℞ Index*
Dermatology	11,200	40	0.70
General Practice/Family Practice	10,900	100	1.70
Pediatrics	9,000	100	1.40
Osteopathy	8,000	100	1.25
Internal Medicine	6,700	80	0.85
Allergy	5,800	40	0.35
Otolaryngology	5,100	40	0.30
Obstetrics/Gynecology	4,500	80	0.55
Urology	3,200	40	0.20
Psychiatry	2,900	30	0.15
Surgery	2,200	40	0.15
Ophthalmology	2,900	40	0.20
Dentistry	500	100	0.10
Average Practitioner	6,400	—	—

Source: Smith, H.A.: Sale or purchase of a pharmacy practice: your price or mine. *Tile and Till, 65*:2–4, 1979.
  *Rounded to nearest 0.05.

not statistically derived, they do reflect available data. These values are then used to estimate the relative strength and the adjustment necessary for each pharmacy in the trade area.

EVALUATING SUSCIPIENT LOCATIONS

The evaluation of suscipient locations requires special techniques. For example, the potential of a clinic pharmacy is estimated by ascertaining the number of prescribers by speciality, and multiplying this by the average daily prescriptions written by the respective speciality. Next, the total estimated number of prescriptions is multiplied by the percentage one can expect to dispense in the general market area. See Table 6–4 for these data. The basic factor determining this percentage is the ratio of the patients who are referred to the clinic by physicians from other communities. This, in turn, is related to the ratio of the number of specialists in the clinic to the number of primary care specialists, such as internists, pediatricians, and general practitioners.

The prescription index in Table 6–4 was calculated by dividing the mean number of prescriptions generated annually by each specialist and generalist by the overall mean (6,400) and multiplying the quotient by the percent filled in the local market. Thus, a GP has a weight of 1.70 and an internal medicine physician has a weight of 0.85. Then the number of each type of prescriber is then multiplied by the respective weights to calculate a score for a cluster of physicians in a clinic. If one is interested only in the number of potential prescriptions, do not divide the annual number of prescriptions generated by the prescriber by the overall mean, but simply multiply the annual number of prescriptions by the percentage filled locally. The validity of the data in Table 6–4 was essentially confirmed by Fassett's study.[3] If there is no competition in the immediate trade area, then a pharmacy located in the clinic or physician's building could expect to dispense nearly all of the new prescriptions of primary practitioners. The percentage of refills is considerably lower in clinic pharmacies.

Other special suscipient locations, such as airports, require still other special techniques. Basically, these consist of estimating the number of people in transit and then estimating the percent of these people making purchases of pharmaceutical products and the average transaction value. Multiplying the latter two statistics by the daily average number of people in transit provides an estimate of the average daily sales.

EVALUATING INTERCEPTIVE LOCATIONS

This method applies primarily to interceptive locations near a clinic or a cluster of physicians but not in or adjacent to the clinic or physicians' building. The value of an interceptive location near a clinic will depend on the following: (1) The larger the clinic and the number of prescribers, the more likely there will be ''spill over'' prescriptions. (2) The quality of pharmaceutical services, both conventional and clinical, within the clinic is important but not likely to prevent ''spill over'' completely. (3) The professional and/or business relations between the prescribers and pharmacists within the clinic is very important, but will not preclude some ''spill over'' prescriptions, especially in large clinics. (4) The accessibility of the interceptive pharmacy must be excellent and be located on and be visible from the main traffic artery leaving the clinic. (5) The pharmacy must develop outstanding professional and promotional programs in order to attract significant numbers of patrons. The general principles embodied in these five specific principles apply to interceptive pharmacies generally.

CALCULATING AN EXAMPLE

A location in a small, convenient shopping center is used to illustrate the calculations for estimating the potential of a location site.

Step 1—Delineating the trade area. A large, regional shopping center located $3\frac{1}{2}$ miles southwest includes a chain pharmacy. Another chain pharmacy is located three miles west in a community shopping center. A medium-size, independent pharmacy is located in a small, neighborhood shopping center $1\frac{1}{2}$ miles to the north. There is no other pharmacy located east or south, and the residential area extends about two miles in either direction. Shoppers in each shopping center were interviewed during random periods within one week. It was found that the pharmacies in each location drew patrons throughout the trade area under study; however, many indicated that they would prefer to purchase prescriptions and drug items closer to home *if* the services and prices were right. Based on this analysis, a trade area was drawn on a city map extending two miles east and south and one mile southwest, west, and north from the proposed site.

Step 2—Estimating sales potential. First, the trade area was identified, which approximated a trapezoid. The area as determined by $A = h\,(\frac{1}{2}b_1 + b_2)$ was almost 5 square miles. The population density for the area as determined from a map of census tracts was just over 1,800 persons per square mile. Part of the area had not been completely developed. Thus, approximately 9,000 people live in the area. The per capita income for the area was $10,050 ($830 above national average). The pharmacist planned to stock a wide variety of products in all the usual departments except food and beverages, tobacco products and hosiery. Therefore, he selected 1.815 percentage figure from Table 6–3. The calculations were carried out as follows:

1. Area $= 2.1250\,[\frac{1}{2} \times (2.8125 + 1.4375)] = 4.52$ sq. mi.
2. $4.52 \times 1,800$ population/sq. mi. $= 8,136$ population.
3. Personal income $= \$10,050 \times 8,136 = \$81,766,800$.
4. $\$81,766,800 \times 0.01815$ (% spent in pharmacies) $= \$1,484,067$, $1,500,000 rounded.
5. Alternatively, $8,136 \times \$167.80$ spent in pharmacies $= \$1,365,220$, $1,400,000 rounded.

Thus, the "vacuum" potential was between $1,500,000 and $1,400,000. The upper figure was selected for further projections.

Step 3—Adjusting for competition. Because of the special geography of the trade area and the conservatism used in delineating the area, its sales potential will probably not be shared proportionally among the four pharmacies. Based on the results of the survey, it was assumed that the new pharmacy would attract one-third of the potential pharmacy sales: $1,500,000 $\times \frac{1}{3} = \$500,000$, estimated sales potential for the new pharmacy.

An alternate method would be to delineate a larger trade area, encompassing that of all four pharmacies; to find the population and sales potential for this area; to estimate the sales volume for the three existing pharmacies, and to subtract these values from the previous value. This determination is difficult because of the large trade area of the two chain pharmacies, especially the one in the regional shopping center.

When to Relocate Your Pharmacy

A change of location for any firm will depend on many factors, a number of which are obscure and difficult to assess. The pharmacist should always be sensitive to changes in the marketplace that affect the potential of his present site in relation to other possible locations. All managers should periodically consider the desirability of a change in location. A formal analysis on an annual basis might be advisable. Relocation would be beneficial when: (1) growth or shift in the population within the market area, especially in older sections of a city, may not be benefitting the pharmacy at the present site; (2) recent site developments and new locations may provide opportunities not previously available; (3) upgrading of the present pharmacy by sizable capital expenditures to achieve a proper operating environment may be better accomplished at another site; (4) relocation may preclude or eliminate the possibility of increased competition in the market; and (5) change in location may be a stimulus for the improvements in business and professional operations that otherwise would be delayed or never achieved.

If a pharmacist—proprietor is considering relocating his pharmacy for any of the foregoing reasons, he should appraise both his present location and any new proposed site along the lines indicated in the preceding sections. In addition, he should investigate the area of the community that is the source of his present trade in order that he may choose a location where he may best serve those patrons. This investigation can be accomplished by an analysis of the prescription files or charge accounts. Also, he may determine his potential trade area by obtaining names and addresses of patrons on slips deposited for a "drawing" for selected item(s) of merchandise. The following sections describe the procedures for determining both present and potential trade areas for established pharmacies.

ANALYSIS OF PRESCRIPTION FILES

A statistical analysis of a sample of new prescriptions will assist the pharmacist in determining the trade area of patients purchasing prescriptions in his pharmacy. Although a discussion of statistical methods is beyond the scope of this text, the following procedure is recommended for such an analysis.[6]

First, the pharmacist should randomly select a sample of new prescriptions purchased during the past 12 months and plot the patients' addresses on a map.* The term "randomly selected" means that each new prescription, or combintion of prescriptions, dispensed during the past 12 months has an equal probability of being a part of the sample selected. For example, the eighth new prescription dispensed on the tenth day of November must have exactly the same probability of being selected as any other new prescription dispensed during the time period under study. Selecting a sample in a random manner is important because all other methods introduce a possible bias, thus limiting their usefulness or statistical validity. Also, the pharmacist must have a large enough sample to be confident that the results obtained will represent the entire population within an acceptable range of error. In our example, this

---

*Stated in statistical terms, a sample is defined as a limited number of units selected from the total group. The entire group of items is called the population or universe. In our example, the population or universe would be all new prescriptions dispensed during the past 12 months.

means the trade area found by using the sample will be approximately the same as the trade area found if the pharmacist used all new prescriptions dispensed during the past 12 months.

The sample size will vary based on how confident we desire to be that the sample represents the population and the percent of error we are willing to tolerate. The more confident we wish to be that the sample represents the population and the less error we are willing to accept, the greater the number of prescriptions which must be included in the sample. Of course, if we would accept no error and desired to be 100 percent confident, the sample would have to include all prescriptions dispensed during the time period under study. However, reviewing all new prescriptions would be a long and expensive task and should be avoided by the use of a random sampling technique.

Although statistical formulas are available to determine the proper number of prescriptions to include in the sample for various confidence limits, allowable errors, and variances, experience using these formulas indicates that reasonable results will be obtained if the pharmacists will review at least 400 prescriptions in a random manner.

A table of random numbers may be used to select the first prescription in a random sample of prescriptions. Alternatively, the following procedure may be used:

1. Determine the total number of new prescriptions dispensed during the past 12 months and number each prescription consecutively. All prescriptions, including drugs controlled by the Drug Enforcement Agency (DEA), should be included in this group and assigned a number.
2. Determine the percentage of prescriptions to be selected so that a minimum of 400 prescriptions will be included in the sample, and use this percentage to determine the number of prescriptions, consecutively numbered, that you should skip (omit) between each prescription you will review.
3. Place consecutively numbered slips of paper of equal size in a box. The number of slips to be used should be equal to the number of prescriptions you will omit between those selected, *plus* one slip for the prescription selected. After thoroughly mixing all the slips of paper, select one number. Beginning with the prescription represented by the assigned number, select each assigned prescription thereafter until all chosen prescriptions have been selected.

The following example will clarify the statistical procedure used to determine a trade area:

STEP 1—Determine total number of prescriptions dispensed during the last fiscal year.

Regular ℞ Nos. 398,621 to 408,615 = New Regular Prescriptions   =   9,995
DEA Nos. 112,134 to 116,205 = New DEA Prescriptions   =   4,072
Total new prescriptions   = 14,067

STEP 2—Assign the number ''1'' to the first prescription dispensed during the fiscal year and number the 14,067 prescriptions consecutively. NOTE: The prescriptions need not actually be numbered, but you must be aware of the number each prescription has been assigned.

STEP 3—Divide the number of new prescriptions dispensed by 400.

$$14{,}067 \div 400 = 35.2$$

(For this analysis the number may be rounded to 35)

STEP 4—Choose a number between 1 and 35 using one of the procedures outlined for selecting a random starting point. For this example the number "5" was chosen.

STEP 5—Starting with the prescription assigned number "5" (acutal ℞ No. 398,626), select every 35th prescription filled during the year. This will result in a total sample of 402 prescriptions.

STEP 6—Plot the address from each prescription selected on an area map.

The above procedure will ensure that each new prescription dispensed in the past 12 months will have the same probability of being selected. Also, the sample is large enough to ensure that the trade area determined represents the *true* trade area. These data can assist greatly in the decision to relocate and also in the selection of a new site that will still be convenient to current prescription patrons. It is strongly suggested that all managers, regardless of their present plans concerning relocation, complete this process on at least an annual basis to determine shifts in the patient population being served.

ANALYSIS OF CHARGE ACCOUNTS

The same sampling procedure may be used to determine the present trade area of persons maintaining charge accounts at a pharmacy. Although experience indicates the trade area for charge customers usually does not differ greatly from the patient population trade area, both groups are extremely important to the success of the enterprise, and thus, an occasional analysis should be completed for both groups and the results compared. If a major difference is found, the reasons for this difference should be determined and the proper adjustments made. Such adjustments may include a change in emphasis or method of future promotional programs.

SPECIAL EVENT TO DETERMINE POTENTIAL TRADE AREA

A manager may obtain a good indication of the *potential* trade area for an established pharmacy using the "special event" technique. Plan a major event, such as a weekend sale, and offer a special gift or prize. Advertise the event consistently using all feasible media to ensure excellent penetration to all parts of the potential trade area. Have all persons sign their names and addresses on special cards of equal dimensions. Thoroughly mix the cards and draw a name for the prize. Then, randomly choose at least 400 of these cards and plot the addresses on a map. If a major difference exists in this potential trade area and the present trade area, a decision to relocate or change promotional and merchandising practices may be made. The results, together with those of previous surveys of prescriptions and/or charge accounts, may indicate a shifting of the population served, which would in turn indicate relocation.

Summary

The pharmacist should screen several potential locations by comparing the basic variables affecting choice of location. After the choice has been narrowed to one, or possibly two or three locations, a more detailed analysis should be made. The method to be used depends largely on the class or type of location, the type of pharmacy, and the amount of time and money available for analysis and evaluation. More than one method should be used as a double check on the estimates. The importance of location analysis and evaluation is such that time and money should not be the major consideration in the choice of methods.

The potential pharmacy proprietor should be aware of the social and economic changes that are taking place in many of the older neighborhood or residential areas as well as the rural areas. The quality of life and standard of living are deteriorating in many of the older sections of our cities, and consequently, these locations should be evaluated carefully and periodically. Also, the commercial potential of many of the central business districts is not as lucrative as it was in former years. This trend is largely the result of the development of the shopping centers. Urban renewal, Medicaid, and other Federal programs, together with the building of "high rise" apartment houses in the central portions of cities, serve to militate against the deteriorating force of the social and economic changes, and these locations may once again be profitable.

The analysis should proceed logically as follows: (1) several locations are screened; (2) the trade area is delineated; (3) the population of the trade area is determined; and (4) the potential total sales volume for the scope of lines of goods and services to be offered is estimated by use of the appropriate expenditure percentage or the appropriate per capita expenditure; (5) allowance must be made for drug competition; and (6) the relative drawing power of the competing pharmacies is estimated and the potential sales allocated on this basis.

Special techniques should be used for suscipient locations and for certain types of pharmacies such as the pharmaceutical centers. Also, an evaluation of the location of established pharmacies may require other methods and techniques. Finally, it should be recognized that the procedures that have been suggested provide only estimates and not precise measurement. Judgment must be exercised in all phases of these procedures.

REFERENCES

1. *1970 Census of Population, Vol. 1, Characteristics of the Population*, Washington, D.C.: Dept. of Commerce, Bureau of Census, pp. x–xv.
2. Kottas, M.J.: Locational determinants affecting the sales volume of retail pharmacies. Master's Thesis, University of Texas at Austin, 1980.
3. Fassett, W.E.: Investigation of marketplace and site characteristics affecting prescription volume in clinic pharmacies in the Puget Sound area. Master's (MBA) Thesis, University of Puget Sound, Seattle, WA, 1983.
4. Shannon, G.W., Cromley, E.K., and Fink (III), J.L.: Pharmacy patronage among the elderly: Selected racial and geographical patterns, *Soc. Sci. Med., 20*(1):85–93, 1985.
5. Deiner, C.H.: *The Lilly Digest*, Indianapolis: Eli Lilly and Co.
6. Huffman, D.C., et al.: *Community Pharmacy Management and Development.* Memphis: University of Tennessee, 1973, pp. 38–45.

REVIEW

1. Discuss the importance of location evaluation in terms of changing socio-economic conditions, frequency of tacit or actual evaluation, and business failures.

2. What is the simple and basic principle of location choice?

3. Classify locations into their various geographic and functional classifications.

4. Define and describe each type of location, including shopping centers.

5. Describe the four types of locations based on the nature of the location and scope of commercial services and functions found in the larger cities.

6. Contrast the differences among suscipient, interceptive, and generative location.

7. Describe an "island" location.

8. Discuss the variables or factors affecting location choice, and the significance of each.

9. Discuss the strength and weaknesses of each technique of location analysis.

10. Outline the necessary steps used in the "vacuum" calculation technique.

11. When provided with the appropriate data, evaluate the sales potential of a location using the "vacuum" calculation technique.

12. Discuss each of the following factors and the means of assessing these in the evaluation of the market strength of pharmacies.
    - (a) Size
    - (b) Shape
    - (c) Front
    - (d) Parking
    - (e) Traffic
    - (f) Proximity to merchants
    - (g) Proximity to physicians
    - (h) Proximity to other health facilities
    - (i) General appearance

13. Given the appropriate data, calculate the trading area in square miles using Reilly's Law of Retail Gravitation.

14. Discuss the techniques used in analyzing and evaluating the trading area of an established pharmacy.

15. When provided the appropriate data, analyze and evaluate the trade area of an established pharmacy; outline the necessary steps to evaluate such a location.

7 | Planning the Layout Design of a Pharmacy

The location of a pharmacy, its management, and sufficient capital are major factors contributing to a pharmacy's success. Another major factor in determining the success of a pharmacy is its general appearance, including the layout design of the pharmacy and the arrangement of the individual departments. Before a pharmacist undertakes to design a layout or modernize a pharmacy, he should consider the objectives of the layout design, the type of pharmacy, the classes of consumer goods and purchases, and the principles of layout design.

Objectives of Layout Design

The *major objective* in the design of the *exterior* of a pharmacy is to attract more patrons into the pharmacy. The overall *objective* of *interior layout design* is to increase the amount of the total purchases of each person who enters the pharmacy.

In addition to the above general objectives, there are *six specific objectives:* (1) to enhance the general appearance of the pharmacy and to project a professional image; (2) to control payroll expenses through convenience and efficiency of the layout; (3) to improve patrons' satisfaction and convenience; (4) to maximize the utilization of space; (5) to disperse and control the traffic pattern within the pharmacy; and (6) to provide surveillance and reduce pilferage.

One other important factor to consider is the philosophy of the pharmacist-owner. Many pharmacists prefer to practice in a specific type of setting. Thus, the design required by a service-oriented pharmacist would differ from that needed by the pharmacist interested in using mass merchandising techniques.

130

Types of Community Pharmacies

PHARMACEUTICAL CENTER

The pharmaceutical center, designed and developed by McKesson & Robbins and the American Pharmaceutical Association, is similar to the prescription-oriented pharmacy, but it must conform to certain standards as described in Chapter 3. The layout design of this center is not so critical as with the other types because no merchandise of any kind is displayed. The inventory is confined to legend and non-legend medication and few convenience goods. The decor, the atmosphere, and the uncluttered floor space are the hallmarks of the pharmaceutical center. The pharmaceutical center usually has a separate room for fitting orthopedic and surgical appliances.

PRESCRIPTION-ORIENTED PHARMACIES

This type of pharmacy usually occupies 500 to 1,000 square feet and is so designed that the patrons will have a comfortable waiting area near the prescription department. Health-related items, including drugs, home health care appliances and supplies, and prescription accessories, are displayed near this vicinity. The pharmacy may have a separate room for fitting trusses and other orthopedic and surgical appliances. Cosmetics, gifts, and a limited number of other items are displayed in the other areas of the pharmacy.

TRADITIONAL PHARMACIES

The traditional or conventional pharmacy usually occupies between 1,000 and 6,000 square feet. The major objective of the layout design for this type of pharmacy is to disperse the customers and expose them to all areas in the pharmacy. These pharmacies also should have a pleasing appearance, project a professional atmosphere, be convenient for both consumers and employees, and provide the opportunity for maximum sales at minimum expense. Of course, surveillance for shoplifters must be included as one objective in the design and layout process.

Although traditional pharmacies vary in design, it is generally agreed that the best traffic flow can be achieved with a 2.5:1 length-to-width ratio.

THE SUPER DRUGSTORE

The super drugstore occupies more than 6,000 square feet, generally 10,000 square feet or more, with the design approximating a square. The basic objective in a super drugstore is traffic control rather than traffic dispersal, which is achieved by the merchandising techniques used. Many lines of goods are sold in this type of drugstore, and the layout design is usually of the self-service type to facilitate traffic control and to provide maximum sales at minimum cost.

Consumer Goods and Purchases

CLASSIFICATION OF CONSUMER GOODS

Definitions of the classes of consumer goods are included to provide an understanding of the relationship between consumers' activity in the purchase of various goods and good layout design principles. In addition to the classification of consumer goods, the manner in which consumers purchase them is very important to the success of a layout design.

Convenience Goods. Convenience goods normally have a low unit value and are purchased frequently, with little effort on the part of the consumer. Convenience goods make up the large majority of the stock of grocery stores, variety stores, and pharmacies.

Shopping Goods. Goods in this class normally have a high unit value, are purchased infrequently, and require considerable effort on the part of the consumer. For such purchases the consumer will compare prices, quality, special features, and required services among other features. Shopping goods are found mostly in department, furniture, clothing, and similar stores.

Specialty Goods. Specialty goods normally have a high unit value, possess unique qualities or features and are purchased infrequently; consumers exert a great deal of effort to purchase them. Rare antiques and exclusive brands of clothing are examples of specialty goods.

It should be noted that pharmacies stock predominantly convenience goods; however, most pharmacies stock some shopping and specialty goods. The prescription is a special case; it includes attributes of all three classifications. For example, some patients shop for expensive or maintenance drugs, while other patients patronize only one pharmacist even at considerable expense and effort because of the personal and special services provided.

CLASSIFICATION OF PURCHASES

Demand Purchases. When consumers enter a pharmacy, or any other place where goods or services are sold, with the deliberate intent of purchasing a particular item and/or service, the purchase is considered to be a *demand purchase*. A prescription is a classic example.

Impulse Purchases. Impulse purchases are purchases made *after* the consumer has entered the pharmacy to purchase one or more other items, or are purchases made when the customer has entered the pharmacy for no particular purpose. This type of purchase frequently is suggested by an attractive display or price. Cosmetics, toiletries, and sundries often are purchased on impulse.

The percentage of pharmacy sales bought on impulse is estimated to be at least 40 percent.[1] It can be assumed that all prescription and most nonprescription drugs, prescription accessories, surgical and orthopedic appliances and supplies, and other home health care aids are purchased on demand. A high percentage of other types of products is bought on impulse.

It should be noted that classes of goods and purchases are not always mutually exclusive, but may be integrated in varying degrees in the mind of the purchaser.

Classes of Layout Designs

HISTORIC TYPES OF SERVICE-ORIENTED LAYOUT DESIGN

Historically, there are three basic types of layouts: (1) clerk, or personal service, (2) self-selection, and (3) self-service. Each is designed to achieve the objectives of the three basic types of pharmacies, professional, traditional, and super drugstore, respectively.

Clerk Service. The clerk service layout is the old traditional design used in most pharmacies before the trend toward self-service and mass merchandising. It consists primarily of complete clerk service with only a small part of the merchandise exposed for patrons to handle. The modern example of this layout design is the pharmaceutical center in which no merchandise is on display. Traditionally, pharmacists have used the clerk service design because it facilitates maximum interchange between pharmacy personnel and patrons, one of the major reasons many independent pharmacies have survived. Convenience and friendly service are still important factors in the patronage of a specific pharmacy.

However, the quality of clerk service has not been maintained in many instances. In addition, prices for pharmaceutical products have risen and the importance of price in relation to service has also increased. Therefore, this combination of factors has caused many managers to reduce services and seek an alternate type of layout design as a solution.

Self-Selection. In an attempt to provide adequate personal service in a more efficient manner, and thus be more competitive with the larger super drugstores, many independent pharmacists now use the self-selection layout design. This type of layout design dictates that clerk service be maintained at all service-oriented departments, such as cosmetics, photo supplies, prescription and selected nonprescription drugs, surgical and orthopedic appliances and supplies, and veterinary departments. Much of the other merchandise, however, is displayed in a manner that the patrons may see, handle, and select themselves. This layout is most frequently found in the modern conventional pharmacies.

Self-Service. The term self-service is restricted for those layouts that utilize a minimum of clerk service and expose the maximum amount of merchandise for patrons to handle. It is not possible to have 100 percent self-service in a pharmacy because of the prescription department. Central check-out of all purchases is the one criterion most commonly used to identify a truly self-service layout, although some "experts" dispute the appropriateness of this basis of distinction alone. This type of layout is most often used in the super drugstores.

STYLES OF LAYOUT DESIGNS

Styles of layout design emphasize *physical configuration* of the layout rather than the degree of service provided, although variations in services will coincide with several of the styles as shown later. Four distinct styles of layout design have been developed over the past several decades. They include: (1) *center service,* (2) *lobby check-out* or *bull pen,* (3) *off-the-wall,* and (4) *right-rear service.* The latter style is often referred to as the "self-selection" style, but we have chosen not to use this term in order to avoid confusion with the use of the term with regard to the concept of a combination of clerk service and self-service.

Center Service Style. This style features an elongated, two-sided wrapping counter and check-out "island" located in or near the center of the selling area of the pharmacy. Usually convenience goods, as well as things purchased on impulse, such as tobacco, candy, and sometimes magazines and photo supplies, are stocked in the island. The objective is to align the major traffic-generating departments around the perimeter and then pull all of the traffic through the check-out island in the center of the pharmacy. It has been tried in several traditional pharmacies, especially those that are rather wide or approximate a square configuration. The concept is good in theory, but it has been less than satisfactory in practice in most instances (Fig. 7–1).

Lobby Check-Out Style. This approach utilizes a square, clerk service check-out "island" near the front of the pharmacy, but there is enough space between the check-out island and the front window to form a "lobby." Again, candy, tobacco, photo supplies, and men's sundries are stocked in the island, while seasonal and promotional merchandise are displayed in the lobby where the traffic is heavy. Frequently, the check-out island is supplemented by a short wrapping counter in the rear of the store in front of the prescription department.

The major traffic-generating departments are located around the walls and some display counters or showcases are placed in front of the wall shelves. Gondolas are aligned front-to-rear in the center portion of the pharmacy. This style is used in the larger traditional pharmacies with floor space of 5,000 square feet or more. A modification of this style, substituting several check-out lanes for the "bull pen," and self-service for clerk service has been used successsfully in super drugstores. The main disadvantage of this style in the traditional pharmacy is the reduction of the depth penetration of the traffic flow caused by the short wrapping counter and the check-out island (Fig. 7–2).

Off-the-Wall Style. This style features open display of merchandise on the wall shelving without showcases or counters in front of the wall shelves. The

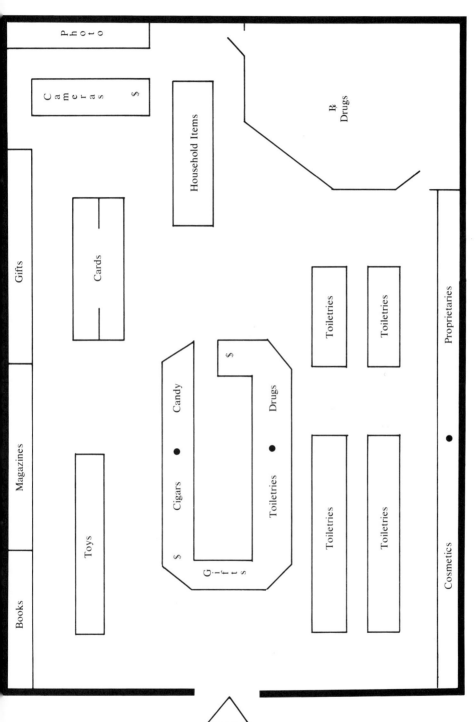

Figure 7-1. Layout design for center service style pharmacy.

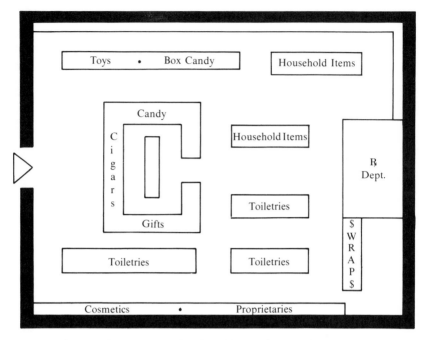

Figure 7–2.   Layout design for lobby check-out style pharmacy.

main wrapping counter, short or long, is placed across the rear of the pharmacy in front of the prescription counter. One or two rows of gondolas are placed in the center of the pharmacy. This style became popular for a time because of the ease and low cost of installing fixtures. It is well adapted to a *very* narrow building, but is not conducive to personal, clerk service (Fig. 7–3).

Right-Rear Service Style. This style frequently is called the self-selection

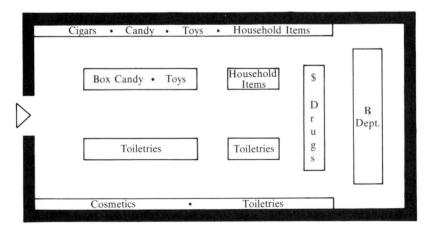

Figure 7–3.   Layout design for off-the-wall style pharmacy.

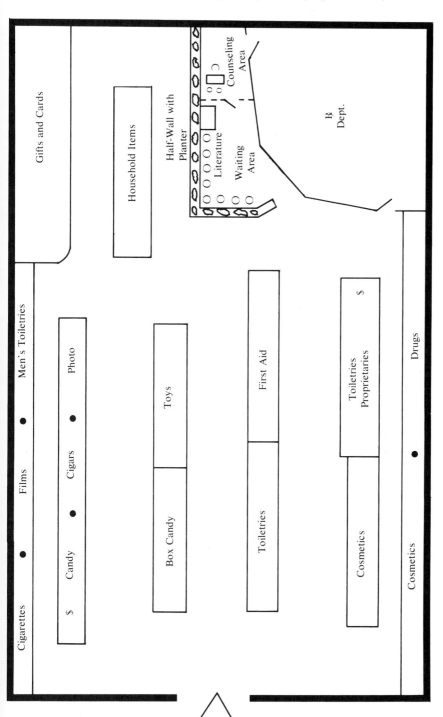

Figure 7–4. Layout design for right-rear service style pharmacy.

style because it accommodates this concept so well. The concept permits self-service where desirable, and thus promotes efficiency and reduces costs. At the same time, it permits personal clerk or professional services as appropriate. When this style is properly designed and implemented, it has the twelve characteristics of optimum design which are discussed below. The right-rear service style is well suited for most traditional pharmacies, especially those that approximate a 2.5:1 length-to-width configuration (Fig. 7–4).

Principles and Characteristics of Layout Design

The principles of layout design include the selection of the appropriate service-oriented design and style best suited to the type of pharmacy and location. They also include the appropriate arrangement of departments and merchandise in order to achieve optimum design characteristics, traffic flow and shopping.

OPTIMUM DESIGN CHARACTERISTICS FOR
THE TRADITIONAL PHARMACY[2]

1. All four corners of the merchandising and service area of the pharmacy should be activated. This is achieved by strategic placement of clerk-activated service or special-skills departments, plus selected ''self-selling'' departments such as greeting cards, gifts, and magazines.
2. All displays are departmentalized and well identified. Related departments and merchandise are grouped adjacent or near similar departments and merchandise.
3. The main wrapping counter with a cash register is placed along the longest clear wall—right side if walls are equal length—and deep to the rear, hence the term ''right-rear'' service style.
4. A selected assortment of the fastest selling nonprescription drugs, dental products, and toiletries are displayed on the main wrapping counter.
5. The prescription department is located in the rear and adjacent to the main wrapping counter. The prescription department is dramatized with commanding identification and a floor elevation of seven inches. There should be a minimum of 150 footcandles of light within the prescription department.
6. An adequate waiting area with comfortable chairs and health-related reading materials should be provided near the prescription department. Sickroom supplies, home health aids, and prescription accessories should be displayed near the prescription department and the waiting area.
7. The cosmetic and toiletry department is aligned with the nonprescription drug and prescription drug departments from front to rear, respectively, along the right or longest wall. ''Pre-sold,'' nationally advertised cos-

metics and toiletries, such as hair care products, lotions, and creams are placed on open display on gondolas across from the cosmetic department.

8. Special skill departments such as photography, imported gifts, costume jewelry, veterinary drugs and pet supplies, and orthopedic and surgical appliances and supplies should be given special treatment and well identified. Clerk service should be provided in these departments.

9. Special care should be given to use of color and special design features so that the pharmacy is a restful, pleasant place to shop and reflects professionalism and pride of ownership.

10. The lighting layout in the pharmacy must conform with the fixture layout, highlighting the merchandise, not the fixtures. A minimum of 100 footcandles should be provided in the selling or merchandising area.

11. The fountain, if one is installed, is located across from the main wrapping counter on the opposite wall deep in the rear of the pharmacy.

12. All clerk service stations must be self-supporting, that is, the service-merchandise departments must produce gross sales at least ten times the weekly payroll.

ARRANGEMENT OF DEPARTMENTS AND MERCHANDISE

The prescription department and other high-skill or specialty departments should be located in the rear or toward the rear of the pharmacy. If the pharmacy has a fountain, it should be placed in the rear of the pharmacy across from the main wrapping counter and the prescription department. Ideally, the fountain should be separated from the prescription department and the prescription waiting area by an attractive planter, a partial partition perhaps made of pegboard on which home health care products can be displayed, health information displays, or other suitable means of separation. This type of arrangement maintains the integrity of the professional atmosphere of the prescription and drug area.

If the pharmacy has a surgical and orthopedic appliance department, a special fitting room is a must. The door of the fitting room and any intermediate door through which a patient must pass should be adequately identified. Separate toilets for men and women should be located near the fitting room because in nearly every instance, the patient will need to use the toilet after a fitting, especially the fitting of trusses.

If the pharmacy does not have a fountain, greeting cards and a gift department are the best choices to replace the fountain in the rear of the pharmacy. A photographic department or a veterinary drug department, if developed into a high-skill department by highly competent clerks, provides another option. A special room located in part of the stockroom in the rear with a separate outside entrance makes an ideal veterinary drug department, provided the entrances are well identified.

The cosmetics, toiletries, and nonprescription drug departments should be arranged as described in characteristic number 7 in the foregoing section. The tobacco, candy, and magazine departments are usually located in the front of the pharmacy across from the cosmetic department. Smoking accessories, photo supplies, and/or men's toiletries are often included in this area to provide greater sales potential, but more importantly, greater gross margin. This is desirable in order to achieve characteristic number 12 mentioned previously. Other major departments can be used to fill the remainder of the wall space opposite the cosmetic and drug side of the pharmacy. Gondolas normally are aligned lengthwise in the center portion of the pharmacy to complete the layout.

Goods and services purchased on demand, and specialty goods, should be placed in or toward the rear of the pharmacy. This arrangement draws the patrons deep into the pharmacy. Convenience goods generally are placed near the front of the pharmacy. Selected convenience goods that are purchased on impulse are displayed near the cash registers. Many shopping goods and most products often purchased on impulse are displayed in the middle portion of the pharmacy. Selected products of both categories are displayed in the front part of the pharmacy and near the cash register. Household products, school supplies, and many sundries are displayed on the gondolas. Promotional merchandise frequently is displayed on gondolas, especially the ends of the gondolas and other "hot" spots.

Traffic Flow Analysis

In each pharmacy there are major traffic flow paths customers tend to take.[3] These traffic patterns should reflect the pharmacy's attempt to display high volume merchandise in a manner that will increase impulse sales. "Over 40% of all buying decisions are made inside the pharmacy while the customer is shopping."[1] Three-quarters of the purchases women make in one week are not planned during the previous week.[3] Therefore, the more the customer can be encouraged to "travel" throughout the pharmacy, the more merchandise she will be exposed to, and the more likely that impulse sales will result. The fundamental objective when making suggested changes in layout is to encourage additional customer purchases by obtaining maximum merchandise exposure and traffic flow through the strategic placement of departments, fixtures, and aisles.[4]

There are two types of traffic flow analyses, qualitative and quantitative. The first is *very* simple to perform and can be done frequently, two or three times annually if desired. The second, quantitative analysis, requires more time and would be performed no more frequently than once each year.

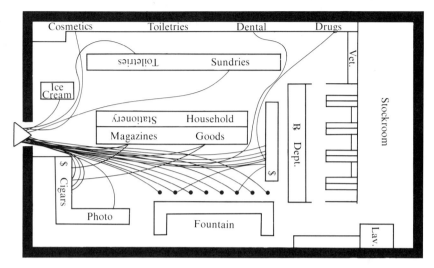

Figure 7–5A. Illustration of qualitative traffic flow analysis to be placed over work sheet in Figure 7–5B.

QUALITATIVE TRAFFIC FLOW ANALYSIS

A qualitative traffic flow analysis is performed by tracing the path of each patron who enters the pharmacy. First, the layout of the floor plan of the pharmacy is drawn on graph or grid paper and several copies made. Several time intervals representing morning, afternoon, and evening traffic, of either 30 minutes or one hour, depending on the amount of traffic, should be selected randomly over a period of a week. The path of each patron is traced on the graph paper from the moment he enters the pharmacy until he leaves. Appropriate marks are made at each point of purchase. It is useful to use three colors for tracing, one representing ladies, another for men, and a third representing children under the age of eighteen (Figs. 7–5A, 7–5B).

The tracings are then compared. Usually, they have similar traffic patterns with some variation due to the different times of day the data were taken. The primary purpose of the qualitative traffic analysis is to identify "dead" areas in the pharmacy where few or no patrons shop. Dead areas are an indication that the pharmacy needs to be modernized with significant changes in the layout design.

The impact that remodeling has on traffic flow is vividly depicted in Figures 7–6 and 7–7.

QUANTITATIVE TRAFFIC FLOW ANALYSIS

The following procedure is used to determine quantitatively whether the present layout of the pharmacy is adequate.[5] At the end of the study you will be statistically confident that the results achieved are correct.

WORK SHEET FOR TRAFFIC FLOW ANALYSIS

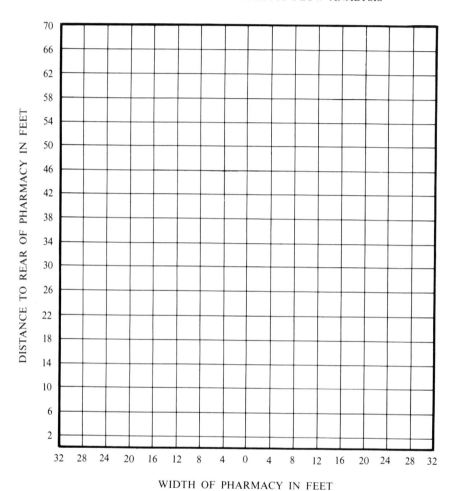

Directions:

1. Sketch floor plan on grid showing department locations.
2. Show each customer's route by colored line.
3. Terminate line at point of final purchase.

Figure 7–5B.   Work sheet for traffic flow analysis.

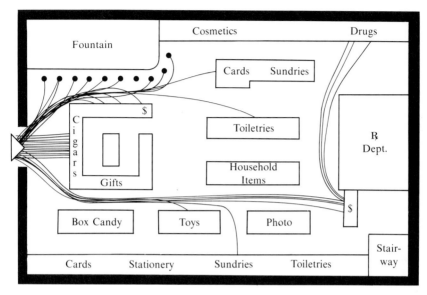

Figure 7–6. Qualitative traffic flow analysis *before* remodeling.

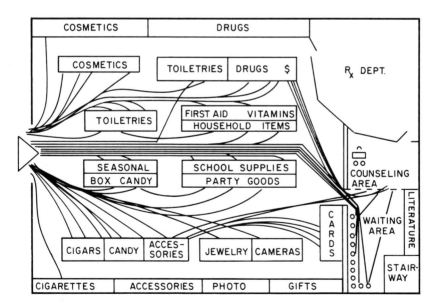

Figure 7–7. Qualitative traffic flow analysis after remodeling.

Step 1— Divide the pharmacy into major departments. In a traditional pharmacy, these departments generally include: (1) the prescription department, (2) nonprescription drugs and health-related items, (3) cosmetics and toiletries, (4) baby department, (5) feminine hygiene, (6) candy, tobacco and accessories, and magazines, and (7) in some instances, veterinary supplies. Pharmacies containing less than 5,000 square feet generally can be divided into fewer than ten departments, usually six or seven. The cash register(s) should be keyed to each of the major departments to record sales and number of transactions.

Step 2— Randomly select enough hours during a one-month period to be assured that at least 400 patrons will be observed. For example, if an average of 40 patrons entered the pharmacy each hour, ten one-hour intervals or 20 one-half hour intervals should be selected in order to conduct a complete and quantitative traffic flow analysis.

Step 3— Record the data from the cash register at the end of each sampling period and label them with date and time of sampling.

Step 4— Total the sales for each department for all sampling periods and calculate the average dollar value per transaction.

Step 5— Conduct a qualitative traffic flow analysis as described previously during the same time interval used to obtain the data in Step 2.

Step 6— Compare the sales efficiency per transaction by department with the qualitative traffic flow to locate "dead" spots within the pharmacy and redesign the layout based upon the data and space needed for each department in order to maximize sales.

The procedure for selecting the times for sampling may be demonstrated with the following example. Assume the pharmacy is open from 9:00 a.m. until 9:00 p.m., Monday through Saturday. The sampling is to be conducted during June. Since the month contains 30 days and five Sundays, the pharmacy will be open 12 hours per day for 25 days, for a total of 300 hours. The number "1" is assigned to the hour beginning at 9:00 a.m. on Saturday, June 1, and each hour thereafter is numbered consecutively. This means that the hour beginning at 8:00 p.m., Saturday, June 29, is assigned the number "300." Assume and average of 40 patrons per hour and 400 observations are to be made. A total of 10 hours should be selected—one hour for each 30 hours the pharmacy is open during June (300 hours ÷ 10 hours = 30 hours).

Next place 30 slips of paper of equal size numbered 1 through 30 into a container, mix them thoroughly, and select one. Assuming number 13 was drawn, the traffic flow analysis would begin at 9:00 a.m. on Monday, June 3. Similar analysis would be conducted each thirtieth hour the pharmacy was open in June.

At the same time a traffic flow study is being conducted, determine the average dollar amount per sales transaction for the entire pharmacy for each time interval and for each department. (The average sales transaction per customer generally will range between $1.00 and $20.00, depending on the merchandise mix and clientele of the pharmacy.) This can easily be accomplished by means of a modern cash register, which shows the number of transactions and sales by departments. Both the number of transactions and the average sales per transaction are important data for the analysis. This analysis will provide a comparison of sales efficiency and the relative space needed for each department when the pharmacy is renovated.

When a complete renovation or any major change is made within the pharmacy, another traffic flow analysis should be completed and the results compared with those before renovation. In addition, it is suggested that the pharmacist complete a traffic flow analysis on an annual basis.

Case Studies

TRAFFIC FLOW ANALYSIS OF A PRESCRIPTION PHARMACY[6]

A traffic flow analysis was conducted on a traditional prescription-oriented pharmacy located in a medical building in a city of approximately 40,000 people. The pharmacy was approximately 40 years old and had not been remodeled for the past fifteen years. In addition to the street entrance in the front of the pharmacy, patients could enter directly by a side door from the lobby after visiting the physicians in the building. Stock was stored in two rooms in the rear of the pharmacy and in several rooms on the balcony level. It was obvious that there was inappropriate use of all the space. The prescription department was located on the balcony level and utilized a dumbwaiter to transfer the prescription orders and the finished prescriptions between the service area and prescription department. Thus, the pharmacist had very little patient contact. The pharmacy generally was cluttered, although it was kept clean. The cosmetic department, which had several prestige lines and a large inventory for this particular size of pharmacy, was kept fairly attractive.

A qualitative descriptive traffic flow analysis was conducted on several occasions before remodeling. These revealed that only minor parts of the pharmacy were not active because large numbers of patrons were forced to circulate throughout the store because of the small waiting area in the prescription department. However, inefficiencies did exist in several areas.

The renovation included the following changes. The prescription department was relocated on the first floor. A first-level stockroom was converted into a surgical and orthopedic fitting room. One of the second-level stockrooms was converted to a physicians' reading lounge where physicians could come to read the most popular medical journals, inspect package inserts of new drugs, and drink free coffee. (This room was entered from the second floor corridor of the building.) The ceiling of the pharmacy was lowered and modern flourescent lighting was installed. All-weather carpeting was placed on the floors. Wood paneling was installed throughout the selling area, the prescription department, the physicians' reading room, and the fitting room. New fixtures were installed throughout the pharmacy. In addition, an individual

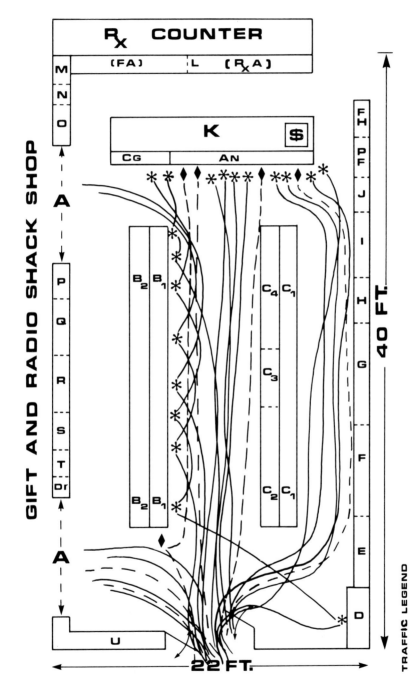

Figure 7–8.   Traffic flow analysis of W and W Pharmacy.

Figure 7–8. Traffic flow pattern in a traditional pharmacy. (Orientation is facing the rear of the pharmacy.)

Departmental Legend:

A —Doorways to Gift Shop and Radio Shack
B_1 —L Gondola: Right Side—Box Candy and Promotional Goods
B_2 —L Gondola: Left Side—Greeting Cards
C_1 —R Gondola: Right Side—Baby Goods
C_2 —L Gondola: Left Side—Dental Care
C_3 —Black Cosmetics
C_4 —Deodorants
D —Magazine Rack
E —Skin Care
F —Hair Care
G —Baby Department
H —Suntan
I —Men's Toiletries
J —Candy, Gum, Tobacco
PF —Photography Department—Film
FH —Feminine Hygiene

$ —Cash Register
K —Check-Out Counter with Selected Fast Moving Impulse/Convenience Goods
A_n —Analgesics
C_g —Humidified Cigar Case
L —First Aid and ℞ Accessories
M —Veterinary Products
N —Topical, Ointments
O —Antacids above; Wets and Drys below
P —Ophthalmics above; Laxatives below
Q —Vitamins
R —Cough and Cold
S —Oral Care
T —Foot Care
D_t —Dermatologics (External Analgesics and Antiseptics)
U —Clocks

patient medication record system was implemented and the APhA Health Education Center was installed. A professional fee for pricing prescriptions was also put into effect.

A quantitative traffic flow analysis was performed before and after the renovation and revealed the following data: Using random samples of time intervals, approximately 31 percent of the patients entered the pharmacy from the lobby through the side door before renovation. After renovation, 56 percent of the patients entered the pharmacy by this entrance. This difference was statistically significant at the 0.01 confidence level—in other words, the investigator was 99 percent confident that the difference was not a result of chance. Each patron entering the pharmacy before renovation made an average of 1.2 purchasing stops. After renovation, each made an average of 1.4 purchasing stops.

The annual sales increased by 14 percent over the previous year, taking into consideration the sales decline rate of the previous year. Prescription sales increased an effective 16 percent on an annual basis—reversing a 14 percent decline trend, in addition to a net 2 percent absolute increase. Most significant of all was the increase in *new* prescriptions, which reversed a downward trend of 15 percent annually in addition to an actual increase of 37 percent over the previous year.

TRAFFIC FLOW ANALYSIS OF A TRADITIONAL PHARMACY[7]

This case study involved an analysis of the traffic flow patterns in a pharmacy in Western Kentucky. An overview of W & W Pharmacy revealed a building 40 feet long from the front to the prescription counter and 22 feet wide. The central entrance allowed patrons to move freely to either left or right and enter into and exit from a gift shop. A sign identified the gift shop above the rear entrance on the pharmacy side. Shoppers may pay for their purchases either at the register in the gift shop or in the pharmacy. The layout of the pharmacy and a two-hour traffic flow pattern are shown in Figure 7–8.

The pharmacy is departmentalized based on therapeutic or intended use of the product and includes such health related departments as vitamins, analgesics, antacids, cold and cough remedies, and laxatives. The non-drug departments include hair care, make-up, men's items, and other specialized groups.

End-cap displays, which are most suitable for new products or for price specials, promotional and discount items are not dispersed throughout the pharmacy and this may be one factor in unevenly dispersed traffic through the pharmacy.

Methodology. A qualitative traffic flow analysis with progressive two-hour time intervals was conducted over a period of six days. Data were gathered as follows: Monday from 8:00 a.m. to 10:00 a.m.; Tuesday 10:00 a.m. to 12:00 a.m.; Wednesday 12:00 a.m. to 2:00 p.m.; and so on. These observations entailed "tracking" the patrons as they entered the pharmacy and

Table 7–1.   Summary of the Traffic Flow Analysis by Group and Time

				Totals	
	Time	*Women*	*Men*	*Children*	*Number*	*Percent*
Monday	8–10	22	5	4	31	17.4
Tuesday	10–12	25	3	4	32	18.0
Wednesday	12–2	24	7	5	36	20.2
Thursday	2–4	17	6	1	24	13.5
Friday	4–6	22	18	2	42	23.6
Saturday	6–8	7	5	1	13	7.3
TOTAL		117	44	17	178	100
Percent by Group		65	25	10		

noting where they stopped to shop. The investigator observed the traffic from a strategic spot in the front of the pharmacy in order to have a complete view of all the sections of the pharmacy. Patterns of patron traffic were classified into three categories: women, men, and children (under 18 and unaccompanied by adults.) Distinctive lines represented women, men and children.

Results. A summary of the traffic flow data is shown in Tables 7–1 and 7–2. No major "bottlenecks" were detected in the pharmacy's traffic flow

Table 7–2.   Summary of Traffic Flow to Floor Areas

	Traffic Count[a]		Purchasing Stops[b]	
Area	*No.*	*%*	*No.*	*%*
Right Wall	12	5.9	12	8.5
Right Gondola	9	4.5	11	7.7
Left Gondola	27	13.4	40	28.2
Left Wall	4	2.0	5	3.5
Gift Shop, Front	45	22.4	U[c]	—
Gift Shop, Rear	30	14.9	U[c]	—
Check-out, ℞	74[a]	36.8	74[d]	52.1
Check-out, Total	(107)[d]	(53.2)	(107)[d]	(43.0)
Total	201	100	249	100

[a]These numbers represent the number of people who traveled to the various areas; in some instances, they traveled to more than one area and were counted for each of these areas; however, the actual unduplicated number of customers was 178 wtih 201 incidences of traffic count.

[b]The number of purchasing stops exceeds both the number of customers and traffic count because a customer might have stopped and purchased two or more times at a wall or a gondola. This number does not represent the actual number of purchases because a customer might have selected two or more products at a given stop.

[c]The number of purchasing stops within the gift shop is unknown.

[d]The number 74 represents those customers who did not stop and select a product on the way to the rear counter and were presumed to be prescription patrons. The 107 count represents all of the people who stopped at the rear counter for all purposes.

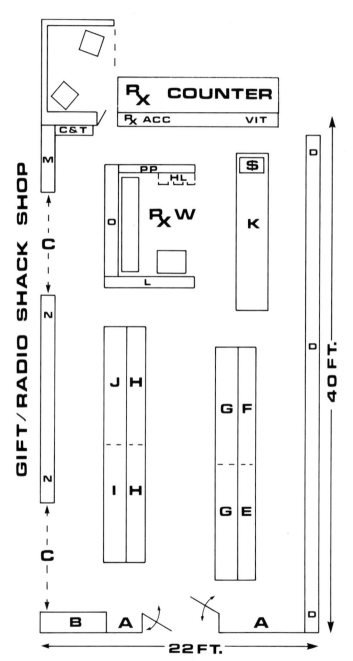

Figure 7-9.

Figure 7–9. Redesigned pharmacy layout. (Orientation is facing the rear.)

Departmental Legend:

A	—Special Promotional Goods	RxW	—Prescription Waiting Area
B	—Party Goods	HL	—Health Literature
C	—Entrances to the Gift Shop	RxACC	—Prescription Accessories
D	—O-T-C Drugs	Vit	—Vitamins
E	—Baby Department	PP	—Professional Products under Pharmacist's Control
F	—Dental Care	CR	—Counseling Room
G	—Box Candy and Seasonal	C&T	—Candy and Tobacco (or Soft Drink Dispenser—see text)
H	—Greeting Cards	M	—Men's Toiletries
I	—Deodorants	N	—Ladies' Toiletries
J	—Hair Care	O	—Cosmetics
K	—Selling Console		
$	—Cash Register		
L	—First Aid		

patterns. However, there were only 16 stops made at the shopping areas along the walls, and 10 of these were made by children at the candy section along the right wall.

The large majority of the patrons were women (65 percent); 25 percent men, and 10 percent unaccompanied children. A majority (61 percent) traveled through the center aisle; 12 percent used the right aisle; 3 percent, the left aisle, and 24 percent entered the gift shop through the front entrance. Of those who traveled to the rear via the center aisle, 57 percent went directly to the rear check-out counter, presumably with prescriptions.

Of the 178 patrons tracked during the 11 hours, 74 (42 percent) traveled directly to the rear check-out counter, presumably with prescriptions, and this represented 37 percent of the total traffic count. Also, the gift shop attracted a similar number of patrons, 75 or 42 percent, and traffic count (37 percent). These two departments accounted for over 80 percent of the patronage and 74 percent of the incidences of traffic count.

Merchandise on the right wall attracted about 6 percent of the traffic and 9 percent of the purchasing stops. The right gondola fared worse, only 5 percent of the traffic and 8 percent of the purchasing stops. The left wall was the least productive—2 percent of the traffic and 4 percent of the purchasing stops. Only the left gondola was reasonably effective, with 13 percent of the traffic and 28 percent of the purchasing stops.

Recommendations. In establishing a layout to achieve maximum traffic flow throughout the pharmacy, physical facilities and their design are paramount. With the advice of an experienced layout design specialist, a plan for the redesign of W & W Pharmacy was developed as shown in Figure 7–9. The new recommended design featured relocating the rear check-out counter, building a small counseling room for special counseling of patients who need indepth advice or the fitting of surgical support and a patient waiting area with health literature displayed.

New gondolas and optimal merchandising techniques were also recommended. The recommended gondolas would be 18 feet by 3 feet at the base designed for the space available. They would be used to complement the merchandise on the respective two walls. The rear check-out counter would be brought over to the right wall and replaced by a multi-tier ''selling console'' and cashier counter. The selling console would feature a selected assortment of high demand O-T-C drugs in popular small to medium sizes plus an assortment of convenience goods and promotional items. The remainder of the O-T-C drugs would be displayed on the right wall. Products in high demand and/or requiring the professional advice of the pharmacist would be placed toward the rear and in front of the prescription department. The first aid department would be placed optimally on the front side of the patient waiting area. Good lighting and attractive departmental identifications would showcase the departments along the wall.

The ''end-caps'' of the gondolas were recommended to be used primarily for seasonal and promotional items. It was also recommended that the magazine rack be replaced by O-T-C drugs. Also, the two areas to the right and left of the front door could be used for special or promotional goods, for example, party goods to the left would complement the greeting card section on the right side of the left gondola. The left side of the right gondola is well suited for box candy and certain seasonal or promotional merchandise, for example, Valentine's Day gifts. Further recommendations are detailed in Figure 7–9 and may be identified with the aid of the legend.

Summary. Although no major "bottlenecks" were detected, several opportunities for improving the traffic flow, enhancing the appearance and efficiency of the pharmacy and rendering more effective professional services were identified. The objective is to make the most use of the facilities we have available.

REFERENCES

1. Slater, R.: *Over the Counter Effective Merchandising.* Kansas City: Marion Laboratories, 1978, p. 2.
2. Adapted from materials distributed by McKesson Drug Co. (part of Foremost-McKesson Drug and Health Care Group), San Francisco, CA.
3. McMahon, J.L., Baldwin, J. and Sawyer, W.E.: *Space Management Manual.* New Brunswick, NJ: Johnson and Johnson, 1972, p. 15.
4. Baldwin, J.: "Space Management" in *Effective Pharmacy Management.* Kansas City: Marion Laboratories, 1979, p. 85.
5. Adapted from Huffman (Jr.), D.C. *et al.: Community Pharmacy Management, Planning and Development.* Memphis: University of Tennessee, 1973, Section IV.
6. Huffman (Jr.), D.C.: The feasibility of modern managerial systems and innovative professional services in a community pharmacy. Doctoral Dissertation, The University of Mississippi, 1971.
7. Adapted in part from Forsythe, M.E. and Smith, H.A.: Traffic flow in the pharmacy: Its impact on purchasing. *Current Concepts in Retail Pharmacy Management,* 2(4):16–19, 1984.

REVIEW

1. What is the major objective of the exterior design of a pharmacy?
2. What is the basic objective of the layout design of the interior of a pharmacy?
3. What are the six specific objectives of the layout design of the interior of a pharmacy?
4. Describe the four major types of pharmacies.
5. Distinguish between the three basic service-oriented layout designs.
6. Describe the four styles of layout design and include the advantages and disadvantages of each.
7. Define and distinguish the characteristics of convenience goods, shopping goods, specialty goods, and demand and impulse purchases.
8. Describe the 12 optimum design characteristics.
9. Outline the most appropriate arrangement of departments and merchandise according to classes of consumer goods, and impulse and demand purchases.

10. Perform a qualitative and a quantitative traffic flow pattern analysis of a traditional pharmacy.

11. Draw to scale an ideal layout design for a traditional pharmacy and identify the departments with the aid of a legend.

12. Discuss the notion that people are drawn to people in reference to good layout design.

8 | Capital Planning for a Pharmacy Practice

Before discussing capital planning, two very important questions should be explored: (1) Why should a pharmacist want to own his practice in contrast to working for someone else? (2) What is the best method of entering the private practice of pharmacy or entrepreneurship?

Why Should a Pharmacist Want His Own Practice?

A partial answer to this question was given in Chapter 3. To those reasons given in Chapter 3, the following five reasons are especially relevant. (1) A pharmacist can practice his clinical skills unencumbered in his own private practice. (2) The pharmacist will be compensated, either directly or indirectly through continuing patronage, in proportion to the *quantity* and *quality* of clinical services provided. This, of course, includes patients' perception of the quality of personal relations and professional services provided. (3) Total annual income generally will exceed the salary of a staff pharmacist or manager, on the average, by $20,000 and $15,000, respectively. (4) The private practice of pharmacy serves as a standard for other forms of practice to emulate. This will be true to the extent that pharmacists with high level skills enter private practice. (5) Private practice provides the opportunity for innovation and creativity not generally provided in other forms of practice. Thus, the pharmacist can bring prestige and status to himself and the profession.

Methods of Entering Private Practice

There are three major ways of entering the private practice of pharmacy.

155

PURCHASING AN ESTABLISHED PHARMACY

Advantages. (1) In general, the purchase of an established pharmacy entails less risk than does the establishing of a new pharmacy. Because the financial records are available for study, the buyer is dealing with a known quantity to a large degree. (2) If all other economic factors remain equal, the purchase of an established pharmacy has the advantage of not increasing the number of competing pharmacies in a given market. If the location is a good one, this fact supports the general proposition of less risk and better chance of success. (3) Related to these two concepts is still a third advantage, namely, no lag time before attaining a profitable status, barring some unusual economic or market upheaval.

An established pharmacy has an established clientele with entrenched shopping habits or patterns, which is a fourth advantage. Habits are not easily changed; therefore, one can expect to retain most of the patrons. The set of charge accounts or accounts receivable is a closely related but separate factor. If the pharmacist purchases the accounts receivable with the pharmacy, then he has the opportunity to begin a sound professional and business relationship if he meets the patrons when they pay their accounts. If the accounts are paid by mail, an appropriately composed letter can accomplish similar results, since the ledger of accounts receivable provides an excellent mailing list. The third item in this category is the prescription files. The prescription files are of definite value because an average of 51 percent of all prescriptions dispensed are refills. Frequently, prescription files are sold to another pharmacist when a pharmacy discontinues its operations.

Collectively the aforementioned make up the concrete aspects of goodwill, the fifth advantage. *Goodwill* is an illusive asset and can be readily overpriced. It is considered to be an *intangible* asset representing the potential earning capacity of the pharmacy. As already indicated, this intangible asset can have, and should have, some of the tangible items in support of its valuation. "Goodwill," if overpriced, can be a disadvantage.

Disadvantages. (1) As previously indicated, one disadvantage in purchasing an established pharmacy is the possibility of paying too much for goodwill. This factor should be studied critically before reaching an agreement on its value. A more detailed discussion of evaluating goodwill will be discussed later.

(2) Other specific disadvantages include used fixtures and equipment, which may require replacement in the near future. Although the old fixtures and equipment may have served the purposes of the former proprietor, they may simply be inadequate for the style of pharmaceutical practice you envision. This, of course, will require additional capital outlay.

(3) Also, the inventory of merchandise may be too large in relation to sales; it may contain items that will not sell; or it may be unbalanced generally, meaning quantities of various goods out of proportion to their sales potential. This problem can be avoided by having a third party take the inventory and

make corrections for unsaleable or deteriorated merchandise. He can identify certain merchandise which may be eligible for return to the supplier for credit.

(4) Two other related disadvantages, which are interrelated, are inadequate policies and procedures and undesirable personnel. The former owner may not have been diligent in formulating and implementing good policies and procedures or in the hiring and training of employees. Like bad habits, bad precedents are difficult to rectify. Dismissal of an old employee can have repercussions in the community, creating ill will among the friends and family of the dismissed employee, and it may have an unfavorable effect on employee morale, although in some instances the reverse may be true.

(5) There is yet one other potential disadvantage in purchasing an established pharmacy—and this can be critical—namely, the lease for the building. The lease may be near its termination and the former owner may have failed to protect himself adequately with the appropriate renewal options. The landlord may have ideas of increasing the rent substantially, or even leasing the building for some other purpose. Related to this problem are such other considerations relative to the building as meeting the fire and sanitation codes and appropriate insurance coverage, which could affect the operation.

ESTABLISHING A NEW PHARMACY

Advantages. In considering both the advantages and disadvantages of establishing a new pharmacy, one is confronted to a large degree with a "mirror image" of the advantages and disadvantages of purchasing an established pharmacy. The advantages of one are the disadvantages of the other, with certain exceptions. For example, in a new pharmacy one: (1) can purchase new fixtures and equipment and a model inventory; (2) develop sound policies and procedures; (3) employ and train personnel of his choosing; (4) check the terms of the lease carefully; and (5) avoid the problem of purchasing goodwill. (6) One other advantage is the potential for finding a superior location with greater potential earnings for the new pharmacy in view of expanding suburbia, the development of shopping centers, and the relocating of many physicians.

Disadvantages. As a general rule, establishing a new pharmacy involves greater risk, basically because (1) the entrepreneur is dealing with unknown quantities, such as shopping habits and possible new competition, and (2) new pharmacies, as a rule, are larger, requiring more capital. (3) It may be more difficult for a young independent pharmacist to borrow the necessary capital for a new pharmacy in a new location. In fact, it is becoming more difficult for an individual pharmacist to obtain a lease in a large shopping center because the developers of the center rely upon lessees with large amounts of capital and a superior credit rating to finance the cost of developing the center. (4) The most obvious disadvantage is the lag time before the practice reaches a profitable level of operation. This lag period can range from approximately one year to three or four years. If it requires more than four years to reach a profitable status, the cause is either poor management or a poor location in a competitive market. If the location is not a good one, relocating should be considered.

JUNIOR PARTNERSHIPS

As indicated previously, a pharmacist has a choice of seeking employment in a pharmacy or owning his own pharmacy. As an employee, he may receive a straight salary, a salary plus a share of the profits, or either of the above two arrangements with an option to purchase an interest in the pharmacy. Under this latter arrangement, a preliminary period of one or two years is stipulated to determine mutual compatibility. Following the preliminary period, a purchase agreement is drawn, usually specifying a percentage of the pharmacy's valuation to be sold to the junior partner annually up to a designated percentage. Frequently, this is accomplished over a period of time when the senior pharmacist is phasing into semiretirement and finally into full retirement. He may retain an interest in the pharmacy after his retirement for a retirement income, or he may sell the entire pharmacy and invest the proceeds along with other savings to provide a retirement income. Payments may be spread over a longer period of time for tax advantages for the retiring pharmacist.

Advantages. First, there is little risk involved in this method of becoming a proprietor. The pharmacist has ample opportunity to evaluate the potential and the risk of investing in a pharmacy with which he has been associated for a year or more. Generally, the initial capital is relatively small, and part of the increments of the investment over time can be derived from the pharmacist's share of the earnings. This type of arrangement provides for immediate profit in addition to the salary in almost every case.

In addition, there are nonmonetary advantages in this arrangement. These include incentive, professional pride, self-esteem, and self-fulfillment. The profession, and society as well, are benefited from the stabilizing influence this arrangement has on pharmacists' employment. There is a greater likelihood that a pharmacist will remain in a permanent location. This saves money in retraining pharmacists in new operations, and the pharmacist can better serve patients whom he has known over a period of years. In summary, there are less risk, less initial capital required, a profit in addition to a salary usually, greater incentive and self-fulfillment for the pharmacist, and greater stability in pharmacists' employment with this type of arrangement.

Disadvantages. Some critics have stated that this arrangement has many disadvantages. They include investment without any real authority in the decisions, the potential of personality incompatibility, the difficulty of disposing of the minor interest without assuming at least some financial loss, and finally, the potential legal entanglements in a partnership. This latter criticism is very real and is discussed in more detail in the chapter on legal organizations. The other criticisms are potential disadvantages, but only if appropriate steps have not been taken to prevent or mitigate these disadvantages. Compatibility should be determined in advance of the purchase agreement. Participation in decisions can be expected to be at least proportionate to the interest owned and will probably exceed this level since the intent is for the junior partner to assume an equal or senior status in the future. Disposing of the minor interest can be prearranged under specified conditions in the purchase agreement.

The reader is reminded of the concept of partnership practiced by the accountancy and legal professions. This concept of partnership incorporates four levels of employment relationship: staff pharmacist, an "associate" status, a junior partnership status, and finally a full partnership status. Promoting and establishing this practice as a professional institution can be of real benefit to the pharmacist, the profession, and society.

Evaluating an Established Pharmacy

What is a fair price for a pharmacy? An owner's concept of the value of his pharmacy usually is considerably higher than that of a prospective buyer. The seller naturally wishes to recover his total investment and to retain all of the accumulated profits remaining in the business. The buyer, of course, is earnestly intent upon obtaining his money's worth in all particulars and in preserving the maximum opportunity for making future profits. There are at least four methods used to approximate the value of an established pharmacy. If the reader is unfamiliar with basic accounting concepts and definitions, he should consult the two sections on the subject on pages 166 to 169.

CAPITALIZATION METHOD

One method, which is a realistic approach, is the *capitalization of the return on the investment method*. This method probably is the most valid of all methods for estimating the value of a highly profitable pharmacy or during an inflationary period. This method is best explained by example. Assume the pharmacy's net profit or net return for the past year was $10,000 before taxes and assume further that you are willing to pay a price that will yield a 20 percent return, before taxes, on the investment or purchase price. If we let X equal the purchase price, we can express the relationship of the above assumptions as follows:

$$(0.20)(X) = \$10,000$$
$$X = \frac{\$10,000}{0.20}$$
$$X = \$50,000\text{—the purchase price}$$

To project further what an enterprising pharmacist may expect, let us make

Table 8–1.   Amortization of Bank Note, 10 Percent Interest on Unpaid Balance Computed Annually

Year	Unpaid Balance	Payment on Principal	Interest Charge	Total Payment
1	$40,000	$ 8,000	$ 4,000	$12,000
2	32,000	8,000	3,200	11,200
3	24,000	8,000	2,400	10,400
4	16,000	8,000	1,600	9,600
5	8,000	8,000	800	8,800
Cumulative Value	0	$40,000	$12,000	$52,000

a few more assumptions and determine the outcome. Let us assume the proprietor's salary is $30,000, giving a total income of $40,000. Assume that the income tax and social security liability is 25 percent per year, leaving an income after taxes of $30,000. If we assume the young pharmacist can save approximately $12,000 annually, he could pay for the pharmacy in five years. Let us assume he had made a 20 percent down payment and had financed the remainder ($40,000) with a bank note at 10 percent simple interest on the unpaid balance and renewable annually for five years. The debt would have been amortized as shown in Table 8–1.

SALES PROJECTION METHODS

Two other methods of estimating the value of a pharmacy utilize *projections from the sales volume.* These are more arbitrary than the other methods. One method is simply taking *one-third of the annual sales,* and the other is *100 times the average daily sales.* To illustrate these two methods, let us use an annual sales volume of $300,000. The respective estimates of purchase prices are $100,000 and $82,192 ($300,000 ÷ 365 × 100 = $82,192.) The first of these two methods tends to overestimate the value of the pharmacy, whereas the latter method sometimes underestimates the value of the pharmacy.

SUMMATION METHOD

The fourth, and perhaps the most valid method, is the *summation of the relevant factors method.* Relevant assets can best be described by taking a typical balance sheet and selecting those assets and liabilities used in this method (Figure 8–1).

A few common-sense observations will identify those items on the balance sheet that normally would not be transferred. These include cash and long-term notes payable. In our particular example, these two items were equal and thus cancel each other in considering the purchase price. If we total the rest of the assets and liabilities and subtract the liabilities from the assets, we

ASSETS

Current Assets:

Cash	$12,000	
Accounts receivable	17,700	
Inventory	55,500	
Total Current Assets		$ 85,200

Fixed & Other Assets:

Fixtures, equipment & leasehold improvements (net after reserve for depreciation)	$12,000	
Prepaid expenses, deposits, etc.	2,800	
Total Fixed & Other Assets		14,800
Total Assets		$100,000

LIABILITIES & NET WORTH

Current Liabilities:

Accounts payable	$17,000	
Notes payable (within 1 yr.)	3,000	
Accrued expenses	7,000	
Total Current Liabilities		$ 27,000

Long-term Liabilities:

Note payable (over 1 yr.)	$ 9,000	
Total Long-term Liabilities		9,000
Total Liabilities		$ 36,000
Net Worth (Equity)		64,000
Total Liabilities & Net Worth		$100,000

Figure 8–1. Balance sheet for pharmacy X.

get a difference of $64,000, which *coincidentally* is the same as the net worth. This is not the purchase price, because the seller will want a reasonable price, to say the least, for the goodwill associated with the pharmacy. In reviewing the profit and loss statement, we find the net profit last year was $12,800 on $325,000 sales volume. A "rule of thumb" valuation for goodwill is a year's net profit, $12,800 in this example. The estimated purchase price is $76,800. The capitalization of the net profit method, using a 15 percent return on the investment, yields a purchase price of $85,300. One-third of annual sales and 100 times the average daily sales yield purchase prices of $108,333 and $89,000, respectively. These four methods provide a range of $76,800 to

$108,333 as an estimate of the value of the pharmacy. This provides ample opportunity for negotiation to arrive at a fair price near the $80,000 figure.

These four methods of estimating the value of a pharmacy can be refined by projecting the next year's sales volume or profit, depending on which method is used, to correct for the trend effect. The projection can be made by using a straight line equation and the middle year as the origin to determine the projected values for each year from the straight line equation. Data for a five-year period should be used.

After a purchase price has been agreed upon, the buyer must determine what sources of financing are available and select the one best suited to his situation. Bank financing similar to the example illustrated in Table 8–1 is probably the best choice if the buyer has a sufficient down payment and a good bank credit. It is a good idea for a young pharmacist to develop a good bank credit by dealing primarily with one bank and meeting his payments regularly on loans to purchase an automobile or other property.

Financing a New Pharmacy

The cost of establishing the pharmacy must be estimated before financing arrangements can be made. The cost will be directly related to the size of the pharmacy, the estimated sales and thus inventory, and the quality and type of the fixtures, furnishings, and equipment. All of these factors, in turn, depend upon the location analysis. The type and sales potential of the location will determine the type and size of the pharmacy. The eight factors that influence the type and size of the pharmacy and the required capital outlay are discussed here.[1]

FACTORS INFLUENCING THE INVESTMENT

Socioeconomic Class Served. A pharmacy serving a number of persons in exclusive residential districts will require a more spacious and prestigious pharmacy, finer fixtures and equipment, broader assortments of merchandise, the offer of generous credit, delivery, and various special services. Farmers, dependent upon the yield of a single crop, or workers for an industrial plant subject to seasonal or cyclical irregularity, may create the necessity for furnishing credit over long periods and to unusually large proportions of patrons.

General Economic Climate. Poor or depressed conditions can reduce the volume of sales and slow the stock turnover while requiring approximately the same inventory investment, with its inherent expenses of insurance, interest, taxes, storage costs, and deterioration.

Expected Sales Volume. Even though a larger pharmacy can make more efficient use of its personnel and buy in larger than "normal" quantities that provide quantity discounts, additional capital will be required to carry a wider range of merchandise and services.

Table 8–2. Capital Requirements

Item	Total Cost	Down Payment	Balance
Inventory	$50,000	$12,500	$37,500
Fixtures	32,000	8,000	24,000
Sign	1,000	1,000	—
Cash Registers	4,000	4,000	—
Card Racks	No charge		
℞ Equipment & References	500	500	—
TOTALS	$87,500	$26,000	$61,500

Distance from Suppliers. A pharmacist receiving more rapid delivery from suppliers should be able to maintain the same sale volume with less investment in inventory.

Purchase Terms. Special purchase terms, e.g., 2 percent cash discount or quantity discount will allow a decrease in the amount of funds required to maintain the necessary inventory level.

Managerial Expertise. The pharmacist trained to analyze financial reports and utilize other managerial tools should be able to make more effective use of his capital.

Competition. The competitive situation may create the need for additional funds to finance a high level of advertising and other promotional activity, selling numerous products at low margins, maintenance of a larger sales force in order to provide prompt service, including prompt and frequent delivery service.

Professional Relations. In a pharmacy dispensing prescriptions written by a large number of prescribers, expanded capital will be required to maintain a wider variety of products necessary to meet the demand, including duplicate lines from many manufacturers.

CALCULATING CAPITAL REQUIREMENTS

There are three major categories of capital requirements for a new pharmacy: (1) inventory; (2) fixtures, equipment, and furnishings; and (3) necessary working capital to sustain the operation until the pharmacy generates enough sales to meet these needs.

Let us take an example of a typical traditional pharmacy and estimate the capital requirements. The pharmacy is in a moderately competitive market. The dimensions are 80 feet long and 40 feet wide, providing an area of 3,200 square feet. The estimated sales volumes for the first five years, based on the location analysis, are $300,000, $400,000, $450,000, $500,000, and $550,000, respectively.

Capital for Inventory. Since prescription sales are slower in developing, a lower than average percent gross margin should be estimated for the first year—probably 33⅓ percent. Thus the estimated cost of goods sold (CGS) for the first year is $200,000 ($300,000 × .66⅔). The *initial inventory* may be estimated by dividing the CGS by the turnover rate (TOR). There are two schools of thought relative to this step, but both reach approximately the same estimate. One school assumes a TOR of at least four because the pharmacy is carefully stocked with saleable merchandise. Thus, $200,000 ÷ 4 = $50,000, which would be the initial inventory.

The other school states that sales volume will reach a modest figure the first year, yet a sufficient assortment of merchandise must be offered the public. The result is a lower TOR, about 3. Dividing $200,000 by 3 gives an *average* inventory of $66,666. However, the proponents of this school assert that the initial inventory can be carefully selected, and by restricting initial quantities of many product lines, only three-fourths of the *average* inventory or $50,000 will be necessary for the *initial* or model inventory. This rationale is probably more realistic, but the results are the same.

Capital for Fixtures.[2] The cost of the fixtures, equipment, and furnishings can vary considerably, depending on the quality, source of supply and size of the pharmacy. For example, the cost of the fixtures may vary from $5 to $12 per square foot, the average being $7.50 for large pharmacies of 10,000 sq. ft. and $10 for smaller pharmacies of 3,000 sq. ft. Carpeting cost may range from $7 to $20 per square yard, with $12 being a typical figure. A small fountain, if one is to be installed, will cost about $18,000. These and other costs have been summarized in Table 8–2.

The fixtures, equipment, and furnishings may be financed through a bank or through the various suppliers. In either case the method of financing fixtures that usually is available is the ''add-on'' interest charge, which is considerably more than simple interest. The interest rate will normally be 1 percent to 2 percent above the prime interest rate—the rate banks charge preferential customers, those with large amounts of assets and high credit ratings. Depending on the money market, the prime interest rate, in turn, ranges from 1 to 3 percent above the discount rate set by the Federal Reserve Bank System. The discount rate is used by the federal government to regulate the availability of money and set monetary policy consistent with the needs of the economy.

A pharmacist can expect to pay an interest rate of 10 to 20 percent based on recent history. The computation below illustrates how the add-on interest works. Using 12 percent interest rate and a five-year repayment period, the interest rate is multiplied by the number of years (.12 × 5 = .60), this percentage is multiplied by the principal ($24,000 × .60 = $14,400), and the product is added to the principal, making a total obligation of $38,400. This sum is paid in 60 equal installments of $640.00 per month.

Working Capital. The enterprising pharmacist should have sufficient *working capital* to cover the expenses for at least three months in addition to the installment payments. Figure 8–2 provides a projected cash flow account for the first three months, which indicates the necessary extra working capital of $13,000.

Sales		$60,000
Purchases		50,000
Gross Margin		$10,000
Expenses:	$6,000	
Proprietor's Salary		
Employee Wages	5,000	
Rent	3,000	
Heat, Light, & Power	1,300	
Licenses & Permits	100	
Insurance	2,400	
Fees, Legal & Accounting	500	
Delivery	500	
Advertising (Grand Opening)	1,000	
Depreciation	noncash	
Bad Debts	none	
Telephone	700	
Miscellaneous	1,500	
Total Expenses		22,000
Profit (Deficit)		($12,000)
Add Estimated Accounts Receivable Accumulation		1,000
Total Required Working Capital		$13,000

Figure 8–2.   Projected cash flow for first 3 months.

Table 8–3 summarizes the initial capital requirements in addition to funds for three payments.

The sales estimate for the first three months was conservative, which is a realistic approach. Some additional working capital may be required, perhaps as much as $2,000 to $3,000. If better credit terms can be obtained for the inventory purchases, this will reduce the initial capital requirements substantially and perhaps the monthly payment as well.

Table 8–3.   Summary of Capital Requirements.

Item	Initial Capital	3 Monthly Payments
Inventory*	$12,500	$ 9,375
Fixtures, etc.†	13,500	1,920
Working Capital	13,000	——
TOTALS	$39,000	$11,295
Total capital requirements for 3 months: $50,295		

*One-fourth down payment required on the inventory with remainder due in 12 monthly payments with no interest.

†Pay $13,500 down and the remainder in 60 monthly payments.

Capital Planning and Assessment

There are two major functions or tasks of capital planning, viz. (1) analysis and evaluation and (2) procurement of funds. The first is utilized most often in the context of evaluating the progress of a firm and/or investment opportunities. The second task includes assessing capital needs, sources, cost, terms of borrowing, and developing good relations with various financial institutions. The second function is the primary emphasis of this chapter.

Before we discuss capital planning, there are basic concepts that need to be defined or explained, and that is the purpose of the next two sections.

BASIC ACCOUNTING CONCEPTS

The basic unit of an accounting system is the *account*. However, business transactions are not recorded directly in accounts; rather they are first entered in a journal. There are two types of journals, viz., the *general journal* and *special journals*. For example, cash sales may be recorded (journalized) in the cash sales column of a sales and cash journal, a specialized journal. Periodically, usually daily, the subtotals of columns are *posted* to the appropriate account for accumulating the data. This negates the necessity of recording every transaction, e.g. each sale, in the general journal and then posting it to the sales account. Thus, business data are accumulated and accounted for through a system of journals and accounts.

Each account has two sides, the credit or right side and the debit or left side. Additions to assets accounts are posted to the left or debit side of the account, whereas deductions from asset accounts are posted to the right or credit side. The opposite is true for the liabilities and net worth accounts. See Figure 8–3. Note the balance of each account is shown by the underscored figure. The balance is determined and so indicated at the end of an accounting period, e.g., a month, unless the *ledger of accounts* has a special column to show the running balance. Also note that the sum of debit balances must always equal the sum of credit balances.

Periodically, usually monthly or yearly, the data in accounts are subjected to a process called *adjusting* in order to take into account certain changes that are not automatically recorded in the accounting systems. Examples of these include depreciation of fixtures and change in inventory. Even if the pharmacy has a perpetual inventory control system, there may be pilferage or soiled goods which changes the value of the inventory.

Another process called *closing* follows immediately after the adjusting process, and it is designed to close out each account by transferring the account balances to the appropriate columns in the *worksheet*. Then the worksheet is used as the mechanism by which the *balance sheet* and *income statement* are generated. See Figures 8–1 and 8–2 for an illustration of the balance sheet and a modified income statement.

The above brief overview of the accounting system was designed to provide

	ASSETS				=	LIABILITIES		
+	Cash	−	+ Inventory −	+ Accounts Receivable −	=	+ Accounts Payable +	− Note Payable +	− Net Worth +
	3,000		20,000	5,000		10,000	15,000	10,800
	500			9,000		9,000		
	1,000		2,000			6,000		
	300		5,000	8,000		7,000	2,000	2,000
				8,000		8,000		
				5,000		8,000	13,000	12,800
	1,800		23,000			4,000		
				5,000				
	1,800	+	23,000 +	5,000	=	4,000 +	13,000 +	12,800
			29,800		=		29,800	

Figure 8–3. Illustration of the relationship of accounts on the balance sheet.

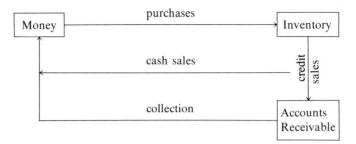

Figure 8–4. Schematic diagram of the working capital cycle.

an appreciation and ''a feeling'' for accounting data, their source and meaning. The purpose is to provide the manager with the necessary data to make decisions. A few definitions will provide the student with additional tools for capital planning.

DEFINITIONS

Capital is the wealth, or *tangible assets,* used in a business enterprise to produce income. Its various forms include actual cash, bank deposits, notes, and property, either real or personal. Capital may be classified in several ways for various purposes. In terms of capital resources, the first classification that comes to mind is equity capital and borrowed capital. *Equity capital* or *net worth* is defined as tangible assets owned free of financial obligations or debts, whereas borrowed capital or *liabilities* are terms applied to assets obtained from outside sources such as banks, other firms, or individuals.

Classified according to the manner in which it is to be used, capital may be either working capital or fixed capital. *Working capital* consists of cash on hand or in the bank, accounts receivable, and inventory; in other words, it is the capital that is working for the firm. The capital is transformed from one form to another through the transactions of the working capital cycle as shown in Figure 8–4.

On the other hand, when funds are committed to long-term or continuing investment for a fixed purpose, such as the purchase of equipment and fixtures, they are no longer available for other purposes. Thus, capital so committed is called *fixed capital* or *fixed assets.* In contrast, working capital may be shifted, to a degree, for alternate purposes: variation in quantity or lines of merchandise, expansion or decrease in accounts receivable, or a corresponding decrease or increase in cash. A more thorough discussion of the management of the working capital cycle is included in later chapters.

Liabilities may be classified further as short-term and long-term. Short-term or *current liabilities* are those debts that become due within one year or less; *long-term liabilities* or *funded debt* are those debts for which payment takes longer than one year. In general, it is better to use short-term liabilities to finance working capital, if necessary, and to use long-term debts to fund fixed assets. Review Figure 8–1 to see the relationships of these terms.

The *balance sheet* or *statement of financial position* summarizes the assets, liabilities and equity or net worth. It reflects the financial condition of a firm *at a particular point in time,* the date of closing the accounts and compiling the balance sheet. The *statement of income and expenses* or *profit and loss statement* summarizes the revenue generated and the expenditures incurred incidental to the generation of the revenue *over a stated period of time.* There are other accounting statements that link these two statements, but we will forego these at this time.

Capital Leverage[3]

Generally, it is the ideal situation when the pharmacist has all the capital he needs to purchase or establish a pharmacy. There would be little or no financial strain on the firm and no interest charge to decrease profits. This situation is seldom the case. Supplying all the capital by the owner(s) may not be the best approach because of loss of the advantage provided by financial leverage. *Financial leverage* is the ratio of net return on investment with leverage (borrowed capital) to the return on investment without leverage (no borrowed capital). The following examples will illustrate this.

Downside Example

Equity (NW)	$100,000—no leverage
Return (NP)	15,500

$$\frac{\text{Net Return}}{\text{Equity}} = 15.5\%$$

Long-term note	$ 30,000	—with leverage
Interest charge	3,000	
Equity	70,000	($100,000 – $30,000)
Return (NP)	12,500	($15,500 – $3,000)

$$\frac{\text{Net Return}}{\text{Equity}} = 17.9\%$$

Financial leverage ratio $\dfrac{17.9}{15.5} = 1.15$, a 15 percent increase in net return.

Upside Example

Equity (NW)	$100,000—no leverage
Return (NP)	15,500

$$\frac{\text{Net Return}}{\text{Equity}} = 15.5\%$$

Long-term note	30,000—with leverage
Interest charge	3,000
Equity (NW)	100,000—(total investment = $100,000 + $30,000 note)

Return (NP)   17,150   ($20,150 – $3,000)
(Assumes the same efficient use of the borrowed capital as with equity.)

$$\frac{\text{Net Return}}{\text{Equity}} = 17.15\%$$

Financial leverge ratio $\frac{17.15}{15.50}$ = 1.11, an 11 percent increase in net return.

Although the leverage ratio is less in the second example, the absolute net profit figure is greater by $1,650.

From a purely risk perspective, supplying all of the capital is a good thing, whereas the use of financial leverage is good from the perspective of maximizing return on the investment. This distinction also illustrates the advantage of purchasing an established practice, which normally reduces risk and provides financial leverage.

Source of Capital

Where does a pharmacist borrow funds and how much should he borrow? The answer to the second part of the question is "as little as possible." The answer to the first part is more difficult and depends on the sources available to him and the route of entry into entrepreneurship he is taking.

If a pharmacist is purchasing an interest in a pharmacy in increments over time—a junior partner as it were—the senior partner or a bank note with a co-signature of the senior partner may be the most logical source of borrowed capital. The junior partner should have a significant amount of his own capital to invest in the pharmacy, ranging from 10 percent to 30 percent of the purchase value.

Relatives or friends are another source of borrowed funds. This source has come under severe criticism because of potential entanglements and disputes. These can be avoided with appropriate advice and arrangements. First of all, the lender should view the loan as a business proposition as well as an opportunity to assist the pharmacist to get a start in business. The lender should not offer to provide the funds unless he has confidence in the pharmacist and has reasonable expectations that the venture will succeed. A business life insurance policy should be purchased by the borrower to protect himself, his family, and the person lending the money. Appropriate interest rates should be charged. Finally, a mutual understanding and the necessary legal arrangements are a must to avoid unnecessary disputes or liabilities.

Banks and other financial institutions are the logical source of borrowed funds because this is the purpose of these institutions. There is a degree of security in using this source because a bank will investigate the potential of success of the pharmacist and the pharmacy to safeguard its loan. In general, banks are the preferred source of borrowed funds. Usually the person borrowing the capital, normally in the form of money, executes a note indicating the amount borrowed, the interest rate, and the date(s) the note or fractions thereof is/are due. Such notes or any form of borrowed capital are commonly referred to as debts, and in the language of the accountant, they are called liabilities.

Another potential source of borrowed funds is the suppliers, generally the full-service wholesaler. This source was the one most frequently used in the past. This is no longer true today. Most wholesalers would rather see the pharmacist obtain the necessary borrowed capital from a bank, and they will gladly assist through such efforts as location evaluation, layout design, and other services. These services assist the bank in making a decision on credit extension.

Suppliers will still provide restricted credit for inventory. The prevailing practice is to sell a "model" opening inventory with a down payment of 25 percent and the balance due in 90 days or longer, net of cash discounts. The rationale is that the "model" inventory will be turned or sold in 90 days or perhaps a longer period, thereby generating enough cash to pay for the opening inventory and replenish the inventory stock. This rationale would have to be based on the assumption that the "model" inventory was minimal and that additional stock would be added as demand indicated it was needed.

As a general rule, it is best to purchase inventory with your own funds or from funds provided by relatives or friends. Banks are reluctant to lend money to purchase inventory. Fixtures can be financed through banks, drug wholesalers, or the fixture company with long-term financing.

An Innovative Capital Structure Plan

It is a well-known fact that independent pharmacists are at an economic disadvantage compared to chain pharmacies. The primary area is finance or capital structure. There are other management areas in which independent pharmacists are at a disadvantage, but these pale into insignificance compared to the financial issue. There is a way to overcome this disadvantage in large measure, of course not entirely. The concept in mind may best be termed capital aggregation. *Capital aggregation* is a means of increasing the total amount of available capital via cooperative effort while retaining control within a defined group of investors. The plan discussed below meets the four criteria of capital structure management about as well as any financial plan. The four criteria are flexibility, control, cost and risk.

The *capitalization plan* would, in the typical case, be organized by five to 10 successful independent pharmacies as a holding company. Their individual pharmacies would form the first five to 10 units of the new enterprise. Alternatively, the holding company could operate as a joint-stock company with individual contracts in respect to each of the original pharmacies, specifying the percent of stock held by the holding company and other mutually agreed upon financial arrangements. The original owners of the holding company would develop the plans for the *on-going functions* and for *expansion* of the enterprise, which would include market (location) analysis, general requirements of new manager-entrepreneurs, broad operational philosophy and guidelines, and a logo for both the old and new operational units. The specific site, size, design, featured departments and motif of each new pharmacy would be determined based on the market analysis data.

The board of directors would employ an executive-manager for the holding company, who along with consultants in the various areas of management would assist in the development of additional plans and strategies, and would *implement* these on behalf of the holding company. Other personnel would be hired as needed. Each pharmacist-manager-entrepreneur, new and old, would manage his/her pharmacy as he or she desired within the broad guidelines developed for all units.

Each new unit would require a total investment in the range of $75,000 to $150,000 depending on the market analysis. The initial investment could be approximately 50 percent of this figure with the remainder financed by appropriate financial instruments. Each new pharmacy would occupy space consistent with the market analysis. Each unit would have the authority to issue 100,000 to 500,000 shares at par value of $1.00. The initial issue would range between 25 percent and 50 percent of the maximum allowed. The pharmacist-manager would be required to purchase a minimum of 5,000 shares initially. She or he and other key employees would be able to purchase up to 49 percent of the total number of outstanding shares at a specified price keyed to the current book value of the stock, but initially at par value, through a stock purchase agreement. The holding or joint stock company would retain 51 percent of the outstanding shares of stock of each new pharmacy.

Assuming 10 original investors, each with a typical pharmacy and collectively equivalent to 10 *Lilly Digest* "average" pharmacies, the initial economic base would be substantial: Sales of $5,000,000, purchase budget of $3,350,000, total assets of $1,500,000, net worth (capital) of $750,000, net working capital of $700,000, inventory of $650,000 and annual net profit of $160,000. A total of 300,000 prescriptions would be dispensed annually. The purchasing power would enable the holding company to negotiate very good prices for most of the additional inventory. Also, the capital or financial leverage would enable the group to obtain expansion capital at competitive (low) interest rates. The group could take advantage of cooperative advertisements and other cost saving programs. In short, the group could be relatively competitive with chains and mass merchandisers with their own strategic design.

Turning briefly to the *marketing* and *management* aspects, the following outline illustrates an appropriate *strategy*. Feature prescription services with full range of clinical services (patient counseling using complete patient— medication profiles, monitoring and screening for hypertension, blood glucose levels, etc.), counseling room where feasible (at least a "semi-isolated corner"), durable medical equipment where the market indicates, the usual HBA's and convenience goods found in most pharmacies and selected, featured "departments with class" (cosmetics, pet supplies, veterinary drugs, cards, gifts, paintings of local artists, etc.) and selective promotional goods—again based on the individual market.

In summary, ten innovative, enterprising and cooperative pharmacists, using their existing pharmacies and capital as a base, can develop the means not only for survival but to expand—to double their current number of pharmacies in five to 10 years! At the same time they could assist 10 other innovative, enterprising and cooperative pharmacists to become successful entrepreneurs. All 20 pharmacists could practice in an environment essentially the same as independent pharmacy and be financially successful. In addition, 20 other pharmacists' could work in the same environment and own a "share of the action." The group as a whole would be sufficiently secure, economically, that they could practice their clinical skills unencumbered and know they would reap the financial rewards from their endeavor. All that is required are 20 (10 initially) innovative, enterprising pharmacists who do not want to be "too" independent, but who want to be in *private practice of pharmacy.*

REFERENCES

1. Adapted from Swafford, W.R., Huffman, D.C., Ryan, M.R., and Watkins, J.R.: *Community Pharmacy Management, Planning and Development.* Memphis, Tennessee: University of Tennessee, 1973, pp. 112, 113.
2. Mudd, F.M., Manager of Professional Services, Begley Drug Co., Richmond, Ky., personal communication, June 20, 1985.
3. Adapted from Mock, E.J. Schultz, R.E., Schults, R.G., and Schuckett, D.H.: *Basic Financial Management.* Scranton, PA.: International Textbook Co., 1968.

REVIEW

1. What are the five advantages of owning your own private practice?

2. What are five advantages and four potential disadvantages of entering practice as a junior partner?

3. What are the five advantages and six potential disadvantages of purchasing an established pharmacy?

4. What are six potential advantages and four potential disadvantages of establishing a new pharmacy?

5. Using the four methods of estimating the purchase price (value) of an established pharmacy, calculate a "fair" price of a pharmacy using *Lilly Digest* data.

6. What are the methods for estimating the value of goodwill?

7. Discuss the eight factors that influence the amount of required capital to establish a new pharmacy.

8. Discuss the three major categories of capital requirements for a new pharmacy, and from appropriate data provided, be able to calculate the initial capital requirements in each category.

9. Given the appropriate data, calculate the annual payment on principal and interest on a bank note with simple interest on the unpaid balance.

10. Given the appropriate data, solve a problem involving the "add-on" interest rate concept, including total obligation and monthly payments.

11. Given appropriate data and other necessary information, estimate via a cash flow chart the amount of working capital necessary to sustain a new pharmacy for three months, including payments on principal and interest.

12. Calculate and summarize the total capital required to establish a new pharmacy.

13. Define each of the following: account, general journal, special journal, ledger, adjusting accounts, closing accounts, balance sheet, statement of income and expenses, worksheet, capital, tangible assets, liabilities, net worth or equity capital, borrowed capital, working capital and fixed capital.

14. What are the various sources of capital? Discuss these in terms of matching best source with the use of the capital.

15. Liabilities are classified as short-term and long-term. Which of these is more appropriate for financing working capital and fixed capital, respectively?

16. What is capital or financial leverage?

17. Given appropriate data, calculate the capital leverage ratio, for a downside and upside example, respectively.

18. What is the purpose of capital leverage?

19. Discuss the innovative capital structure plan.

20. What is the purpose of the innovation capital structure plan?

SECTION III

SECTION III

ORGANIZATION

This section includes four chapters: Macro-organizational Theory and Practice, Micro-organization Theory and Practice, Legal Organization and Personnel Administration. The first chapter deals with the gross aspects of organizations such as schools of thought on the subject, relationships between an organization and its socioeconomic environment, organizational design within the constraints of the above relationships, social control, organizational structure, work groups (including Quality Circles), organizational change and development, an attempt to lay a foundation for an integrated theory, and a summary of applied principles. The second chapter treats the organization at a micro level and focuses on motivation and leadership/supervision with a summary of applied principles. The third chapter on legal aspects of organizations is very much traditional. The income tax liability of the various forms including subchapter S corporations is very much unsettled for the future. The fourth chapter, personnel administration, includes elements of organization and direction of human resources. We have chosen to include it in this section because human resources must first be organized before directing takes place.

9 | Macro-Organizational Theory and Practice

In the past, pharmacists have not given much attention to organizational theory and practice. As we move into a more complex health care delivery system, it will be important for the pharmacist to understand how organizations, subgroups, and individuals interact and behave in the manifold roles and interrelationships of a large organization. This understanding is especially important to the pharmacist who wants to assume a leadership role, or even to have any significant impact on the direction(s) the organization may take.

It is important that students understand the nature of organizations generally and business organizations specifically. An organization is not mere abstract concepts used to describe an inanimate object or a set of connecting lines to depict relationships. One of the meanings of the root word "organic" is living or pertaining to living matter. The proper view of organizations is as a living, functioning entity with component parts that must function in concert to be effective. As with any living organism, an organization must be in harmony with its environment; it must be nurtured and cared for, and it should not be abused or neglected. This is true with both large and small organizations as with an elephant or a partridge in a preserve.

Much of the information in this and the next chapter is designed to provide an understanding of the nature of organizations, how they behave and perform, and how they can be developed as instruments to serve our personal and professional needs more effectively. Understanding the nature and complexities of organizations is important in order for pharmacists to be able to function optimally in any type of practice situation. Pharmacists must be acutely aware of the changes taking place in the social and economic environment in order to make adjustments in their respective organizations and practices. Changes may take the form of new competition, population shifts, decreased demand for a service, e.g., delivery, heightened interest in personalized services, e.g., blood pressure monitoring among the many possible changes.

Organizational theory and practice may be classified according to a macro-perspective and a micro-perspective. The first deals with the design of an organization in respect to its environment, its structure and its overall development. It includes the relationships between the organization and social and economic systems; the relationships between various components within the organization especially groups, departments and foci of interests, and the relationships within the hierarchy. Primary domains of interest include environmental factors, technology, organizational structure, work groups, and organizational change and development. The micro-perspective involves the domains of interpersonal relationships, leadership, supervision and motivation. This division into two classes is somewhat artificial since there is, of necessity, interactions between elements in both classes.

In addition, the subject may be studied from the point of view of various schools of thought on organizational theory and practice. This will be dealt with in a cursory manner only.

Organizational Schools of Thought

There are three schools of organizational theory—classical, behavioral and management science.

CLASSICAL SCHOOL

There have been several schools of thought and attempts to explain how organizations behave. The first, the *classical school of organizational theory,* grew out of the "scientific" or classical school of management. This school of thought can best be described as a management control approach to organizational theory. The proponents of this school were concerned with such principles and concepts as (1) division of labor or work, (2) clear lines of authority and responsibility, (3) scalar chain of delegating authority, (4) unity of direction and command, (5) centralization of power and authority, (6) span of control, (7) order, (8) discipline, (9) equity, (10) initiative, (11) stability of tenure of personnel, and (12) esprit de corps.

These concepts and principles were first formulated by Fayol in 1925.[1] His 12 principles were developed from a practicing manager's perspective. More recent American contributors include Mooney, Urwick, and Barnard.[2-4] With his formulation of objectives, Barnard may be considered a forerunner of Drucker, and with his emphasis on communication and cooperation and his caution on relying wholly on authority and rigorous structure, he harbingered the behavioral school of management. Massie has provided one of the best overviews of the contribution of the classical school.[5] The most enduring contribution of this school is the formulation of the five functions of management: (1) planning, (2) organizing, (3) directing, (4) coordinating, (5) controlling and evaluating.

BEHAVIORAL SCHOOL

The behavioral school is actually composed of two related developments or schools of thought. The first was the human relations branch, which began with the Hawthorne studies (1927 to 1932)[6-8] and gained wide recognition in the 1940s and early 1950s. The human relations school emphasized the humanistic aspect of work and productivity and the role of the individual in the organization. The foundation for this school was a combination of the results of scientific discovery and maxims, with a preponderance of the latter. The second branch of this school involved the *application* of *behavioral sciences* that began in the early 1950s and continues to be popular today. However, there have been "inroads" and modifications made by persons with different backgrounds and perspectives. The difference between human relations and behavioral science is that the latter is more concerned with the application of the scientific method and empiric data to organizational behavior and theory.

The contributions of the human relations school were mostly modifications in the classical concepts. The negative consequences of the division of labor— such as the feeling of anonymity, social isolation, and the lack of the feeling of task completion because of the never ending production line—were explored. They sought ways to minimize or to nullify these negative consequences. The playing of music, group activity, group goals, and group social functions were among the various remedies suggested.

The human relations writers believed that the scalar principle (carefully defined and distributed authority) and the functional processes were sound, but that their callous use was counterproductive. The writers were especially concerned with the proper balance of authority and responsibility and with the delegation of the appropriate amount of authority.

The human relations proponents tried to solve the problems associated with the rigidity of the structure of the organization and the concomitant rigid span of control. They pointed out that both the structure and the span of control should be designed to fit the particular nature of the work to be done and the personalities and the abilities of the persons involved—in other words, to consider individual differences.

The behavioral science advocates continued the work of the human relations school. Industrial psychologists had been involved earlier, to some degree, in the classical school as well as in the human relations movement. They, with the reinforcement of social psychologists, were the leaders of the behavioral science movement, although sociologists contributed as well. Organizational problems were subjected to empiric study using the scientific method. This movement gained momentum in the 1960s and flourishes even now. The fruit of their endeavor constitutes the bulk of organizational theory and practice, which is in use today.

MANAGEMENT SCIENCE SCHOOL

Management science is known by several names—operations or operational research, quantitative analysis for decision-making, operations analysis, and systems analysis. Practitioners of management science may belong to either Operations Research Society of America, established in 1952, or the Institute of Management Science, established in 1953. The management science school is the latest in terms of recognition and wide application, but its origin can be traced to Eli Whitney in the eighteenth century. The accounting equations, Assets = Liabilities + Net Worth (Capital), as one form of mathematic models, can be traced as far back as the Middle Ages.

The main emphasis of the management science school is the application of mathematic models to management problems. The two major areas of application are production, either products or services, and operations. The models may be based on the accounting system, statistics, matrix algebra or calculus, and, in some cases, simply diagrammatic or schematic models, as well as combinations of these methods. For our purposes, a mathematic model may be defined as a simplified representation of the relevant aspects of a real system or process.

The reader may ask why management science is considered in organizational theory and practice. The answer is simply that this subject contains the theory and methods of describing and predicting much of the behavior of an organization viewed from a broad perspective. Management science provides the tools for sophisticated analysis of management problems, the prediction of the outcomes from a given set of input variables, and the basis of sound decision-making. Because of the complex nature of some of the models, the computer is often required to carry out these operations.

Design of an Organization

The design of an organization is the product of a series of interactions among three major variables—the environment, technology and structure. There are two major schools of thought on how these interaction processes take place. One school states that the process is externally initiated and controlled primarily by forces within the environment, viz., economic, political, social and technical forces. The other school places the locus of the process within the firm itself in the form of strategic choices in the planning function. Most likely it is a combination of the two sources with the proportion of control determined by the intensity of the respective sectors.

Considerable research has been conducted on the nature and forces of organizational design. This body of data was reviewed, analyzed and resynthesized by Randolph and Dess in a paper titled The Congruence Perspective of Organizational Design: A Conceptual Model and Multivariate Research Approach.[9] Much of this section was adapted from their paper.

ENVIRONMENTAL FACTORS

Whenever *organizational environment* is mentioned, there are two possible entities in view, the internal work environments and the external environment.

The latter is the one that is primarily involved in the process under consideration. The former is associated with the organizational design and is determined largely by the same process.

The external environment is not a self-determining or self-directing entity, and therefore, there must be an initiating act to begin the process. This is accomplished when a firm decides on the product and market it will pursue. Within our realm of interest, this could be a pharmaceutical manufacturing firm, a drug wholesale firm or a pharmacy. If it is the latter, it could be a chain, independent, institutional, traditional or prescription pharmacy, or a pharmaceutical center. It is apparent that this decision will elicit a range of environmental factors in response. This response, as well as the entire process, is depicted in Figure 9–1. The decision could involve a new firm, a new product and/or service, a line of products or a new department. In either case, the process is similar but will vary in scope.

The environmental factors include *complexity* and *dynamism* (variability) which collectively provide *uncertainty* or the *risk* variable, *resources* which collectively provide the *munificence* (generous benefits) variable, and the *market* or demand variable (including competition). All of these may be represented by data in some form. The role of research, either product or market, is to determine the feasibility of the enterprise, i.e., the fit between what the firm wants to do and what the environment will accommodate. The product-market decision determines the configuration of environmental variables which will be translated into the particular TASK for the firm. See Figure 9–1.

TECHNOLOGY

Technology has been defined in numerous ways. The one used here is simply the application of knowledge to accomplish the task efficiently. The emphasis is on "how to do" work efficiently and usually involves machinery, but not necessarily, men and materials. There are three aspects of technology that are derived from or determined by the task, viz., task predictability, problem analyzability and task interdependence. By *task predictability* is meant the sameness of the task reflecting a high division of labor in the process, which, in turn, is determined by the product-market variable. By *problem analyzability* is meant the ease by which problems arising from the process can be identified and dealt with. These two aspects together represent a routine—nonroutine continuum. The third aspect, *task interdependence,* is the measure of the degree one component activity is influenced by or dependent upon another component activity and ranges from low to high.

The configuration of technology that should be used is largely determined by the task to be done. Thus, if the product-market is such that the task is nonroutine and highly interdependent, and if the product-market elicits highly uncertain, complex and dynamic environmental and market characteristics, then the technology must be designed to perform that kind of task. This

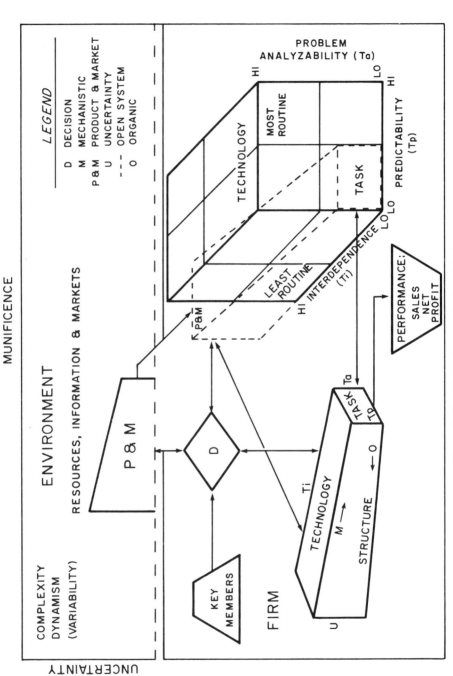

Figure 9–1. Model for organizational design.

implies that "high" technology and highly skilled personnel should be employed. This situation is depicted in Figure 9–1. Of course, the configuration may be just the reverse or some point between these two extremes.

STRUCTURE

Stucture is defined as the hierarchial relationships among members of the organization. This is "where" the respective organizational components accomplish their work. For the present purpose, structure may be divided into five dimensions: (1) division of labor; (2) impersonality; (3) formalization; (4) hierarchy of authority; and (5) participation in decision making. The reader will recognize the first four dimensions as characteristics of the classical approach to organizations, and the fifth as being quite different from the others, a characteristic of the nontraditional or neoclassical approach. The first four dimensions may be summarized in a word, mechanistic, whereas, the fifth may be labeled organic. Thus, we have a mechanistic—organic quasi-continuum representing structure. An *organic structure* is defined as less of the first four dimensions and more of the fifth, whereas, a *mechanistic structure* is defined as just the opposite.

It must be apparent to the reader that technology and structure should match. Indeed, considerable research indicates that nonroutine technology is associated with a more organic structure among successful firms. Also, a direct relationship between task interdependence and organic structure appears to exist. These relationships may be curvilinear and not linear.

LINKAGES

Randolph and Dess formulated linkages among the three primary variables. The *technology-structure linkage* and the *environment-structure linkage* have been subjected to considerable research. In either case, the more complex, uncertain or nonroutine the characteristics or dimensions are, the more likely the structure will be organic in nature among successful firms. The opposite characteristics, i.e., a simple, static environment and routine technology, are associated with mechanistic structures in many successful firms. There has been little research relating munificence with structure; however, it is postulated that munificence is positively associated with organic structure.

There has been little research on the *environmental-technology linkage*. If the product-market choice elicits a highly uncertain environment, the technology should be nonroutine and highly interdependent. In the same vein, environmental dynamism suggests low task predictability, and environmental complexity suggests low problem analyzability. It would be necessary that flexibility be designed into the organization in order for managers to be able to search for solutions of the manifold problems inherent in such a work environment.

ORGANIZATIONAL PERFORMANCE

Organizational performance may be measured in various ways. The measure(s) selected would depend largely on the goals of the organization. For most economic organizations, economic measures are most appropriate including sales, profit, return on investment, growth and market share. For pharmacies, the above measures of performance could be expanded to include incidences of therapeutic-interventions of various types, referrals of patrons with suspected pathologies via screening programs, and related activities. Organizational performance is the *dependent variable* for the ultimate testing of hypotheses derived from the above linkages.

MODEL AND HYPOTHESES

The model is portrayed within Figure 9–1. It is unnecessary to select the primary variables and link them neatly in a separate model. Also, it is beyond the scope of this text to formulate a long list of hypotheses or to operationalize all the various constructs. Randolph and Dess identified 10 constructs and formulated 13 hypotheses. To complete the picture of how all these variables fit together, a set of constructs and hypotheses was formulated in Figure 9–2.

The reader may not be familiar with multiple regression equations as shown in Figure 9–2. Multiple regression is a statistical procedure for relating a set of independent variables to a dependent variable shown as the variable on the left side of the equation. The independent variables may be associated with the dependent variable in a linear (additive) fashion, or inversely (reciprocal), or curvilinearly in which one or more independent variables is/are raised to some power. Also, the reader may wonder how both T_{n-r} and T_i may be defined apparently by the same equation. In either case, the coefficients (b_o, b_1, b_2, etc.) have unique values and thus define the respective constructs by the same terms but with different relationships.

It should be noted that the five equations in Figure 9–2 do not exhaust the many possible relationships. There is one other difference between this treatment and the one described by Randolph and Dess. They defined several constructs both subjectively and objectively, whereas the present approach is to use one or the other whichever seemed most appropriate.

SUMMARY

Organizations do not ''just happen,'' they are designed, either poorly or well. Pharmacists should understand the various factors and their relationships that constitute organizations whether they be primarily economic or social, for profit or not for profit, public or private in purpose. Pharmacy is both a socioeconomic and a scientific occupation. Its contribution to society as well as its continuing existence as an independent quasi-autonomous profession

CONSTRUCTS AND HYPOTHESES

ENVIRONMENTAL CONSTRUCTS:

1. *Perceived risk*[a] (R) is the probability of a return less than a target amount but not ruinous loss, which is avoided at all cost and thus places a limit on the degree of perceived risk that will be assumed.
2. *Munificence* (Mμ) is measured by the ratio of the return on the investment of the industry to the mean return on all of the other comparable industries.
3. *Market*[b] (M$_a$) is measured by demand for the product-service.

TECHNOLOGICAL CONSTRUCTS:

4. *Technology*, nonroutine to routine (T$_{n-r}$) is the application of knowledge to tasks and is measured on an ordinal scale of 1–10.
5. *Technology, interdependence* (T$_i$) is the application of knowledge to tasks that are highly interdependent and therefore require sophisticated technology and probably human skills. It is also measured on a 1–10 ordinal scale.

STRUCTURAL CONSTRUCTS:

6. *Structure, organic* (S$_o$) is the degree the structure is sensitive to people's needs, and changes as needed, and it is measured on an ordinal scale of 1–10.
7. *Structure, mechanistic* (S$_m$) is the opposite of organic structure and is measured on a 1–10 ordinal scale.

PERFORMANCE CONSTRUCTS:

8. *Performance* (P$_o$) of an organization is measured by return on total investment (% NP on TI): TI is net worth plus long-term loans.

HYPOTHESES:

1. $T_{n-r} = b_o + b_1 (R) + b_2 (M_u) + b_3 (M_a) + E$ where b$_o$, b$_1$, b$_2$, b$_3$ are constants with different values in each equation and E is a unique error term in the multiple regression equations.
2. $T_i = b_o + b_1 (R) + b_2 (M_u) + b_3 (M_a) + E$
3. $S_o = b_o + b_1 (R) + b_2 (M_u) + b_3 (M_a) + E$
4. $P_o = b_o + b_1(T_{n-r}) + b_2 (T_i) + b_3 (S_o) + E$
5. $P_o = b_o + b_1(R, M_u, M_a) + b_2 (T_{n-r}) + b_3 (T_i) + b_4 (S_o) + E$

NOTE: Apply all combinations of all variables, both original variables (R, M$_u$, M$_a$) and derived terms T$_{n-r}$; T$_i$; S$_o$) but avoiding redundance, as additive models. These are the minimum explorative, descriptive models. See Randolph and Dess[9] for thorough explanations.

[a]Perceived risk replaces environmental dynamism or variability in the scheme proposed by Randolph and Dess.[9]

[b]Market demand replaces environmental complexity of the scheme proposed by Randolph and Dess.[9]

Figure 9–2. Constructs and hypotheses of organizational design.

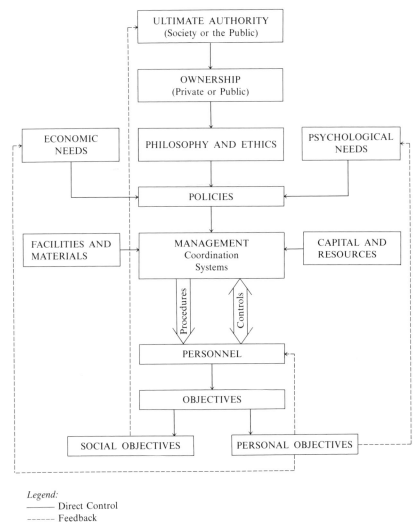

Legend:
——— Direct Control
------ Feedback

Figure 9–3. Relationship between society and an enterprise.

depends, in large measure, on how well pharmacists meet the challenges in both socioeconomic and scientific arenas.

Social Control

Society has devised various mechanisms to control organizations regardless of their purpose. The above discussion focused primarily on how society nurtures and helps shape the design of organizations. This section focuses on how society controls organizations through another set of relationships, which compliment those discussed above. This set of relationships is depicted in Figure 9–3, which was adapted from a similar model designed by Professor R.V. Evanson several years ago.

If one looks at the top echelon of the diagram, it is apparent that in a democratic society, the ultimate authority for any type of professional or business enterprise rests with the public or society. Property rights and professional privileges are derived from and controlled by this authority through two mechanisms, laws and the marketing process. In most enterprises, and this is especially true of pharmacy, both mechanisms function in a real way. A cursory study of pharmaceutical law confirms the degree to which laws and regulations control the practice of pharmacy, and indeed the entire pharmaceutical industry as well. The number of pharmacies that have discontinued business in recent years is indicative of the operation of a competitive free market. Thus a pharmacist-proprietor must comply with the statutory laws and regulations, and he also must conform to a large degree with the "laws" of the marketplace.

The ownership—whether an individual, a partnership, or a corporation—will espouse a set of ethical principles and a philosophy of conduct. When these are combined with the economic and psychologic needs of the owner(s), they provide the basis for the formulation of the policies under which the firm will operate. The necessity of meeting both economic and psychologic needs is probably obvious to both pharmacists and pharmacy students. That these needs permeate throughout the organization, including the lowest level of employment, may not be as well recognized. This principle is one of the basic premises of management by objectives, as previously indicated in Chapter 4.

Beginning with policies as a foundation, a management system is organized to achieve the objectives of the firm. This involves the coordination of capital and other resources and personnel. Procedures and control mechanisms are developed in a systematic way, such as the system of management by objectives. The philosophy of the top echelon of the firm, ranging from a proprietor to a board of directors, is important in determining the style of management and management system that will be implemented. At this point it should be noted that the objectives of all the personnel from the proprietor or chief executive to the clerk and janitor must be met, including both the economic and psychologic components of these objectives. Of course the social objectives must be met if the enterprise expects to thrive or even continue. The pharmacy must meet the needs of the people in the market. The market includes the range of merchandise and services at prices consistent with the type of pharmacy, the affluence of the people, and the needs of the people within the market. The pharmacy must also conform to the laws and regulations applicable to the pharmacy.

Organizational Structure and Charts

The purpose of an organizational chart is to illustrate the lines of authority, responsibility, communication, and span of control throughout an organiza-

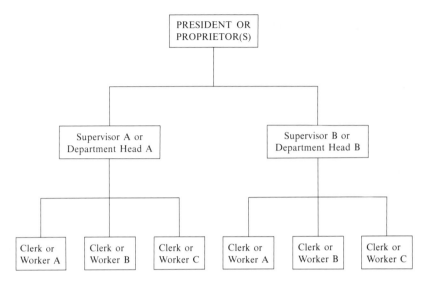

Figure 9–4.   Straight line or scalar organizational chart.

tion, beginning with the final authority at the top. There is limited application of a highly structured organization and complex organizational charts for a small sole proprietorship pharmacy employing only a few people and doing less than $250,000 annual sales volume. However, many of the principles and concepts embodied in an organization structure as depicted by organizational charts are useful even to smaller pharmacies. The four general types of organizational structures are as follows: straight line or scalar, line and staff, functional, and some combination and/or modification of these.

LINE OR SCALAR ORGANIZATIONS

This is the least complicated organizational structure, and it is most useful in organizations with fairly simple, repetitive, and uniform functions and operations. The structure allows for the direct flow of authority, responsibility, and communication from the top authority to the lowest level of work. It was the structure used in most firms during the early days of the industrial revolution and in the military services. The straight line organization is not used as much today, but it is still used with some modification in the military and certain manufacturing firms.

An illustration of this simple organizational structure is shown in Figure 9–4. In the pure line organization, each of the clerks or workers would have the same range of work responsibilities and tasks.

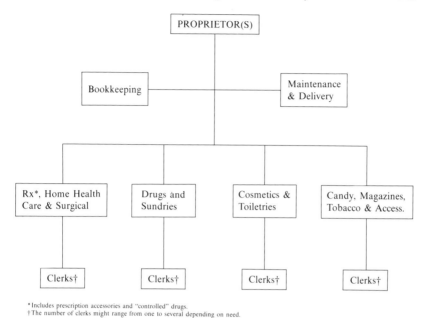

* Includes prescription accessories and "controlled" drugs.
† The number of clerks might range from one to several depending on need.

Figure 9–5. Modified departmental line organization chart.

DEPARTMENTAL MODIFIED LINE ORGANIZATION

A modification of the above structure, which we will call the "Departmental Modified Line Organization," is adaptable to medium and large pharmacies and to other types of organizations or firms. For example, a pharmacy with self-selection layout and annual sales of $400,000 or more, four or five major departments, and twelve or more employees could very well adapt this modified structure. Each department would be directed by a specialist with two to four clerks under his supervision. The department head is responsible for the activities in the department including purchasing, personnel, merchandising, and/or professional services appropriate to the department. Of course, the pharmacist-proprietor(s) should direct and coordinate the activities of the department heads. A system of management by objectives would be applicable to this type of organizational structure. Some writers include this modified departmental line organization as a simple extension of the pure line organization (Fig. 9–5). The responsibilities and duties of each department manager and employee are determined by the system of management by objectives.

LINE AND STAFF ORGANIZATIONS

The line and staff organization was developed as the various management (staff) specialists evolved and were employed to advise management without assuming any direct line authority within the organization. The staff organization supplements the line organization, which has the primary responsibility for the operation of the firm. The staff organization and functions include comptroller (treasurer), purchasing department, real estate, personnel department, legal department, public and professional relations department, operational analysis, and market research.

This type of organizational structure is better adapted to larger firms, such as a chain of drugstores, a very large independent pharmacy, large drug wholesale company, or pharmaceutical manufacturers. The number and type of staff departments vary with the type of operation, but a typical organizational chart for a corporate drugstore chain with 50 units is illustrated in Figure 9–6.

Authority, responsibility, communication, and functions flow downward through the line, to the operational division. The staff serves in an advisory position only. In certain instances, the staff may set guidelines and standards for the entire organization, but communication and enforcement normally proceed through the line organization. Although this form of organization is rather complicated, it provides some of the advantages of the functional organization of specialization in management, with the simplicity of the pure line organization in communication and transmission of authority, responsibility, and duties.

FUNCTIONAL ORGANIZATIONS

The functional form of organization shown in Figure 9–7 is an extremely old concept, albeit not popular today. It dates back to the time of Frederick Taylor and the beginning of scientific management. However, a pharmacist or small businessman must understand the principle of the functional organization, because most small businesses start as functional organizations, formally or informally, and then grow into organizations that are either line or line and staff. What is meant by the functional organization, at least in the traditional sense, is that each supervisor is in charge of a specific function, rather than in charge of specific workers. For example, assuming there are six or eight areas of functions in a pharmacy, six or eight supervisors would be needed, one in charge of each function. You would then find a supervisor who is in charge of all operations having to do with purchasing, another in charge of finances, another in charge of prescription dispensing, and so on. Each supervisor would have the last word with respect to the function he directs.

Normally a pharmacist who is just starting a business has only a few people working for him and he is in charge of all functions. However, when the organization grows—perhaps into a group practice—its character changes to that of a functional organization. Each pharmacist then is in charge of one or more specific functions of the pharmacy. Obviously, this means that as an employee moves from function to function, he works under a different pharmacist each time. And this is the source of trouble with the functional form

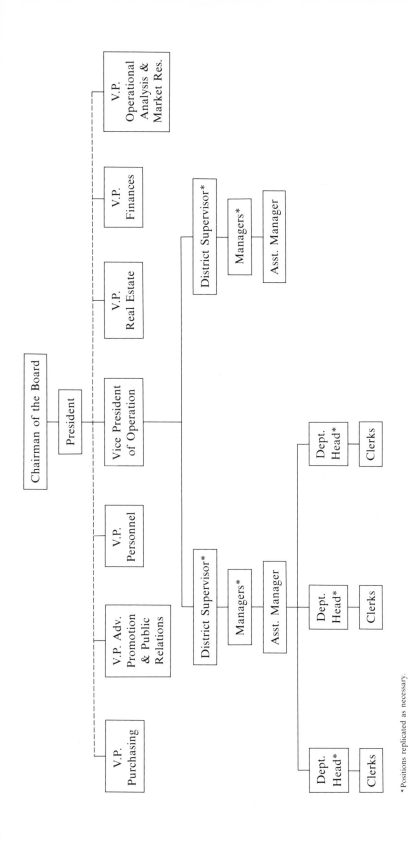

* Positions replicated as necessary.

Figure 9–6. Line staff organization chart: ——represents line operation and departments; - - - represents staff functions and departments.

191

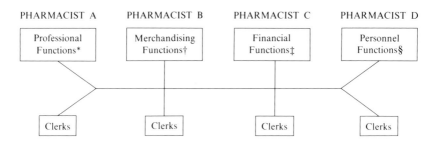

* Professional functions would include prescription dispensing, patient drug record systems, patient consultations, home health aids and surgical supplies, and professional relations.

† Merchandising functions would include purchasing, inventory control, displays, advertising, and personal selling, except prescription and professional goods.

‡ Financial functions would include the general financing, budgeting, accounting, operational analysis and control.

§ Personnel functions would include recruiting, selecting, firing, training, employee performance evaluation, wage determination and other employee relations including fringe benefits.

Figure 9–7. Functional organizational chart.

of organization. People become confused when they work on more than one function and therefore must work for more than one boss. Not only do job responsibilities get extremely confusing, but it becomes difficult for a supervisor to observe the performance of the employee. Therefore, the functional form of organization is only amenable to the small organization. However, because pharmacies tend to start small, pharmacists anticipating a group practice should be aware that in all likelihood, the first kind of organization they will utilize is the functional organization.

INFORMAL ORGANIZATIONS

A discussion of the organization of business would be incomplete without at least passing mention of the phenomenon called the informal organization. The informal organization cannot be seen, but it certainly can be felt by the pharmacist. The reader is referred to the section on work groups for a more complete discussion of the effects of informal organizations.

Work Groups

Ever since people have worked together in large numbers, there have been work groups. Study of work groups date as far back as the famous Hawthorne studies in the 1920s. The reader may wonder just what are work groups. Donnelly, Gibson and Ivancevich define *work group* as "a collection of employees (managerial or nonmanagerial) who share certain norms and who strive to satisfy their needs through the attainment of a group goal(s)."[10] The same authors state that "work groups are inevitable, exert strong influence on the behavior and performance of employees, and may have positive as well as negative effects.'' These are sufficient reasons for studying work groups.[10]

CLASSIFICATION AND CHARACTERISTICS OF WORK GROUPS

There are two general types of work groups, formal and informal. The *formal work* group is one that is designed by management and is often evident in the organizational chart. One type of formal work group is the *permanent work group* sometimes called *command* groups. It has a well-defined structure with lines of communication and authority that are readily recognized, and it is usually permanent. There is one other type of formal work group, viz. the *ad hoc task* group also called simply task group. This is organized by management for a specific purpose or mission. Generally, it is not permanent.

The *informal work* group develops through employee affiliation of some type to achieve a common purpose. These groups are either *economic interest groups* or *psychosocial friendship groups*. The former type of group is organized to fulfill an economic, social, and/or psychologic need on the job. The friendship gorup is strictly social and often functions outside the work environment. See Figure 9–8 for a summary of work group characteristics.

GROUP INTERACTIONS

There are several ways of studying work groups, but one approach particularly has gained considerable recognition. Bales studied groups attempting to reach a decision and found that group interactions could be classified into four types; thus his method is called Bale's Interaction Analysis.[11] The four types of interaction are:

1. Positive human relations that
   (a) show group solidarity, give help and rewards;
   (b) show tension release, joke, laugh;
   (c) understand, concur, and comply.
2. Positive task-oriented, which
   (a) provide direction, suggestions;
   (b) give opinions, show feelings;
   (c) provide goal orientation, repeats, clarify.
3. Negative human relations that
   (a) show disagreement, are passive, show rejection;
   (b) show tension and increase tension;
   (c) show antagonism, are self-defensive.
4. Negative task-oriented, which
   (a) ask for orientation, help;
   (b) ask for opinion, suggestions;
   (c) ask for confirmation, evaluation.

A comprehensive view of work group behavior is shown in Figure 9–8.

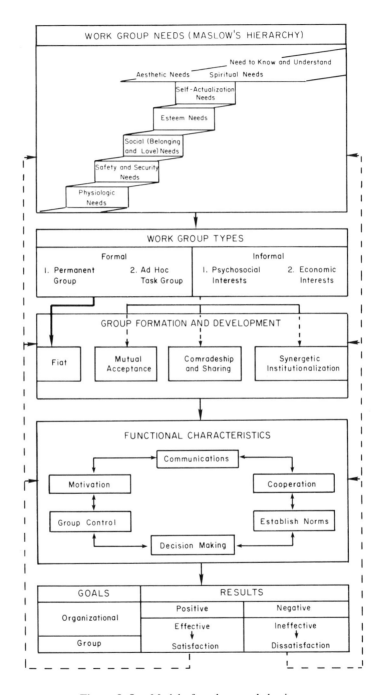

Figure 9–8. Model of work group behavior.

Although most of the features of work group behavior are well described in Figure 9–8, a few additional comments on the characteristics of work groups are appropriate. Although the group leader and other features of the formal group are visible from the outset, the emergent leader, the status hierarchy, norms, and group control of the informal group evolve over a period of time. Informal work groups may not be efficient at first, but they often develop into an efficient and formidable group. Much depends on the solidarity of the group and group leadership. A good leader will have the following characteristics.[12]

1. The individual will have personal attributes that the group members perceive as critical to their needs.
2. The leader embodies the values of the group and is able to perceive the values, to organize and articulate them in an intelligent manner to nonmembers.
3. The leader is able to receive and to decipher communication from relevant groups and to explain the significance to group members.

Groups, especially informal work groups, *exercise control* over their members first by establishing norms and values and then enforcing these, mainly by three mechanisms. The most forceful of these means is *group pressure*. This phenomenon has been demonstrated experimentally by Asch.[13] A second mechanism is *group review* and enforcement, which is more nearly formal than the other two mechanisms. A noncompliant member is confronted, usually by the group leader, in a friendly manner and the deviant behavior is explained to him. A variety of corrective action may be used, ranging from a "soft" approach to ostracizing the person. The third and most subtle mechanism is the personalization or *internalization of the group norms and value system*. This is probably the best method of the three, but its effectiveness is determined by group solidarity, by cohesiveness, and by the quality of norms and values vis-a-vis broader social ones.

SPECIAL GROUPS

Committees. Committees are a special kind of work group. They may be formal, appointed by management, or they may be informal, initiated by workers. They are constituted for one or more of the following purposes: (1) exchanging views and information; (2) generating ideas; (3) recommending action; (4) developing counter proposals; or (5) making decisions. The success of a committee depends on the attitude and effort of its members, but, to a large degree, it also depends on the leadership provided by the chairperson. The following five guidelines will almost assure a good functional committee.[14]

1. Be a careful listener and listen with an open mind.
2. Allow each member to voice opinions and do not place your opinions above others.

3. Get everyone involved in the committee's activities.
4. Display an active interest in the purpose of the committee and in the ideas of the membership.
5. Help the committee focus on the task at hand and on the progress being made.

Quality Circles. Quality circles, or quality control circles, are a Japanese invention, but ironically they have their roots in the participative management and organizational theories of Argyris, Rensis Likert and McGregor, all Americans. Also, the expertise of two American management consultants, Edwards Deming and J.M. Juran, played a large role in the Japanese focus on upgrading *quality and productivity.* The success of Japanese industrial management is due, in part, to the United States' assistance and expertise in post World War II reconstruction. The Japanese were good students; they learned the techniques well and applied them, whereas American industrialists learned the techniques but failed to widely implement them.

A *quality circle* is a small number of employees who work in the same area and who along with their supervisor (usually) voluntarily meet regularly to identify problems and solve them. Quality circles are classic examples of task forces and may be command groups in many instances. The number of members ranges from four to 15. Sometimes the leader is an experienced senior employee rather than a supervisor. They usually meet outside work hours but not always. In most instances, the members are paid for their participation. They are a recognized, formal part of most large Japanese manufacturing firms with a coordinating office and coordinator who reports directly to the plant manager. The company promotes quality circles via fostering competition, prize money and bonuses.

The group will identify a problem, develop a solution and present it to management for review and a decision on whether to implement it. The group with the assistance of management implements the solution, and the results are evaluated by the circle and management. The group makes a presentation of the project for management's review and also for evaluation. Groups compete for special prizes and recognition at various levels up to a company-wide basis on a planned schedule. Competition is vigorous, and quality circles have become an integral part of the Japanese industrial culture. There are 600,000 quality circles involving about 6 million workers in Japan compared to less than 1 percent of those figures in the United States.[15] Success of Japanese industrial management is not due solely to quality circles. An excellent review article of the many theories advanced on the reasons for Japan's widely acclaimed success appeared in the *Academy Management Review* in 1984.[16]

The quality circle technique may be utilized by almost every type and size firm with a critical mass of employees, about 10 or more. It is a neat way of implementing participative management.

Organizational Change and Development

Change is inevitable in any organization. Sometimes there is a need for change that is not forthcoming in an organization. Organizational development is designed to cope with both possibilities. Organizational development (OD) is the systematically planned and executed program of improving the effectivness of an organization through the application of behavioral science concepts, principles, and theory, primarily operant behavior theory. The OD program is a method for facilitating change and development in the *structure* (formal relationships and rules), *people* (attitudes, behavior, and skills), *technology,* and *physical resources* (machines, routines, and work methods) of an organization. It is most often successful where the tasks are relatively simple.

Donnelly, Gibson, and Ivancevich have discussed methods for managing organizational change and development.[17] Figure 9–9 is a representation of a model for managing these changes. The model identifies six phases of OD, and none is more important than the second phase, recognition of the need for change. Management that fails in this important task will be forced to manage by crises, one crisis after another, a situation that is far too common in pharmacy. Some symptoms of this type of management include: (1) an orientation toward the past (the good old days), (2) bemoaning current conditions and not recognizing opportunities and challenges, and (3) holding to rituals and form rather than to substance and direct analysis of an issue or problem.

FORCES OF CHANGE

There are two general types of forces of change, external and internal. *External forces* include changes in the marketplace and the economy, technology, and the social environment, including government policies. The marketplace may change due to competition, new products and services, shifting population, and/or drastic economic changes. Technologic changes have been explosive since World War II. The most important of all technologic changes has been the computer. Business in general could not operate at the present level of productivity without the computer, and this situation is rapidly developing for the practice of pharmacy.

Environmental changes affecting pharmacy are less visible, but nevertheless important. The relationship of environmental conditions to many diseases is well established. Regulatory or governmental impact on the economic/political environment has been pervasive, sometimes for the good and sometimes not. One such change with the enormous impact is the introduction of patient package inserts (PPI). This is a change that pharmacy collectively probably could have prevented by properly counseling and monitoring patients' use of drugs. This is a classic example of a profession's failure to manage change,

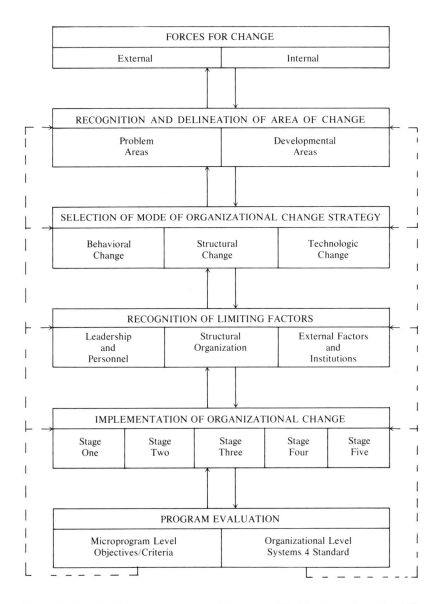

Figure 9–9. Model for the management of change. (Modified from Donnelly, J.H., Gibson, J.L., and Ivancevich, J.M.: *Fundamentals of Management, Functions, Behavior, Models,* 3rd ed. Dallas: Business Publications, Inc., 1978.)

thus letting change manage its members. DRGs and preferred provider organizations (PPOs) are other examples.

Internal forces occur within an organization and can be traced to processes and people, and more specifically to a breakdown in communication, interpersonal relations, and improper policy and/or decisions. Symptoms include low morale, absenteeism, employee turnover, and, eventually, low productivity. Management must be attuned to these symptoms early and must institute proper remedies; better yet is the prevention of these problems through appropriate OD.

RECOGNITION OF THE NEED FOR CHANGE

Management may anticipate change by persistent attention to the signs of change. The foremost source of these signs is the financial statements, but other sources are important. These include market reports, reports of technologic innovations in the current literature, surveys among clients and employees, suggestions from employees, customers complaints, absenteeism, and many others.

Diagnosis of the problem is, of course, important. Management must analyze the signs and decide what is the real problem. Often, signs may be deceiving. After proper diagnosis, the problem should be translated into achievable objectives and criteria. This is one indication that the problem has been properly identified.

DEVELOPMENT OF STRATEGY

When the problem has been diagnosed, identification of alternative OD methods and strategies is the next step. OD techniques will impinge on all the major components of the organization, but they usually will have an impact primarily on the structure, on the people, or on the technology of the organization.

Structural Changes. Structural change focuses on one or more of the following: (1) Formal structure may be modified in terms of span of control, lines of authority and responsibility, and relationship of line and staff positions. A staff position may be converted to line position, or vice versa. (2) The bases for departmentalization may be modified, for example, to a flatter, more decentralized and democratic form, with a large number of persons per unit, or to a higher, more centralized and bureaucratic form, with few persons per unit. (3) The definition and nature of jobs may be altered in one of two directions—work simplification or job enrichment.

Behavioral Changes. Behavioral change is the second major type of OD, and it is designed to improve personnel attitudes, skills, and knowledge, thus leading to a change in behavior and to high performance. Traditionally, this effort was carried on in the form of training programs, with emphasis on conceptual materials and communication. The vehicles for this training include lectures, films, discussion groups, organized collegiate courses, and, more recently, role playing. This approach has had limited long-term effects on behavior.

A more effective approach may be subsumed under the term, sensitivity training. *Sensitivity training,* also called T-group training, focuses on the emotional level rather than on the conceptual, cognitive level. Awareness is the key—awareness of one's own attitudes, biases, and limitiatons, as well as awareness of the needs of others.

Attitude Awareness. Attitude awareness is a well-known executive development program based on the above principles.[18] Usually, this type of training takes place at a site other than the work place, often has no agenda or at least not a rigid format, and has an unobtrusive trainer or group leader. A detailed review of 100 research studies on sensitivity training found the training most effective at the personal level, but not at the organizational level.[19] The review concluded that the training: (1) stimulated short-term improvement in communicative skills; (2) caused the trainees to believe that they controlled their own behavior more than did others; (3) increased the participative orientation of trainees in leadership roles; and (4) improved the perception of others toward the trainee.

Technologic Change. The third area of OD is a technologic change. This category includes any application of science to new ways of transforming resources into products or services. As indicated earlier, the computer is the outstanding example of modern technology. It should be noted that technology is not just machines or hardware. Great care must be exercised in the implementation of any category of OD, but this is especially true of technologic changes. Amadio has written a case study on the negative impact of the improper implementation of tablet-counting machines in the prescription departments of a chain drugstore company.[20]

LIMITING FACTORS

There are limiting factors on the type and scope of OD programs for any given organization. These limiting factors fall into three categories: (1) leadership climate and skills; (2) organizational culture; and (3) formal organization and legal constraints. Leadership climate refers to the style and skills of the leadership. If the leadership is not competent, it probably will not have the self-confidence and openness necessary to nurture successful OD programs. Organizational culture refers to the group norms, values, and informal relationships that exist in the organization. Any OD program contrary to the values, norms, and relationships of the organizational culture probably will not succeed. The formal organizational structure may not be compatible with the envisioned OD program, but the formal structure can be changed. There may be a limitation of OD programs because of legal constraints, e.g., fair labor practices and minimum wage laws.

IMPLEMENTATION

Selection of Strategy. Implementation of the OD strategy and method is the next step in the OD model. Greiner researched a number of OD programs to determine the relationships of OD strategies to the relative success of the programs.[21] He found that the general approach to the implementation or strategy could be located along a continuum of: unilateral authority → shared authority → delegated authority. He also found that those programs at either extreme had little to no success—the first extreme, unilateral authority, because of either passive resistance or deliberate sabotage; the last extreme, delegated authority, because of the lack of leadership. Successful OD programs used the shared authority approach and the process was composed of six phases, according to Greiner. These phases are a replica, to some extent, of the organizational change model. For our purpose, a five-stage implementation strategy replaces Greiner's six phases.

Stages of Implementation. The recognition and arousal stage encompasses the first two components of the OD model for Greiner. Not only must the need for change be recognized, but also management must feel the need deeply and must become committed to the change. The second stage is the circumspect and consultative phase of the process. Someone, either in the organization or outside the organization, who can be objective about the problem should be consulted. This stage includes the second, third, fourth, and possibly, the fifth components of the model. The next stage is participative, in which representatives of all levels of personnel are involved. This stage overlaps the previous ones and includes the third through the fifth components of the model. The fourth stage is the experimental stage, in which the OD program is implemented in one or a few units (products, a product line or some portion or level) of the organization. The results are monitored carefully and are evaluated. This stage corresponds to the beginning of the fifth component of the model. If the change has been successful, the OD program is fully implemented in the final institutional stage, which includes the fifth and sixth components of the model.

EVALUATION

The last component of the model is the evaluation of the OD program. The evaluation process should be conducted at two levels—the micro-program-specific level and the organizational level. For the micro level, the results are compared to the objectives and/or to criteria identified during the diagnosis of the problem. At the organizational level, a broader standard should be used. Likert has provided us with an excellent standard, from a behavioral science perspective, which he called a system 4 organization.[22]

A system 4 organization may be considered to be the ideal organizational type among four types:

System 1—Exploitive-Authoritative

System 2—Benevolent-Authoritative
System 3—Consultative-Group-Oriented
System 4—Participative-Group-Oriented

Likert no longer uses these value-laden labels, but simply refers to systems 1, 2, 3, or 4. Organizations are classified in one of the four types based on the responses of the personnel at all levels (usually all personnel) to a 51-item questionnaire. The items are the Likert-type and may be categorized into eight operating characteristics as follows: leadership, motivation, communication, interaction, decision-making, goal-setting, control and performance. Each of these characteristics is described in detail in reference 22.

A system 4 organization may be generally described by the following three statements. Management: (1) uses the principle of supportive relationships; (2) uses group methods for decision-making and supervision; and (3) has high performance goals.[22] This method of Likert and his system 4 organization provide a good format to evaluate an organization and its OD programs.

Toward an Integrated Organizational Theory

Each of the schools of organizational theory contributed significantly to a better understanding of organizations and their behavior; some contributed more than others. There is not yet a formal integrated theory of organizations. However, efforts to that end may be bearing fruit.[23]

CHRONOLOGICAL DEVELOPMENT

The *classical school* of engineers and managers delineated and described the five traditional functions of management. They developed the concepts of organizational structure, division of work, span of control, scalar (graduated) chain of authority, lines of responsibility and authority, all of which fostered a structured mechanical approach to management. *Organizational control* was probably the most important characteristic of the classical school.

Following Barnard and the Hawthorne studies, the *human relations* school made its mark. This movement came at an appropriate time in our country, when unions were growing rapidly. The humanizing approach to management of this school made it easier to negotiate labor settlements, especially of issues other than wages. Probably the major contribution of this school was the elevation of *human dignity* of the worker and his outlook on work. The behavioral science branch of the behavioral school meshed the scientific method with the human relations approach with remarkable results. The behavior school made a considerable contribution to organizational theory and practice; however, the behavioral science branch contributed much more. Collectively, they gave us a *better understanding* of the *organizational process,* including motivation, work group behavior, leadership, and organizational change and development. The contributions of Maslow, McGregor,

Likert, Herzberg, and others had an enduring effect, yet not all the issues had been settled. Results of their research were certainly not conclusive as to the merits of some of the newer techniques in organizational management.

There was a resurgence of the near mechanical approach to management in the form of bureaucracy. *Bureaucracy* gained respectability as a result of the work of a German sociologist, Max Weber. Rules and structure seemed important to the affairs of organizations, and indeed, there is a place for these. Failure of management was attributed to the failure of following the rules, or to going outside the system. The system was supposed to prevent or to expose and eliminate incompetence, discrimination, payola, and arbitrary authority, for example. It was supposed to compensate expertise and productivity. The problem with this approach was that a tightly controlled organization could be used to cover up malfeasance and incompetence. Also, it stifled initiative and suppressed motivation. The popular book *The Peter Principle*,[24] "blew the whistle" on the *negative effects* of bureaucracy.

Next came the *political scientists*, who began to research the issues of *power* and *conflict* within organizations, especially nonprofit organizations. Resolution of conflicts was a means of organizing and deploying power and influence, and scarce resources as well. Perrow described how the "structionalists" (largely sociologists) and the behavioralists (largely social psychologists) managed to incorporate these newer concepts.[25] Even the economists had little trouble with conflict and conflicting goals, as long as these were associated in some fashion with economic factors. The strict "structionalists," with their preoccupation with bureaucracy, had the greatest problem accepting the incorporation of conflict and its resolution as a legitimate mode of organizational behavior.

Out of the efforts to sort out the areas of conflict and associated factors (people or groups, structure and relationships, influence and power, resources and expertise, and possibly other factors), and the effort to determine how this theory could explain organizational behavior came still another major contribution to organizational theory, namely decision theory. *Decision theory* developed as a means of selecting the best or second-best (most feasible) alternative among many that are available to an organization. This choice required the consideration of so many variables that ordinary methods were unsuitable. The manager, being limited in his capacity to account for all these variables in an ordinary mental process, needed a means to focus on the real issues. Several attention-directing techniques evolved. Two such techniques, control of the premises of the decision and the reward system, were the most useful, but even they were insufficient. Then enter the statistician, the computer, and quantitative methods.

In a sense, organizational theory had gone full cycle and had returned to "hard" science. Each school focused on a particular aspect of organizational theory and behavior. Yet each school contributed, answering a few more questions than it raised.

CURRENT STATUS OF THEORIES

Miner surveyed 100 scholars in the field of organizational theory for their nominations of theories that had made a significant impact on understanding organizations.[23] Each theory had to meet three criteria: (1) the theory should have proved useful in understanding, explaining and predicting the functioning of organizations or the behavior of their members; thus it should have proved to be valid to some degree; (2) the theory should have clear implications for practice in some area of management; thus it should be useful; and (3) the theory should have generated significant research; thus it should have been in existence long enough to have been tested and become established. Altogether 110 theories were nominated involving 350 theorist, i.e., those who had contributed to one or more of the theories. Of the 110, 24 had 10 or more nominations. Miner selected the 24 plus eight others to provide a full range of nomination frequencies for his analysis. Three variables were used to evaluate the 32 theories: frequency of nomination and the first two of the above criteria. The third criterion was also indirectly utilized because the evaluation was based on published research.

The results of the analysis were not very positive in respect to usefulness (7 of the 32 theories), and only moderately positive in respect to validity (11 of the 32). Four of the seven "useful" theories were also valid. A word of criticism is in order. Miner's criterion of "usefulness" was based on published research that *proved* the theory to be useful under rigorous constraints. It may be possible that a theory was useful but not subjected to rigorous research because it lacked "research appeal" or was not amenable to research design. A theory may be so patently useful that no one bothered to subject it to research.

The above line of reasoning is further supported by a critical review of the types of theories that were valid and/or useful. Miner classified the theories into four classes—structure and organizational development (two macro theories), motivation and leadership—supervision (two micro theories). All four of the highly valid and highly useful theories were motivational. Of the other seven highly valid theories, but of questionable or low usefulness, two were motivational and two were leadership-supervision theories. These theories involve constructs that are more easily defined operationally and thus measured. Of the other three highly useful theories, but of low or "mixed" validity, one was motivational and two were organizational development. Miner's analysis was oriented toward easily validated theories. It was not designed necessarily to identify those theories that best explained *how* organizations and their members behave. It did identify those theories that best explained *why* organizations and their members behave as they do.

Miner closed his paper with a plea for developing a *new organizational science*. I believe his plea for a new science goes farther than is necessary. What is needed is a method of integrating or unifying the compatible theories that will explain why and, to the degree possible, how organizations behave.

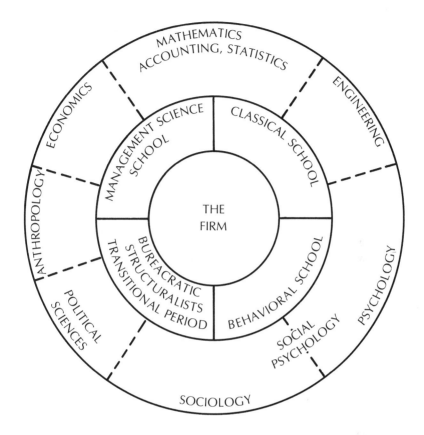

DISCIPLINE	CONTRIBUTION
Anthropology	*Adaptation,* survival, cultural development
Economics	*Choices,* allocation of scarce resources, competition, cooperation
Engineering	*Construction* (structure), transformation, functions, rules
Mathematics (Accounting, algebra, calculus, statistics)	*Relationships* through symbolic representation and rigorous application of rules
Political Science	*Conflict* and *conflict resolution*: goals, power, among groups and/or individuals
Psychology	*Experiential processes,* needs, motives, emotions, thoughts affecting behavior
Sociology	*Group accommodation* leading to group decisions and behavior

Note: There is considerable overlap among the contribution and utility of the behavioral sciences (anthropology, economics, political science, psychology and sociology), and considerable interrelationship among all of the disciplines in the model.

Figure 9–10.　A model of integrated organizational theory.

Miner identified the basic discipline of the 40 theorists who had contributed to the 32 theories.[23] There were 22 psychologists, four "organizational behavioralists," four sociologists, two political scientists, two economists, and one each of the following: industrial relations specialists, management specialist, social scientist, engineer, lawyer and historian. Psychologists constituted 55 percent of the groups. A broad, general framework of how various disciplines can contribute to a unified organizational theory is shown in Figure 9–10.

Randolph and Dess' model for testing the congruence of the components of organizational design (see Figure 9–1) is a first step toward a unified theory. A similar model for relating and testing the primary and congruent constructs of micro-organizational theory is needed. Then a means of interfacing the two models would provide an overall framework for viewing and refining organizational theory that could be useful in practice. However, many of the present theories and systems are useful.

Summary of Practical Principles

In respect to macro-organizational practices, the following principles are useful.

1. The design, configuration of technology and structure are contingent on variables found in the environment and the nature of the products and services that are marketed. Simple products or services produced in mass are suited to a more routine technology and a simple, more highly structured organization.
   (a) The organizational structure tends to be tall in these organizations with a smaller span of control.
   (b) The organizational structure tends to be flat in these organizations with a larger span of control.
2. Organizations generally should be considered open in respect to socio-economic and political systems and sensitive to social trends.
3. Focus on operational participation of small natural work groups is one of the surest ways to harness tremendous brain power and energy, e.g., quality circles and systems 4.
4. Goals generally must be congruent within an organization and with those of society.
5. Bureaucracy and control serve a purpose but they should be sparingly and delicately utilized in most organizations.

REFERENCES

1. Fayol, H.: *General and Industrial Management*. Translated by C. Starrs. London: Pitman Publishing Corp., 1949.
2. Mooney, J.D.: *The Principles of Organization*. New York: Harper and Brothers, 1947. (There was an earlier version by Mooney and Reiley, *Onward Industry*, 1931.)

3. Urwick, L.: *The Elements of Administration*. New York: Harper and Brothers, 1944.
4. Barnard, C.I.: *The Functions of the Executive*. Cambridge: Harvard University Press, 1938.
5. Massie, J.L.: Management theory. In J.H. March, ed., *Handbook of Organizations*. Chicago: Rand McNally and Co., 1965.
6. Roethlisferger, F.J., and Dickson, W.J.: *Management and the Worker*. Boston: Harvard University Press, 1939.
7. Landsberger, H.A.: *Hawthorne Revisited*. Ithaca: New York School of Industrial and Labor Relations, Cornell University, 1958.
8. Carey, A.: The Hawthorne studies: a radical criticism. *Am. Socio. Rev., 32*:403–416, 1967.
9. Randolph, W.A. and Dess, G.G.: The congruence perspective of organizational design: A conceptual model and multivariate research approach. *Acad. Mang't Rev., 9*:114, 27, 1984.
10. Donnelly (Jr.), J.H., Gibson, J.L. and Ivancevick, J.M.: *Fundamentals of Management*. 5th ed., Plano, TX: Business Publications, Inc., 1984, p. 348.
11. Bales, R.F.: *Interaction Process Analysis: A Method for the Study of Small Groups*. Cambridge, Mass: Addison-Wesley, Inc., 1950.
12. Donnelly (Jr.), J.H., Gibson, J.L., and Ivancevich, J.M.: *Fundamentals of Management*. 3rd ed. Dallas: Business Publications, Inc., 1978, pp. 227–242.
13. Asch, S.E.: Opinions and social pressure. *Sci. Am. 193*:31–35, 1955.
14. Prince, G.M.: How to be a better chairman. *Harvard Bus. Rev., 47*:98–108, 1969.
15. Donnelly, Gibson and Ivancevich, *op. cit.*, ref. 10, p. 357.
16. Keys, J.B. and Miller, T.R.: The Japanese management theory jungle. *Acad. Mang't Rev., 9*:342–53, 1984.
17. Donnelly, Gibson and Ivancevich, *op. cit.*, ref. 10, pp. 456–499.
18. Lewter, B.R., Winchester, KY., personal communications, 1979. Dr. Lewter modified the Attitude Awareness Program as a component of the research variable in his Doctoral Dissertation, University of Kentucky, Lexington, KY.
19. House, R.J.: T-group education and leadership effectiveness: a review of the empirical literature and a critical evaluation. *Personnel Psychol., 20*:1–32, 1967.
20. Amadio, A.J.: The technological innovation. In *Case Studies in Pharmacy Management*. Vo. IV. Philadelphia: Merck & Co., 1974.
21. Greiner, L.E.: Patterns of organizational change. *Harvard Bus. Rev., 45*:119–130, 1967.
22. Likert, R.: *The Human Organization*. New York: McGraw-Hill Book Co., 1967.
23. Miner, J.B.: The validity and usefulness of theories in an emerging organizational science. *Acad. Mang. Rev., 9*:296–306, 1984.
24. Peter, L.J.: *The Peter Principle*, New York: William Morrow & Co., 1969.
25. Perrow, C.: The short and glorious history of organizational theory. *Organizational Dynamics, 2*:2–15, 1973.

REVIEW

1. Distinguish between macro- and micro-organizational theory and behavior.

2. Name the three major schools of organizational theory and behavior.

3. Define or explain the following: division of labor and specialization, scalar principle, organizational structure, span of control, and social isolation.

4. What are the two branches of the behavioral school of organizational theory, and what is the essential difference between the two?

5. What is the management science school of organizational theory and how does this "science management" differ from the "scientific management" associated with the classical school of organizational theory?

6. Describe the "design of an organization." What are its three major variables? Differentiate between the two major schools of thought on the interactive processes of organizational design.

7. Describe the environment factors and variables as these relate to organizational design. How are these factors and variables activated in respect to a particular

organization and what determines the scope, force and effects these factors and variables have on organizational design?

8. Describe the task in the context of organizational design.

9. Define technology, task predictability, task interdependence and problem analyzability within the context of organizational design.

10. What is meant by organic and mechanistic organizational structure?

11. What type of organizational structure is best suited to a high tech task? Low tech task?

12. What type of organizational structure and technology would you select for a firm that intended to produce a product that is associated with high uncertainty, high potential for munificence and potentially a short product life span? Identify three such products.

13. How would you describe the organizational design of a typical community pharmacy?

14. Discuss various forms of organizational performance of a pharmacy. Other types of firms.

15. Explain what is meant by the social organization and how this is related to the management of a pharmacy.

16. Explain how the social organization correlates with the philosophy of management by objectives.

17. Compare similarities and differences between legal regulation and market regulation of a pharmacy practice.

18. Contrast ethical precepts and legal precepts.

19. What is the purpose of the organizational chart?

20. Describe and contrast the various types of organizational structures and charts as to form, purpose, application and effectiveness, especially in respect to various types of pharmaceutical firms.

21. Explain how work groups come into existence. Distinguish among the basic types of work groups and give a pharmacy example of each.

22. Can you recall an incident in your experience of each type of Bale's Interaction Analysis? Explain how this affected the group.

23. What is meant by informal organization?

24. Explain how groups exercise control over group members.

25. What is meant by internalizing a group norm or value system?

26. Discuss the guidelines for a functional committee.

27. What is a quality circle? What is the purpose of quality circles? Where did quality circles originate? Who assisted in the establishment of quality circles?

28. Discuss whether quality circles would be productive in various types of pharmaceutical firms.

29. Discuss the concept of organizational change and development with all its ramifications.

30. Explain the forces of organizational change and compare these with the primary factors of organizational design.

31. Describe the six phases of organizational change and development.

32. Differentiate among the three methods of organizational change and development—structural, behavioral, and technologic change.

33. What are the limitations to organizational change and development?

34. How would you evaluate an OD program?

35. Explain what is meant by a system 4 organization.

36. Discuss the integration of organizational theory, how organizational theories evolved, the various "schools," and the application of the various disciplines.

37. What three criteria did Miner use in selecting organizational theories for analysis?

38. What criticism may be made of Miner's approach?

39. What types of theories did Miner find to be more valid? Useful?

40. Summarize by listing and briefly explaining five practical principles of macro-organizational theory and behavior.

10 | Micro-Organizational Theory and Practice

Micro-organizational theory focuses on explaining *why* members of organizations behave as they do as contrasted with macro-organizational theory which focuses on *how* organizations behave. As classified by Miner, micro theory may be categorized into two broad genre—motivation and leadership/supervision.[1] Of the 32 theories analyzed by Miner, nine dealt with motivation and eight dealt with leadership/supervision. This chapter is divided into those two broad divisions: motivation and leadership development.

Motivation

Motivation is a hypothetical construct that cannot be observed directly but may be inferred from some type of behavior. The same may be said of IQ and attitudes. Just as there are three components of the structure of attitudes, there are three stages of motivation.[2] The *first stage* is an *arousal* or a stimulus by which a target behavior is energized. This stage is associated with an inherent need in some form. That which is aroused may be thought of as a *force within* that activates or drives a person to act.

The *second stage* is the *directing* or *channeling* of behavior toward a *target* or *goal*. This stage is, in one sense, a discriminating stage by which the activity or behavior is focused on a goal and not randomly dissipated.

The *third stage* is the *maintenance* stage by which the behavior is sustained by either forces from within, or the environment through a *positive reinforcement* mechanism. In contrast, a *negative feedback* may not sustain the desired behavior, but may either reduce the level of intensity of the behavior or change the behavior entirely.

The various motivational theories and techniques will be discussed within the framework of the three stages of motivation. As we shall see, some theories explain aspects of one stage, whereas other theories explain other stages. Some of the theories explain aspects of two, perhaps three, stages to some

210

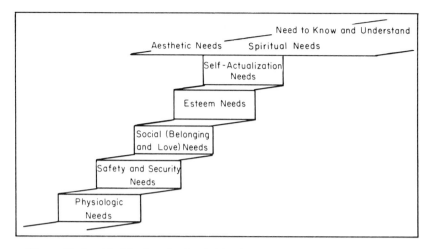

Figure 10–1. Model of motivational drive based on hierarchy of needs theory.

degree. No theory is all sufficient. Motivational techniques, like theories, usually focus on one stage more than other stages, but not exclusively, because motivation is a very complex process.

ENERGIZING HUMAN BEHAVIOR: NEED THEORY

The theory that best explains the basis for energizing behavior is Maslow's *hierarchy of need* theory.[3] Maslow postulated that the *underlying needs* of all human motivation can be organized in a hierarchial manner on five general levels as shown in Figure 10–1. Maslow labeled his motivational theory a synthesis of holistic-dynamic theories. He borrowed concepts from the functionalist tradition of James and Dewey, fused these with the holistic approach of Wertheimer, Goldstein, and Gestalt pyschology and the dynamics of psycho analysis of Freud, Jung and others.

Premises of the Theory. Maslow prefaced his theory on sixteen propositions, many of which were self-evident. The essence of these propositions may be abridged and summarized in several well-chosen statements.

1. An individual functions as an integrated whole and not in parts, and thus his motivations are integrated and not isolated.
2. Hunger is not the paradign or base for all other motivations even though hunger and the sequential behavior can be readily observed and subjected to experimentation. On closer analysis, hunger is seen as more of a special case of motivation than a general one because it is more isolated.
3. The observed, everyday desires and drives may be only a means to an end, which may not be apparent at all. Underlying motivations may actually exist in the subconscious mind.
4. There is sufficient evidence to indicate that desires or motivations are conditioned by cultural and environmental factors.

5. There are so many specific desires or motivations which are not of equal force that they cannot be enumerated and placed into mutually exclusive classes or atomistic lists. There are indeed multiple motivations operating sometimes synergistically and sometimes antagonistically.

6. Motivations are interrelated and may be loosely subsumed into *categories* forming a hierarchy of needs, but they cannot be formed into classes of discrete drives. This interrelationship is manifested by the fact that a person rarely, if ever, reaches a state of complete satisfaction, except for a short period of time. At any given time, the need that is manifested depends upon those needs already satisfied. Because some needs are more basic to survival than others, a hierarchy of needs or basic goals may be constructed, keeping in mind that even these goals are perceived in an integrated fashion by an integrated, whole person. This is the holistic approach to psychology and motivation.

7. People's expectation, motivation, and behavior are influenced, and generally limited, by reality and the possibility of attainment of goals. People may behave in a manner that demonstrates maturity and various expressions of self-actualization without any apparent motivation in the conventional sense.

The Hierarchy of Needs. Maslow's theory may be expressed simply as an integrated hierarchy of five basic needs, the satisfaction of which is preconditioned by cognitive impulses. In addition, he postulated a need to know and understand, and aesthetic needs. This hierarchy is depicted in Figure 10–1.

Physiologic needs form the first order of motivational drives. Satisfaction of the physiologic needs may dominate, but only with total deprivation. When this is the case, hunger is the most prepotent of all, followed by thirst, sexual drive, and other basic physiologic needs.

When the basic physiologic needs are met, higher needs emerge as motivators, and these, rather than physiologic needs, dominate the organism. When these in turn are satisfied, again new and still higher needs emerge, and so on upwardly through the hierarchy of needs. Thus, basic human needs are organized into a hierarchy of relative prepotency. An implication of this concept is that *gratification* becomes as important as deprivation in Maslow's theory. Thus, the prospect of a potential gratification of a met or unmet need may motivate an individual. When a person has learned the relationship between the source of gratification of a higher need and a given behavior pattern, then the prospect of sustaining that gratification may very well trigger a motivational force. In a society such as ours, most people are released from the domination of satisfying the relatively-more-basic physiologic needs, permitting thereby the emergence of other goals. A need that is satisfied is no longer a primary need in respect to motivational theory. The organism is dominated and its behavior energized primarily by unsatisfied needs.

Safety and security needs may be characterized by security, stability, independency and protection, freedom from fear, anxiety, and chaos, and the need for structure, order, law, and limits. Under certain conditions, people are dominated by this set of needs, and this phenomenon may be easily seen in the case of infants. One influence of culture on motivation is that adults are taught to inhibit reactions to the deprivation of safety, that is, to be brave and self-reliant. A broader aspect of seeking safety and security is the common preference for the familiar rather than the unfamiliar and the tendency to fear change and innovations. A highly mature person can cope with and accept change more readily than one less mature. This is an important principle to consider when contemplating innovations in an organization. Management should consider the readiness of the personnel to accept the innovation, and above all, should involve the employees in the decision to implement the innovation. Management should employ the principles of proper organizational change and development and MBO.

Third in the hierarchy is the *social (belonging* and *love) needs*. These encompass, in addition to belonging and love, the need to be accepted, to have friends, to have "roots" in a particular place, to belong to the "in-crowd" or class, and comradeship. All of these are fulfilled on a two-way basis: you must give to receive. Work groups, especially informal work groups, are a manifestation of this motivational need in a special way, although work groups fulfill other needs as well. Management should recognize and, at least, should accommodate, if not capitalize on, this phenomenon.

Esteem needs consist of two subsidiary sets, namely, *self-esteem* and *esteem of others*. The first includes the desire for strength for achievement, competency, confidence, independence, and freedom. The second set includes reputation, prestige, respect, recognition, status, attention, importance, dignity, and appreciation. These are powerful motivators, and the thwarting of these needs produces feelings of inferiority, of weakness, and of helplessness. These feelings, in turn, give rise to either basic discouragement or else to compensatory or neurotic tendencies. Whenever a person becomes overly concerned with these needs, he may become egotistical and eventually an egomaniac.

Most organizations in the United States meet the first three levels of Maslow's five tier hierarchy of needs. The challenge to management is to motivate employees to higher performance through the application of the upper two levels, especially the esteem-needs level. Not every job may fully accommodate the self-fulfillment need, but it should, at least, provide the means of fulfilling esteem needs. This fulfillment should, of course, be tied to performance. Providing unwarranted esteem and prestige is amoral and unfair, and it is an injustice not only to employees who have earned esteem and prestige, but also to the one on whom esteem has been bestowed unfairly. It deludes that employee into believing that he has actually attained a level of prestige when he has not. Eventually, such misapplication of this motivating factor will destroy the effectiveness of an organization.

Self-actualization is the pinnacle of the hierarchy of motivational needs; it is the desire for self-fulfillment. A person must do what he/she can best do in order to fulfill himself and be true to his/her real nature. The emergence of these needs and their fulfillment usually proceeds after satisfying the other more basic needs. However, a good administrator or manager must always strive to provide this means of motivation. Putting square pegs in round holes, as it were, is a weakness of our bureaucratic society, as described in *The Peter Principle*,[4] and makes it impossible for these persons to fulfill themselves. Management has a great responsibility to provide the means, if possible, for every employee to find self-fulfillment in his job. Herein lies the real payoff in productivity and efficiency. To do less is to cheat the manager, his organization, and most of all, his subordinates.

Maslow sees the *noble concepts,* which might better be called precepts, such as freedom to seek knowledge and to express oneself, freedom to do what one wishes to do as long as it does not bring dishonor to himself or God, or harm, injustice or disorder to others as preconditions for satisfying the basic needs. Thwarting these freedoms is a threat to a person and will produce emergency reactions. These freedoms are defended because, without them, the basic needs satisfaction is quite impossible, or at least, severely endangered. These conditions are not ends in themselves, but almost, since they are so closely related to the basic needs.

In addition to the prerequisite, functional role of the desire to know and understand, Maslow postulates a positive, inherent impulse to behave in this manner. He bases his case on observations of the behavior of lower animals that cannot be explained by normal animal instinct patterns, by historic facts, and by many clincial cases of psychopathology. He strongly suggests that one must guard against the tendency to separate the desires to know, to be curious, and to understand from the basic needs. The same caution is given for dichotomizing cognitive and conative needs. It seems practical to assign the need to know and understand as a simple extension of the need for self-actualization. The same is true of the aesthetics needs. To pursue these needs unselfishly is to fulfill oneself more completely. However, helping others fulfill their lives can be even more fulfilling.

Maslow's theory has much support from the research of Argyris,[5] McGregor,[6] Whyte,[7] and Porter.[8] Maslow's theory provides a deeper understanding of personality and motivation, and his model (Fig. 10–1) provides a conceptual framework for supervisors in personnel relations, especially for motivation.

Criticism of Maslow's Theory. The model adopted from Maslow's original five basic needs theory has been criticized by some as being too simplistic on the one hand and too complex on the other, especially the highest level of self-actualization. Some of the criticism arose before the publication of the second edition of his book.[3] For example, McFarland states the "first level needs are satisfied before going to the next level."[9] This is an oversimplification based on Maslow's first edition of *Motivation and Personality*,[10] rather than an appropriate interpretation of either edition.

Other skeptics of Maslow's theory include Sayles,[11] Herzberg,[12] and Vroom.[13] Sayles views the concepts of self-actualization permeated with too much value judgment, reflecting a moral judgment as to how people ought to behave, and not direclty connected with organizational life.

In a review of related research, Wahba and Birdwell found little support for Maslow's model as originally formulated.[14] The data did not confirm the existence of five distinct need categories; rather the data suggested there was a cluster of related lower-order needs and a different cluster of overlapping higher-order needs. Also, Alderfer's research[15] made a case for a three-tier model of needs: (1) *existence* needs; (2) *relatedness* (social) needs; and (3) *growth* (psychosocial) needs.

Lawler and Suttle's longitudinal study[16] provided additional data in support of modifying the hierarchial character of Maslow's model. Their data indicated that lower-order needs (physiologic and security) as a group must generally be met before higher-order needs will surface. However, once the lower order needs have been satisfied, any of the several higher-order needs may become functional as motivators. At this juncture, the higher-order need not operate in a sequential manner.

Need theory is difficult to test empirically and only a few researchers have attempted to do so. Research results support the following points: (1) There is evidence of a hierarchy of needs although it may not be as Maslow postulated. (2) Across all managerial levels, the least satisfied needs are most prepotent. (3) Security and social needs tend to be better satisfied in higher-level managerial positions. (4) Higher-order needs are usually activated and satisfied after lower-order needs are fulfilled.[2]

Miner rated Maslow's model low on scientific validity and usefulness although it received 16 nominations among 35 respondents.[1]

In Defense of Maslow's Theory. Consideration should be given to the purpose and character of Maslow's work. His purpose was to provide a theoretical framework by which behavioral scientists could better understand the nature of motivation and to provide a conceptual framework from which specific hypotheses may be deduced for further research. Much of his data came from clinic encounters with clients as well as the available empirical data, which was meager at that time. He did not concentrate on measurable constructs in the narrow sense. He did, however, provide us with a general theory of motivation, and his work provided a foundation on which others have built.

DIRECTING HUMAN BEHAVIOR

Once the motivating *force* has been activated, how can it be directed toward the intended behavior? The question might be better formulated as why is motivation directed toward a specific end? Three theories provide partial answers to these questions.

Behavior Modification. Behavior modification had its origin in the theory and research of B.F. Skinner.[17] He distinguished between two basic types of behavior, *respondent* and *operant*. *Respondent* behavior is an instinctive, unlearned behavior, such as coughing or the reflex jerk of the knee when tapped with the physician's rubber hammer. *Operant* behavior, on the other hand, is learned through experience, such as a handshake when introduced to a stranger.

In studying the distinction, Skinner introduced the concept of *operant conditioning,* which means that an individual is conditioned to behave in a certain manner because of previous experience. The key is to provide the type of experience that will set up the conditioning effect that fosters operant behavior. Another key concept is *reinforcement,* that is, some type of "pay-off" or reward for a particular operant behavior. The reinforcement may be either positive or negative.

Positive reinforcement occurs when praise is given for increased production. Because of the positive reinforcement (praise), the worker increases his productivity. *Negative reinforcement* occurs if a negative influence or factor is removed when a particular operant behavior occurs. An example might be the transfer of an unpopular supervisor to a less sensitive position to combat poor quality of work by employees. The operant behavior may be either negative (less absenteeism) or positive (increased production). There is yet another reinforcement, viz. *punishment.* Punishment may be the introduction of something that is disliked, or the removal of something that is liked, following a particular behavior. Thus these three types of reinforcement provide three strategies for modifying behavior. Positive reinforcement is by far the most effective and popular strategy, although behavior modification in people has not been widely studied in a scientific manner.

Operant Model. The operant model was derived from Skinner's operant conditioning theory.[17] The primary operational principle is the *contingency of reinforced response,* i.e., the motivational force depends on the reinforcement of the desired response. The model specifies the following sequential events: (1) A *stimulus* (from among many possible stimuli in a given situation) elicits a *response* from the subject. (2) If that *response* is the desired response, then it is *reinforced* by immediate *consequence(s).* (3) The *reinforcement,* if sufficiently powerful and repetitive, will set up an *operant behavior* which is the desired response or behavior. In simple straightforward terms, the model is: stimulus → response → reinforcement (immediate and relevant consequence of the response) → operant behavior. The reinforcement is contingent on the immediate relevant consequence of the response.

Another aspect of the model is the ability of a given stimulus to differentiate among the many potential responses. A stimulus that differentiates, i.e., elicits the desired response, is a "loud and clear" stimulus, and that sets the process in motion. It is the discriminating quality of stimuli and the selectivity of the reinforcement that places this model within the category of "directing motivation." It is apparent that this model and theory explains a certain type of learning process, the original purpose of the theory. It is less apparent how the theory explains directed motivation unless such motivation is a learned process. Another aspect of the model is that the reinforcing consequence must be immediate. This requires the supervisor to be close by to be able to reinforce the desired response of the worker. That may be one reason for the recent popularity of management-by-walking, i.e., frequently walking among the employees. The use of techniques based on this model should not suggest to the workers that they are "being manipulated," rather they should feel the consequences are used to honestly praise them.

Positive reinforcement via the operant model was successfully used at the B.F. Goodrich Company.[18] The operant model received 15 nominations, and it was rated highly for its usefulness but with equivocal validity by Miner.[1]

Expectancy Model. The expectancy model is one of the most popular motivational models having received 24 nominations and a tie for first place.[1] The theory was originally proposed by Tolman in 1932.[19] The underlying principle is ancient and has been expressed as a proverb: "Where there is no vision, the people perish."[20] Without a vision there is little expectation, or it becomes stale. This very basic principle is also the underlying principle of the goal setting theory, to be discussed in the next section.

In essence, the theory states that a person's behavior in a particular fashion is predicated on the *perceived likelihood* that the behavior will lead to a valued outcome or *reward*. Vroom[13] was the first to apply the expectancy model specifically to motivation in the work environment. He hypothesized that a person's choice between alternate courses of behavior depended on the relative strength of the various motivational forces. The relative strength, in turn, can be measured by the product of two variables: (1) degree of preference for a particular outcome, designated *valence;* and (2) the expectancy of the particular outcome expressed as a *subjective probability.* See Figure 10–2.

Vroom viewed motivation as a process of selecting from among alternate patterns of behavior the one that had the greatest potential of achieving a particular goal. Since subjective probability is ultimately controlled by the individual, management can alter this variable only indirectly.

Management can influence subjective probability by administering policies, rules and rewards consistently, evenhandedly and promptly. Pay as well as other rewards should match differential performance. Keeping pay schedules secret can lead to speculations about salaries and cause them to be perceived as being unfair. Workers will reason: "Salaries must be unfair, else why are they kept secret?"

Subjective probability may be differentially evaluated because of differences in self-esteem or self confidence. Management should try to improve the self-esteem of their employees as an indirect way of motivating them. Thus, management can improve the subjective probability component of the model (Pi) through fairness and a nurturing atmosphere, and it can improve the valence component of the model through a well constructed reward system.

Vroom's primary contribution via the expectancy model is the emphasis the theory places on the *individual's perception* of the value and probability of the outcome, not what management may believe the value or significance

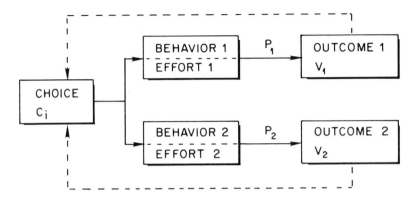

$$C_i \propto P_i V_i$$
$$E_1 : E_2 :: P_1 V_1 : P_2 V_2$$
C_i = choice
P_i = subjective probability
V_i = valence or value of outcome
E_i = effort
C_1 is preferred if $P_1 V_1 > P_2 V_2$
C_2 is preferred if $P_1 V_1 < P_2 V_2$

Figure 10-2.   Model of expectancy theory of motivation.

of an outcome to be. Miner gave the expectancy model a high validity rating but a questionable usefulness rating.[1]

Goal Setting Theory. Although the expectancy theory is the most popular explanation of how motivation is directed in the workplace, the goal setting theory has had more impact on organizational practices. Locke,[21] the author of the goal setting theory, criticized the expectancy theory on the grounds of being basically cognitive hedonism, which posits that an individual choose the course of action that produces the most pleasure or the smallest degree of pain. He also thought the expectancy model was insufficient to account for ones value system. He thought it more accurate to state that people strive to attain goals, values or purposes in life vis-a-vis pleasure. Thus, he substituted goals for expectancy in the model. The model takes the following form. Values → emotions or desires → goals (intentions) → performance (responses) → consequences as feedback → reinforcement.

The goal setting model has two cognitive determinants of behavior: *goals* or *intentions* and *values.* Within this theory, a value is something one acts to gain or retain, and is regarded as conducive to one's welfare. Thus, one's goal directs one's behavior toward achieving the goal which, in turn, has value for the individual. The task for management is to assist the worker to choose those goals that are mutually beneficial within the work environment.

It is apparent that this model fits the MBO style of management. That very likely is the reason it has had such an impact on organizational practices. MBO has been widely accepted; indeed MBO had been practiced for years before there was any research concerning its merits. The first research of this nature was not focused on MBO as such.

There are many goals that may be espoused at any given point in time. Some goals may conflict. Some goals have less perceived value compared to others. Therefore, not every goal will lead to efficacious behavior. The objective then is to select from among the various goals those that will provide the most value taking into account the feasibility of achieving the goals. That is where MBO, when practiced properly, comes into the picture within the workplace. Also, the goal must be internalized, i.e., the person must "buy into" the goal, otherwise it will be a futile exercise.

Research by Locke and associates found that the higher the goals or intended level of achievement among the subjects, the higher the level of performance.[22] Those who tried for goals so high that the goals were rarely, if ever, attained performed better than those individuals who set relatively easy goals. In this regards, it is similar to the Pygmalion effect. (The Pygmalion effect is the enhanced performance by subordinates whose supervisor, teacher or mentor expects more from them.) All the manager needs to do is to determine the goals and rewards the employees cherish and to incorporate these into the system via MBO.

There have been several studies that have established the external validity of goal setting as an important motivational tool. Miner rated the model high on both usefulness and scientific validity.[1]

A Comparison. All three models are *process* models. The operant model looks backwards to the conditioning phase during prior experiences; the other two models look forward, especially the expectancy model. The operant model places more emphasis on previous reinforcement and considerable emphasis on differential stimuli. The goal setting model places emphasis on goals and *values;* the expectancy model emphasizes *probability* and *valence.* It is the only probability model within the area under consideration. It is also one type of decision-making model. Both the expectancy and goal setting models extend the planning horizon, whereas the operant model has a short planning horizon. The goal setting model seems to be more readily applied in the work environment than either of the other two models.

SUSTAINING HUMAN BEHAVIOR

In order to have a well-functioning organization, management must be able to not only energize and direct the behavior of the members, it must be able to sustain those behaviors. There are four primary theories that address this stage of motivation–the operant or behavior modification model, the two factor model (also known as the motivation-hygiene theory), the equity theory, and the attribution theory.

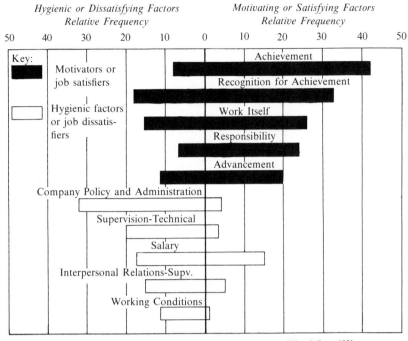

Adapted from Herzberg, F. et. al.: *The Motivation to Work.* New York: John Wiley & Sons, 1959.

Figure 10–3.   Comparison of motivating and hygienic factors.

Operant Model. This model explains this stage of motivation albeit in an attenuated form. The operant model specifies prompt, clear and repetitive reinforcement of the response or effort; otherwise the motivational force is often short-lived. However, by designing a schedule of reinforcements for a protracted period, it is assumed the motivation may be sustained. Research has shown that a variable, intermittent schedule of reinforcement produces more consistent and higher rates of responses which are more resistant to extinction. Thus, motivation may be sustained by an appropriate schedule of reinforcements.

Two-factor Model. Herzberg[12] classified all motivating variables in the work environment into general categories or factors, which he labeled *hygienic factor* or *dissatisfiers* and *motivating factor* or *satisfiers.* See Figure 10–3. The hygienic factor is composed of items that are *extrinsic* to the work but are a part of the job environment, i.e., within the *context* of the job. The motivating factor is composed of items that are *intrinsic* to the work, i.e., within the *content* of the job.

The two-factor model was further described in Herzberg's second book, *Work and the Nature of Man.*[23] His basic work,[12] which consisted of in-depth interviews of 200 engineers and accountants, produced the data from which he derived the motivation-hygiene model. The subjects were asked first about specific events on the job that produced job satisfaction and positive feelings, and then later about those events that produced job dissatisfaction or negative feelings. All events had to meet five objective criteria to be used. The responses were analyzed and coded, and from the coded data, five motivating factors (satisfiers) and five hygienic factors (dissatisfiers) emerged. The length of each bar in Figure 10–3 represents the relative frequency with which the factor was identified among the events as presented in the interviews. Herzberg included another dimension, which is not represented in Figure 10–3, namely the duration of the good or bad feeling represented by the motivators and hygienic factors, respectively. Short duration was defined as two weeks or less; long duration was defined in terms of months or even years. In general, the events that produce satisfaction among all ten factors were of longer duration than those that produce dissatisfaction. The exceptions apparently were recognition for achievement, salary, and perhaps working conditions. Overall, the dissatisfiers produced short-term change in job attitudes and the converse was true of the satisfiers. Note that some factors extend into the opposite category to a degree, especially salary, work itself and recognition of achievement.

Herzberg explained the functional basis of the dissatisfiers or hygienic factors surrounding the job as man's need to avoid pain and discomfort. He related this to the Adamic concept of humanity—the curse placed on man to work and to earn a livelihood. In contrast, the motivating factors inherent in work itself and the closely related factors represent a need to achieve and receive recognition for it. This is the Abrahamic concept of humanity in which man has hope for better things and feels the need to realize his full potential to that end.

Based on these two concepts, Herzberg's basic model consists of a two-dimensional need structure: (1) a need system to avoid unpleasantness, and (2) a parallel need system for personal, psychologic growth. While these concepts are not incompatible with Maslow's holistic-dynamic motivational theory, Maslow could hardly accept the dichotomization and compartmentalization of Herzberg's hygienic and motivating factors.

Criticism of Herzberg's Model. Herzberg's model has been criticized on the basis that it is technique-bound, that is, the results can be confirmed only if identical methods of research are used. Another criticism is that responses represent a defensive mechanism of the respondents. These criticisms have some validity, but the criticisms can be explained for the most part.[24] Herzberg's model does provide a practical tool for supervision and motivation primarily because the model is expressed in terms of the job situation.

Herzberg's theory of motivation has been subjected to a considerable number of tests. Allen found the theory applicable to employees of commercial banks.[25] Myers reported that Herzberg's theory held to varying degrees for several occupational groupings—engineers, female assembly line workers, hourly technicians, manufacturing supervisors and scientists—at the Texas Instrument Company.[26] The company researchers followed up on these findings and as a result, restructured its personnel administration plan to fit the motivation-maintenance theory. Again the Herzberg findings were replicated in public utility firms,[27] a large multi-unit corporation,[28] the Armed Forces,[29] and a large manufacturer.[30]

Vroom has surveyed and analyzed in depth the significant research on motivation.[13] He is critical of Herzberg and related studies on three points. He states the research methods were neither correlational nor experimental in design. He claims the researchers' interpretation of the data was not the only possible one. Finally, he doubts the ability of the subjects to report accurately the conditions causing satisfaction or dissatisfaction, and says that such responses could be the result of a defensive mechanism. House and Wigdor reviewed 31 studies, some of which did not use Herzberg's methodology, and found a general lack of confirmation for the dual-factor theory.[31] They found that lack of achievement and recognition were more frequently associated with job dissatisfaction than were working conditions and relations with supervisors. However, the theory is accepted by a number of practitioners and researchers, and certainly his terminology is well ingrained in modern management literature. Herzberg's dual-factor received 14 nominations but was rated low on both usefulness and validity by Miner.[1]

Equity Theory. Equity theory explains how people interpret social rewards and how this interpretation impacts the maintenance of a given level of work effort.[2] The equity model resembles the input-output economic model in that input and outcome are the primary variables. According to Adams, who is the originator of the theory, people seek social justice in the way they are rewarded for their job performance.[32] First, people take into account the total set of personal outcomes from the job, both intrinsic and extrinsic to the job—pay, benefits, status, pleasant working conditions, recognition of one's performance and the interest and challenge of the job itself. Second, people consider all the inputs they provide to the job—time, effort, experience, skills, sacrifices, stress we experience, loyalty and commitment. We expect the inputs and outcomes to be "balanced" or appropriate to each other. Third, the model specifies that we mentally construct a ratio of outcomes to inputs and then compare this ratio with other relevant ratios. These may be based on similar co-workers, similar workers in another organization, or some other relevant standard.

If our outcome to input ratio exceeds the ratio used for comparison, we may feel we are overpaid or unjustly rewarded. We then may increase our inputs. If the reverse is true, we may feel that we are underpaid and not justly rewarded. We then very likely will take measures to rectify the inequality we feel by reducing our input, seeking a greater outcome from the job, or begin looking for another job. Another possibility is that we may re-evaluate the respective outcome-input ratios to determine whether we may have erred.

Research indicates that most people will tolerate a certian degree of inequity and not attempt to make adjustments. Also, evidence indicates that people generally will increase their efforts when this is necessary to correct the situation. Beyond this (and the above findings are not conclusive), there are little data to indicate just what the behavior will be. The practical implications of this theory is that to the extent people view their remunerations in this light (and certainly many do), the performance evaluation criteria should be made explicit, the type of inputs that are highly valued should be communicated, and secrets should be avoided. This theory received 14 nominations and was rated high on scientific validity but low on usefulness by Miner.[1]

Attribution Theories. There are several theories of this general type, but none of these has proved to be of much practical significance for explaining organizational behavior. In general, the theories attempt to explain why people tend to *attribute* their behavior to external forces (e.g., extrinsic reward) or to their own motivation (intrinsic reward). Kelly termed this approach the *discounting principle* based on the tendency that "the role of a given cause in producing a given effect is discounted if other plausible causes are also present."[33] Although there is considerable research evidence that this principle holds within individual task situations, application to management seems remote. For example, if management wants an external reward, e.g., pay raise, to not be discounted, then management should make it a salient feature of the work environment.

Another variation of this group of theories is the *cognitive evaluation* theory. This theory is based on an *evaluation of causality,* whether a person perceives himself as the *locus* of causality for his behavior or an external influence. These theories seem to posit intrinsic and extrinsic motivation as counter currents, and this is bothersome to organizational psychologists. There does not seem to be any reason to worry about this possibility since the jury is still out. Miner did not include these theories in his analysis.

MOTIVATIONAL PROGRAMS

Organizational leaders and executives have applied the various theories discussed in this chapter to this point in various ways. One of the most significant programs is organizational development (OD) discussed in Chapter 9. OD is sometimes labeled organizational behavior modification (OBM). OD is predicated primarily on Skinner's operant behavior theory.[17] Yet OD does not concern itself with personality nor motivation directly. It concentrates on changing the overall organization, including employees behavior of course, by modifying contingencies and schedules of reinforcement. Enchanced productivity and satisfaction are the goals. Other programs are discussed below.

Job Enrichment/Redesign. This method of improving work performance has been used fairly extensively and it has been reported as fairly successful. The basic premise of this method is that job motivation is sustained largely by the job itself, via the intrinsic rewards generated by the task effort. It should be apparent that this approach is rooted in the theories of Maslow, Herzberg, Argyris and McGregor. It was Herzberg's work, however, that gave the most impetus toward developing this methodology. But all of these approaches, which were spawned by the perceived sameness of work as a result of the classical "scientific" management, made a contribution. Herzberg contended that job *enlargement* was insufficient, but job *enrichment* such that the worker could get a sense of achievement was needed. Argyris pointed to the natural growth and development of people through the various life stages as a philosophical and theoretical basis for job enrichment.

Research by Turner and Lawrence[34] identified some of the job characteristics that were involved in job enrichment. This research was followed by Hackman and Lawler,[35] and later by Hackman and Oldham.[36] Together they discovered five job attributes or core dimensions of a job that should be considered in the enrichment process: (1) variety, (2) task identity, (3) task significance, (4) autonomy, and (5) feedback. The idea is to examine the job in terms of these job core dimensions and to determine which dimensions, if any, can be modified to enrich the job, and also whether the employee is ready for this type of change. For this determination, there are three relevant questions: (1) Can the employee accept more responsibility? (2) Can the employee work with greater autonomy? (3) Is management able and willing to change the job so that more responsibility and autonomy are given to the employee?

Results from the experimentation with job enrichment have been mixed. Generally, the programs have been successful, at least initially. One problem is how to continue to motivate employees, because there is a limit to the desired degree of delegated responsibility, and especially autonomy. This limit was disclosed in the Non-Linear Systems case.[37] After a period of several years, the work teams were unable to make quick decisions, and quality and productivity declined. There is a need for a certain amount of structure, authority, and discipline for groups to function maximally. The objective is to supply sufficient structure and discipline without its becoming burdensome. On balance, the results have been mixed in terms of productivity. There has been more consistent improvement in terms of the quality of finished products. In a majority of instances, there has been improvement in absenteeism and tardiness.

Although job enrichment as a management technique was not an object of Miner's analysis,[1] one of the underlying theories, Hackman's job characteristics theory, was rated high on both scientific validity and usefulness. The theory received 15 nominations.

Management by Objectives. MBO has been discussed rather extensively in Chapter 4, and is mentioned or discussed to some degree in more chapters than any other single managerial concept. Whereas job enrichment is designed primarily for the lower echelon, operative employees, MBO is designed primarily for managers and professionals. MBO involves the whole of the organization, but it focuses on supervisors and employees. MBO, properly conceived and implemented, provides an ideal work environment for both OD and job enrichment, as well as other motivational techniques.

MBO does have limitations.[2] (1) MBO is designed primarily for managers and professionals, although there is nothing logical or theoretical that would hinder its application to any group. (2) Some have criticized the amount of paperwork involved. (3) Some complain that MBO places too much emphasis on tasks or outcomes that are easily measured and thus slighting important aspects of supervision. (4) Others think MBO induces subordinates to feel they are forced to perform at extremely high level and that MBO is used as a "club." This reaction may well be the result of improper application of MBO. (5) MBO does not normally provide for a measure of intrinsically subjective or quality dimensions, although this could be developed.

SUMMARY OF MOTIVATION

1. Motivation is a hypothetical construct of a psychologic process that takes place in three stages: *arousal* by a stimulus within the environment, *directional* by a discriminating stimulus and by selective reinforcement or feedback, and *maintenance* by a selective reinforcement schedule and selective rewards (those that have long duration of effect, intrinsic).

2. The arousal stage may be termed energizing behavior and is best explained by one or more need theories. The operant conditioning theory may have a place within this stage because the theory includes an initiating stimulus. This stage is critical because without this stage the other stages are inoperative.

3. The directional stages may be explained in varying degrees by one or more of the following: behavior modification (operant conditioning), expectancy model and goal setting theory.

4. The maintenance stage may be explained by one or more of the following: operant model, hygiene—motivational (two-factor) model, equity theory and attribution theory.

5. Motivational programs and techniques may be designed based on one or more of the various theories and/or models of motivation, but generally these have been one of the following: job enrichment/redesign, management-by-objectives, or as a part of an organizational development program.

Leadership Development

Leadership is thought to be one of the most important aspects of organizational behavior and organization theory. Just what is leadership? Many definitions have been advanced, but one of the simplest yet most complete is Stogdill's: "Leadership is the process of influencing the activities of an organized group in efforts toward goal setting and goal achievement."[38] The key word is "influencing," and this word is included or implied in every definition reviewed. The setting and attainment of goals appear in most definitions, and an organized group is usually included or implied in the definition.

BASES OF INFLUENCE

The real issue or question is, how does a leader influence others? French and Raven have provided one of the best explanations, among several, in terms of power.[39] They have proposed five different bases of power:

1. *Coercive power.* This power is based on fear. A subordinate perceives that failure to comply with the wishes of the superior will lead to some type of punishment.
2. *Reward power.* This is the opposite of coercive power, in that compliance will lead to a reward of some type.
3. *Legitimate or position power.* This type of power comes from the position of the superior in the organization.
4. *Expert power.* This type of power is accrued to an individual because of his expertise, special skills, or knowledge.
5. *Referent power.* This power is based on the subordinate's identification with the leader because the leader is admired for one or more personal traits—physical attributes, intelligence, or personality, for example.

The first three of these bases of power are anchored in some type of formal relationship, usually an organization. The last two bases may or may not have their roots in a formal relationship or organization. Thus the organization controls the first three bases of power, whereas persons control the last two power bases. Of course, a combination of several of these bases provides a greater level of power, thus influence and leadership.

There are three basic views of leadership: psychologic, sociologic, and mutual sharing of responsibility and influence. The *psychologic view* is primarily a motivational view, and the Maslow hierarchy of need theory provides an effective model for this view. Leaders should include expertise and referent power bases when developing motivational programs. The *sociologic view* holds that leadership is a facilitating function through which the leader establishes group goals and reconciles organizational conflicts—between group members or between group members and management hierarchy, for example—and removes organizational barriers of all types, thus facilitating the achievement of goals. Social status, hierarchal stratification, communication network, and roles are elements of the sociologic view. The *mutual sharing view* recognizes the purpose and place of legitimate power, but sees advantages in sharing influence and responsibilities with subordinates. Management-by-objective and participatory management systems are based on this view of leadership. Another view of leadership classifies it as a type of social role. In this respect, it would take on even greater status than simply a supervisor.

THEORIES OF LEADERSHIP

There are many theories of leadership and leadership development. These may be grouped into the following classes: trait theories, personal behavioral theories, and contingency or situational theories.

Leadership Paradigm. Before discussing leadership theories, it is useful to look at a paradigm for leadership theories.[2] The *dependent variable, i.e.,* the effects or results which are considered measures of leadership, most frequently is subordinates' productivity or satisfaction or a combination of these. Such behavior as tardiness, absence or personnel turnover is sometimes used, but these generally are considered overt evidence of employee dissatisfaction. Many factors other than leadership affect these measures, especially productivity. The *independent variable, i.e.,* the cause or antecedent of the somewhat nebulous concept, leadership, usually is thought to be either an *attribute* (skills, personality traits, or physical traits, etc.) or a *dimension of behavior.* Some theories postulate *intervening variables* that link the independent leader variable to the dependent (effect) leader variable. These intervening variables may be motivational, attitudinal, expectative, exemplary or other possible variables.

Trait Theories. These theories state that leadership can be developed by improving personal traits such as physical attributes, personality traits, intelligence and motivational traits. In addition to intelligence, personality traits include self-assurance, assertiveness, decisiveness, initiative, maturity, extrovert-introvert, masculinity-femininity, to name some that are commonly recognized. The motivational traits are reflective of the Maslow hierarchy of needs and other theories discussed already in this chapter. Some of the advocates and researchers in this area include Stogdill,[40] Ghiselli,[41] and Fiedler.[42] There are several weaknesses as well as utility in the trait theory. Stogdill[40] reviewed 124 empirical studies of leadership for the period 1904–1946. He found 27 attributes that had been studied by three or more researchers. The criterion (dependent) variable was status of leadership, i.e., the 27 attributes consistently distinguished between the leader and the group. Stogdill found that these attributes could be categorized into three broad dimensions: (1) physical attributes, primarily height; (2) intelligence, a large number of more specific traits, e.g., originality; and (3) a broad category that might be labeled "energy" or "activity."

He found that emotional stability and extraversion to be unreliable predictors of leadership status. The *most important finding* was that 19 studies found the profile of leadership traits varied with the situation, especially group composition and group tasks. This discovery caused the emphasis in leadership research to shift from leadership traits to leadership behavior, and still later to the contingency (situational) model. Miner[1] did not include any of the trait theories in his analysis. For a more comprehensive treatment of the trait theory of leadership, the student should consult Stogdill[40] and Ghiselli.[41]

Personal Behavior Theories. Since 1950, research on leadership and the practice of leadership development have shifted to leadership behavior (P-B). P-B theories focus on what the leader does in carrying out the managerial function. Most, if not all, of these theories mesh well with the MBO approach to management. Indeed this approach was ushered in by Stogdill's discovery and Drucker's book, *The Practice of Management,* which established MBO.

As we shall see, several of the theories under this rubric are similar to the leadership model depicted in Figure 4–1.

The *continuum of leadership behavior* was postulated by Tannenbaum and Schmidt, based on opinions and observations derived from the literature.[43] This theory can be described best by a model as shown in Figure 10–4. Compare this with Figure 4–1. Although the continuum of leadership behavior provided a good conceptual framework for viewing and classifying leadership style, the underlying "leadership pattern choice" theory was rated low on scientific validity and usefulness. It received only two nominations!

Likert and co-workers advanced the *job-centered: employee-centered theory* of leadership, based on extensive research at the University of Michigan beginning in 1947.[44] The job-centered supervisor structures the jobs of subordinates, closely supervises them, makes use of time studies, and uses incentives to spur productivity. In other words, he uses theory X. The employee-centered supervisor focuses attention on the needs and problems of his subordinates while keeping performance goals in view. This is, of course, theory Y in action. These researchers found employee-centered supervisors generally to be more effective, as measured by a series of job-related indices: productivity and less absenteeism, for example. Although Miner[1] did not analyze Likert's job-centered:employee-centered theory, he did rate Likert's expanded theory of systems 4 and 4T (an organizational development theory, see Chapter 9) high on usefulness and low on validity. The theory received 14 nominations.

During the same period, researchers at Ohio State University (Stogdill, Fleishman, et al.) were engaged in both in-depth and extensive research of what constitutes effective leadership.[45] Based on this research, a *two-dimensions theory* of leadership was formulated. Two dimensions, "consideration" and "initiating structures," were isolated. These two dimensions roughly parallel the employee-centered and job-centered qualities of the Michigan studies. The researchers assessed how supervisors think they should behave, and subordinates' perception of supervisors' actual behavior was ascertained. These measures provided a "high" and "low" score for each of the two dimensions for each supervisor. In addition, the supervisors were rated for their proficiency by plant managers. Also, objective measures such as unexcused absenteeism, accidents, formally filed grievances, and employee turnover were used to evaluate the work of the supervisors.

High "consideration" scores and low "initiating structure" scores and vice versa were the independent measures, while the proficiency ratings and objective measure of employee satisfaction were dependent measures. In production departments, there was a positive correlation between proficiency ratings and high initiating structure scores, and a negative correlation with high consideration scores. Conversely, in nonproduction departments, the reverse was found. Thus, this two-dimension theory has elements of the personal-behavior model and elements related to the situational model to be discussed later. Miner did not include the two-dimensions leadership theory in his analysis.[1]

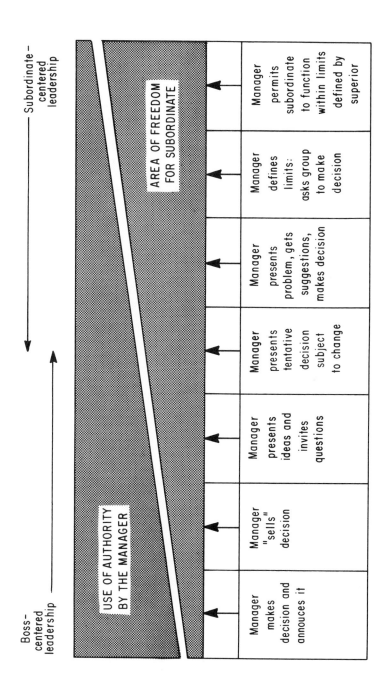

Figure 10–4. Continuum of leadership behavior. (From Tannenbaum, R., and Schmidt, W.H.: How to choose a leadership pattern. *Harvard Bus. Rev., 51:*164, 1973.)

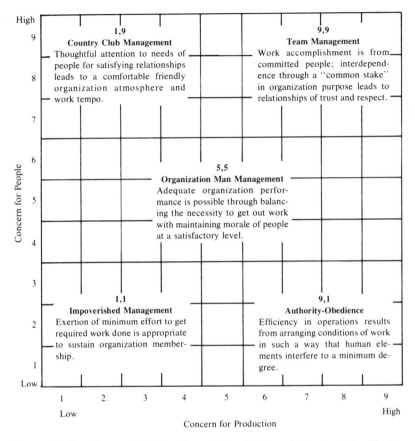

Figure 10–5. Managerial Grid. (From Blake, R.R., and Mouton, J.S.: *The Managerial Grid.* Houston: Gulf Publishing Company, 1974.)

The P-B approach to leadership has culminated in the Managerial Grid theory developed by Robert Blake and Jane Mouton.[46] The Managerial Grid is made up of a two-dimensional plot—concern for people and concern for production, as shown in Figure 10–5. These two dimensions are similar to those of the "two-dimensions" theory and the "job-centered: employee-centered" theory. The unique feature of the Managerial Grid theory is that the various combinations of the several levels of the two planar dimensions lead to five basic leadership styles.

1. *Apathetic*—a minimum of effort or concern for the job, with regard to both people and production—position 1,1.
2. *Low-pressure; easygoing*—focus on the concerns of persons with low level of effort on production—position 1,9.
3. *Task-oriented*—foucs on the production function with little regard for concerns of people—position 9,1.
4. *Balance approach*—even-handed, or balance of adequate emphasis and

effort for production and people, but less than full potential in either direction—position 5,5.

5. *Full production, team effort*—high level of motivation and productivity with genuine concern for both people and production—position 9,9.

Blake and Mouton emphasized the potential of leadership development through a six-phase program.[47] This program is much in tune with the MBO approach to management. All P-B theories of leadership have several characteristics in common and may be integrated in a general theory of two dimensions: (1) the concerns of people and (2) job structure, with a dipolar continuum describing each dimension. Thus the four general P-B leadership styles are (1) low structure, low concerns; (2) low structure, high concerns; (3) high structure, low concerns; (4) high structure and high concerns. Miner did not evaluate the grid version of the two-dimensions leadership theory.[1]

The literature on P-B leadership with special emphasis on "consideration" (people concern) and "initiating structure" (close supervision, directing and structuring work) was reviewed by Korman[48] and Fleishman.[49] In general, leadership consideration (concern) appears to be a consistent and reliable predictor of employee satisfaction-dissatisfaction and various indices of this, but there is little evidence that initiating structure influences satisfaction, measured objectively by employee turnover, grievances filed, etc., *until* the initiating structure reaches very high degrees. However, the relationship between either dimension and productivity is nebulous. Leadership influence on subordinates' performance is either (1) negligible or (2) dependent on the situation— a view to be discussed later. Because there are so many variables (technology, resources, production efficiency, relative production capacity, group composition, group's effect on the leader, etc.) that influence productivity it is very difficult to measure the influence of the leader on productivity.

Contingency Theories. The situational or contingency theories add a new dimension, the situation or set of conditions that surrounds the leader and the subordinates. Fiedler has conducted considerable research from which he developed one contingency theory.[50,51] The model used three dimensions— (1) leadership-group relations, (2) task structure, and (3) position power— from which eight combinations of situations, based on high-low scores, were derived.

This research has been criticized by several persons.[52] The conceptual model as outlined above is sound. The primary issue is the measure of the independent variable—the "Esteem of the Least Preferred Co-worker" (LPC)—which Fiedler stated measured the leader's view of subordinates as a person vis-a-vis a worker. A high score on the instrument indicated a nondirective, concerned relationship-oriented manner toward group members. A low score indicated a task-oriented, controlling manner. In addition to the issue of the validity of the instrument, there was the obvious confounding of the scores on the instrument and the measure of one situational variable, leader-group relations. Fiedler's theory was rated equivocal on scientific validity and questionable on usefulness. It received 20 nominations.[1]

Another version of the contingency model was developed by Vroom and Yetton,[53] which is a decision tree theory or model. In addition to the situational approach to participative leadership, the theory is actually a *normative* (standard to be followed) *decision tree model*. The authors specified five levels of group participation in management decisions, ranging from one extreme of the supervisor making the decision based on the information at hand, through various levels of participation, to the other extreme of involving the total group throughout the decision process. Thus a continuum of participation similar to Tannenbaum and Schmidt[43] was employed. Based on the nature of the problem to be solved in terms of desirability and feasibility of group input, the authors generated 14 types of problems-decisions. The decision tree embodied sequential questions, as branches, to ask in identifying the type of problem, which in turn, specifies the level of group participation that is most desirable. This theory was rated high for scientific validity and questionable on usefulness with 10 nominations.[1] However, Organ and Hamner[2] (p. 415) concluded there was limited evidence of its validity.

In summary, situational or contingency theory includes an important variable, the organizational or job situation, yet the results of research, which included this variable, do not provide easily recognizable and applicable principles beyond those revealed by older theories.

Path-Goal Theory. House's path-goal theory combines some aspects of the P-B theory, expectancy theory and contingency theory.[54] Emphasis is placed on the behavior of the leader/supervisor, but equal emphasis is placed on the nature of the task (situation) to be performed. He posits the behavior of the leader, whether he should initiate structure for the task or manifest consideration (concern) for subordinates, depends on the nature of the task. If the task is highly structured already, and probably dull, the supervisor should manifest consideration. If, on the other hand, the task is unstructured and varied, the leader should initiate structure in the job.

To provide a formal guideline for this approach, House constructed a five-component model: (1) intrinsic rewards from *work itself* (doing the job); (2) intrinsic reward from *accomplishing* (finishing) *the job;* (3) extrinsic rewards based on *achievement* of the *task(s);* (4) the *clarity of the path* or plan to achieve the task or goal, and (5) the *subjective probability* of achieving the goal. In practice, components 2 and 3 are emphasized if component one is absent. If the task is unstructured and/or is ambiguous, component 4 becomes very important. Component 4 is the key for increasing component 5. Components 2 and 3 should have salience, without being used as a club, to move toward productivity. Basically, the leader attempts to help subordinates to find the best path, to set challenging goals, and to remove stressful barriers along the way. These efforts have produced readily applicable principles or concepts.

Several researchers have investigated this theory with mixed results.[54,55] Miner rated this theory low for usefulness and equivocal on validity, but it received 15 nominations.[1]

HOW SIGNIFICANT IS THE LEADERSHIP ROLE?

Research of the role, posture and effectiveness of leadership has provided mixed results at best. That is not to say leadership is not important or unnecessary. However, Pfeffer has challenged the accepted premise that leadership is causally related to organizational performance.[56] He based his conclusion on the following: (1) organizations tend to limit the range of attributes and styles in the leadership role. For example, the statement by Wright of General Motors that GM didn't want a flashy individualistic type of executive was cited in support of this point. (2) The leader is further restricted by his perception of the expectation of others in the organization. (3) The success of the organization is determined largely by external forces, which Pfeffer thought was the most important consideration. Pfeffer's point is not that leadership makes no difference, but that we have exaggerated that difference. Also, the effects of leadership are difficult to measure. Most students of the subject would not go as far as Pfeffer suggests.

Another aspect of the overall relationship between the leader and the group is one of reciprocal causality (relationship). Lowin and Craig proposed such a hypothesis and their findings supported it to a degree.[57] The research was experimental in design utilizing a role player, Charlie, and applicants for a temporary supervisory position. When Charlie performed well, the supervisors displayed more consideration and initiated less structure. Conversely, when Charlie performed poorly, the reverse behavior tended to be demonstrated. When consideration was displayed, more group participation was encouraged.

Greene[58] utilized time lag correlation approach to the reciprocal relationship issue. He found that consideration directly affected subordinates' job satisfaction. His findings also suggested that causal relations between supervisor and subordinates run in the opposite direction, i.e., the supervisor initiated job structure *following* poor performance. When subordinates performed well, the supervisor decreased emphasis on structure and increased emphasis on consideration.

In a similar vein, Kerr and Jermier[59] have argued that certain attributes of the *group,* the *task* and the *organization* can function as a substitute for much of the leadership role in many circumstances.

Perhaps the focus of leadership-subordinate relationship should be a one-on-one approach. Dansereau, Graen and Haga[60] have proposed a vertical dyad linkage (VDL) model based on this perspective. Their data indicate that leaders practice two types of roles with two general types of employees. One type of employee does just what he has to do; the other type will do more and are critical to the overall group performance. The leader will practice *contractual exchange*[2] with the former group, i.e., he will provide the necessary support to fulfill his minimum role as their supervisor for their minimum contribution. The leader will find ways to provide more support, especially consideration and less structure, for members of the latter group on a one-to-one basis. This arrangement may be labeled *noncontractual relationship*.[2] There are several similarities between this approach and House's path-goal model. Miner[1] rated the VDL model high on validity but low on usefulness. The model received four nominations.

The various leadership theories and models, with their similar and overlapping dimensions, may be confusing to the beginning student. To overcome some of this confusion, an *integrated model of leadership* has been constructed in Figure 10–6. An examination of Figure 10–6 shows the interrelationship among the several components, the basic elements of each component, and the interactions between the major components. As the model suggests, the particular leadership mode is determined by the interaction of the several components. Concern for people and the participation of workers are parallel dimensions, whereas job structure and concern for production are parallel dimensions. Group satisfaction is related to the former; productivity may or may not be related to the latter. Parallel dimensions will normally be considered in a similar manner by a supervisor. However, the adoption of a high level of concern for people suggests a low level of concern for production, but this may not necessarily be true. A particular leader may select different levels of the several components in different situations.

SUMMARY OF THE LEADERSHIP ROLE

The four studies, cited immediately above, seem to confirm what could be deduced from a number of other studies discussed in this chapter. Therefore, the following points may be abstracted from research on leadership.
   1. Students of and experts in this field have all but abandoned the attribute (trait) approach to identify leadership status or skills.
   2. The behavior approach is still valid using the two major dimensions of consideration and initiation of job structure.
   3. Empirical research has demonstrated consistently the causal relationships between supervisor's consideration and subordinate's job satisfaction measured by employee turnover rate and number of grievances processed.
   4. There is mixed evidence of a relationship between supervisor's initiation of structure and subordinate's job satisfaction, except that it tends to be negative.
   5. The evidence of a causal relationship between initiation of job structure and either group performance or subordinates' satisfaction is equivocal. However, as Greene[58] indicated, there may be a reverse causal relationship between group performance and supervisor's behavior.
   6. The contingency model provided another important variable, the situation or environment, to explain much of the variance which had not been explained with other models. Unfortunately, Fiedler's LPC measurement has come under serious criticism.[2] A different, more valid measure of the supervisor's role, behavior and attitude toward subordinates is needed.

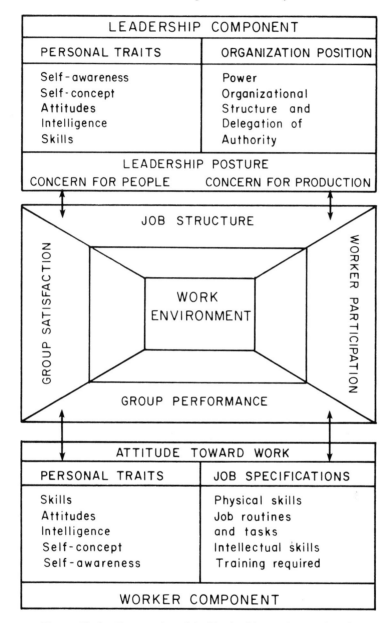

Figure 10–6.   Integrated model of leadership, workers and work.

7. House's path-goal theory[54] provides us with the most comprehensive model of leadership behavior, incorporating three types of rewards (incentives) with goal in view in two of these, the leader as a facilitator or pathfinder, and subjective probability. There appears to be less emphasis on the leader per se. If the evidence provided by Greene, Lowin and Craig is true, then this model becomes even more valid, especially if "path" includes the total environment of leader-subordinate interaction.

REFERENCES

1. Miner, J.B.: The validity and usefulness of theories in an emerging organizational science. *Acad. Mangt. Rev., 9:*296–306, 1984.
2. Organ, D.W. and Hamner, W.C.: *Organizational Behavior an Applied Psychological Approach.* Plano, TX: Business Publications, Inc., 1982, pp. 158–215.
3. Maslow, A.: *Motivation and Personality,* 2nd ed. New York: Harper and Brothers, 1970.
4. Peter, L.J.: *The Peter Principle.* New York: William Morrow & Co., 1969.
5. Argyris, C.: *Understanding Organizational Behavior.* Homewood, Ill.: The Dorsey Press, 1960.
6. McGregor, D.: *The Human Side of Enterprise.* New York: McGraw-Hill Book Co., 1960.
7. Whyte, W.H.: *The Organization Man.* New York: Simon and Schuster, 1956.
8. Porter, L.W.: *Organizational Patterns of Managerial Job Attitudes.* New York: American Foundation for Management Research, 1964.
9. McFarland, D.E.: *Personnel Management: Theory and Practice.* New York: The Macmillan Co., 1968, p. 382.
10. Maslow, A.: *op cit.,* 1st ed., 1954.
11. Sayles, L.R.: *Individualism and Big Business.* New York: McGraw-Hill Book Co., 1963.
12. Herzberg, F., et al.: *The Motivation to Work.* New York: John Wiley & Sons, Inc., 1959.
13. Vroom, V.: *Work and Motivation.* New York: John Wiley & Sons, Inc., 1964.
14. Wahba, M.A. and Birdwell, L.G.: Maslow Reconsidered: A Review of Research on the Need Hierarchy Theory. Proceedings of the 1973 Academy of Management Meeting, Boston, via Organ and Hamner, *op cit.,* p. 161.
15. Alderfer, C.P.: An empirical test of a new theory of human needs. *Organ. Behav. Human Performance., 4:*142–75, 1969.
16. Lawler (III), E.E. and Suttle, J.L.: A casual-correlational test of the need hierarchy concept. *Organ. Behav. Human Performance. 7:*265–87, 1972.
17. Skinner, B.F.: *Science and Human Behavior.* New York: Macmillan, 1953; *Contingencies of Reinforcement.* New York: Appleton-Century-Crofts, 1969, and *Beyond Freedom and Dignity.* New York: Alfred A. Knopf, 1972.
18. Fry, F.L.: Operant conditioning in organizational settings: of mice and men. *Personnel, 51:*17–24, 1974.
19. Tolman, E.C.: *Purposive Behavior in Animals and Men.* New York: Century, 1932.
20. Proverbs 29:8, *Holy Bible,* A.V., 1611.
21. Locke, E.A.: Personnel attitudes and motivation. Working paper, University of Maryland, 1976, via Organ and Hamner, p. 167.
22. Locke, E.A.: Toward a theory of task motivation and incentives. *Organ. Behav. Human Performance, 3:*157–89, 1968.
23. Herzberg, F.: *Work and the Nature of Man.* Cleveland: The World Publishing Co., 1966.
24. *Ibid.,* pp. 130, 131.
25. Allen, G.R.: Testing Herzberg's Motivation-Maintenance Theory in Commercial Banks. Unpublished doctoral dissertation, Arizona State University, 1967.
26. Myers, M.S.: Who are your motivated workers? *Harvard Bus. Review., 42:*73–87, 1966.
27. Schwartz, M.M., et al.: Motivational factors among supervisors in the utility industry. *Personnel Psychol., 16:*45–53, 1963.
28. Schwartz, P.: *Attitudes of Middle Management Personnel.* Pittsburgh: American Institute for Research, 1959.

29. Hahn, D.: Dimensions of job satisfaction and career motivation. In Schwarts, *ibid.*
30. Gibson, J.W.: Sources of Job Satisfaction and Job Dissatisfaction as Interpreted from Analyses of Write-In Responses. Doctoral Dissertation, Western Reserve University, 1961.
31. House, R.J. and Wigdor, L.A.: Herzberg's dual-factor theory of job satisfaction and motivation: A review of the evidence and a criticism. *Personnel Psychol., 20*:369–89, 1967.
32. Adams, J.S.: Toward an understanding of equity. *J. Abn. Soc. Psych., 67*:422–36, 1963, and wages inequities in a clerical task. Unpublished study for General Electric Co., New York, 1961.
33. Kelly, H.H.: *Attribution in Social Interaction.* New York: General Learning Press, 1971.
34. Turner, A.M. and Lawrence, P.R.: *Industrial Jobs and the Worker.* Cambridge: Harvard Graduate School of Business Administration, 1965.
35. Hackman, J.R. and Lawler, (III), E.E.: Employee reaction to job characteristics. *J. Applied Psych., 55*:259–86, 1971.
36. Hackman, J.R. and Oldham, G.R.: Development of the job diagnostic survey. *J. Applied Psych., 60*:159–70, 1975, and *Work Redesign.* Reading, MA: Addison-Wesley, 1980.
37. Malone, E.L.: The non-linear systems experiment in participative management. *J. Bus., 48*:52–64, 1975.
38. Stogdill, R.M.: Leadership: memberships and organization. *Psychol. Bull., 47*:1–14, 1950.
39. French, J.R.P., and Raven, B.: The bases of social power. In D. Cartwright and H.P. Zander, eds.: *Group Dynamics,* 2nd ed. Evanston, Ill.: Row, Peterson and Co., 1960, pp. 607–623.
40. Stogdill, R.: Personal factors associated with leadership: A survey of the literature, *J. Psychol., 25*:35–71, 1948.
41. Ghiselli, E.E.: *Exploration in Management Talent.* Pacific Palisades, Cal.: Goodyear, 1971.
42. Fiedler, F.: The leader's psychological distance and group effectiveness. In D. Cartwright and A.F. Zander, ed.: *Group Dynamics,* 2nd ed. Evanston, Ill.: Row, Peterson and Co., 1960, pp.. 586–605.
43. Tannenbaum, R., and Schmidt, W.H.: How to choose a leadership pattern. *Harvard Bus. Rev., 51*:162–180, 1973.
44. Likert, R.: *New Patterns of Management.* New York: McGraw-Hill Book Co., Inc., 1961.
45. Fleishman, E.H., and Peters, D.A.: Interpersonal values, leadership attitudes and managerial success. *Personnel Psychol., 15*:127–143, 1962.
46. Blake, R.R., and Mouton, J.S.: *The Managerial Grid.* Houston, Texas: Gulf Publishing Co., 1964.
47. Blake, R.R., and Mouton, J.S.: Utilizing the managerial grid to ensure MBO. *Organizational Dynamics, 2*:54–65, 1974.
48. Korman, A.K.: ''Consideration,'' ''initiating structure,'' and organizational criteria—a review. *Personnel Psychol., 19*:349–361, 1966.
49. Fleishman, E.A.: Twenty years of consideration and structure. In Fleishman, E.A., and Hunt, J.C. (eds.). *Current Developments in the Study of Leadership.* Carbondale, Ill: So. Ill. Univ. Press, 1973.
50. Fiedler, F.E.: *A Theory of Leadership Effectiveness.* New York: McGraw-Hill Book Co., 1967.
51. Fiedler, F.E., and Chemers, M.M.: *Leadership and Effective Management.* Glenview, Ill.: Scott, Foresman and Co., 1975.
52. Graen, F., Alvaris, K., Orris, J.B., and Martella, J.A.: Contingency model of leadership effectiveness: antecedent and evidential results. *Psychol. Bull., 74*:285–296, 1970.
53. Vroom, V., and Yetton, P.: *Leadership and Decision Making.* Pittsburgh: University of Pittsburgh Press, 1973.
54. House, R.J.: A path-goal theory of leader effectiveness. *Administrative Sci. Quart., 16*:321–338, 1971.
55. Filley, A.C., House, R.J., and Kerr, S.: *Managerial Process and Organizational Behavior.* Glenville, Ill.: Scott, Foresman and Co., 1976.
56. Pfeffer, J.: The ambiguity of leadership. In McCall, M.W. (Jr.) and Lombardo, M.M. eds: *Leadership: Where Else Can It Go?* Durham, N.C.: Duke University Press, 1978.
57. Lowin, A. and Craig, J.R.: The influence of level of performance on managerial style: An experimental object-lesson in ambiguity of correlational data. *Organ. Behav. and Human Performance, 3*:440–458, 1968.
58. Greene, C.N.: The reciprocal nature of influence between leader and subordinate. *J. Applied Psychol., 60*:187–193, 1975.

59. Kerr, S., and Jermier, J.: Substituting for leadership: their meaning and measurement. *Organ. Behav. and Human Performance, 13*:375–403, 1978.
60. Dansereau (Jr.), F.D., Graen, G. and Haga, W.J.: A vertical dyad linkage approach to leadership within formal organizations: A longitudinal investigation of the role-making process. *Organ. Behav. and Human Performance, 13*:46–78, 1975.

REVIEW

1. Define motivation and describe the three steps of motivation.

2. How does motivation and motivational technique affect organizational behavior?

3. Discuss Maslow's hierarchy of need theory, its various categories or stages and their interrelationships, the criticisms of the theory and the defense of the theory.

4. What are the seven premises of Maslow's theory? Explain each premise.

5. Discuss behavior modification, operant model, respondent behavior vs. operant behavior, operant conditioning, positive and negative reinforcement, punishment as a type of reinforcement, schedule of reinforcement, discriminating stimulus, and model's application to motivation.

6. Describe the expectancy model, its application to motivation, its strengths and weaknesses.

7. Describe the goal setting theory and compare it with the expectancy model, and how it fits into the MBO scheme of management.

8. Compare all three process models of motivation.

9. Discuss the two-factor (hygiene-motivational) model of motivation, contrast the two factors, and compare it with Maslow's hierarchy of need model.

10. Discuss the criticisms and the defense of the two-factor model.

11. What is the equity theory and how does it relate to motivation?

12. What are attribution theories and how do these relate to motivation?

13. Compare those motivational theories and models reviewed by Miner in terms of scientific validity, usefulness and frequency of nomination for the review. What was the weakness (perhaps a fallacy) of Miner's approach to his review?

14. Discuss the various motivational programs and techniques. Which do you think offers the greatest potential for success? Give examples or explain how each may be applied in pharmacy.

15. Define leadership. What are the characteristics of a good leader?

16. What are five bases of influence? Compare these as to source, potency and applicability to pharmacy.

17. What is the leadership paradigm? How can the independent variable, leadership, be measured? The dependent variable? What is an intervening variable and how does it operate? Give some examples.

18. Discuss trait theories of leadership. What are the three categories or dimensions of traits as classified by Stogdill? What was the one most important finding of Stogdill's review of trait theory research?

19. Discuss personal behavior theories of leadership and compare these with the trait theories.

20. Describe the continuum of leadership postulated by Tannenbaum and Schmidt.

21. What is meant by job-centered leadership? Employee-centered leadership? What are some indices of each leadership style?

22. Disucss the two-dimensions theory of leadership and compare it with the job-centered: employee-centered theory of leadership.

23. Describe the Managerial Grid theory of leadership and the five leadership styles derived from this theory.

24. What is the contingency theory of leadership? How does it differ from previous leadership theories? What is meant by the least preferred co-worker (LPC)? What are the criticisms of LPC?

25. Describe Vroom and Yetton's version of the contingency theory. How does it differ from other contingency theories? How valid is the theory according to Miner? According to Organ and Hamner?

26. Discuss the path-goal theory of leadership. Explain how it differs from other leadership theories. What are the five components of the model?

27. Discuss the significance, or lack of it, of the leadership role. What reasons can be advanced that mitigate the significance of the leadership role?

28. What did Green discover concerning the leadership role with his time lag correlation approach?

29. Describe what Dansereau, Graen and Haga discovered in the manner that leadership is practiced. What is VDL? Contractual exchange? Noncontractual relationship?

30. Compare all the theories and model of leadership according to Miner's criteria. Describe an integrated approach to leadership theory. Summarize leadership research and the application of the results to pharmacy—independent community, chain community, institutional and industrial.

11 | Legal Organizations

Any time a person decides to go into business, he is faced with the decision of doing so alone or of joining with one or more other people in this venture. A second and equally important decision is the form of business enterprise which will be utilized.

There are three forms of legal organizations which are available to the owner(s) of a pharmaceutical firm, including a community pharmacy. These are the sole proprietorship or single ownership, the partnership or co-partnership, and the corporation. Each of these has advantages and limitations which the individual(s) should consider in choosing a particular form for his/their pharmacy. Certainly the nature of the business, the number and philosophy of the people involved, capital, and other factors will determine the type of organization required. In most situations, the basic factors of the operations are known or can be anticipated, and thus will provide the basis for deciding on the legal form that best meets the requirements of the firm.

The sole proprietorship is the oldest, simplest and the most common form of legal organization. The number of sole proprietorships among pharmacies is decreasing as the number of chain units is increasing, most of which are almost always incorporated. Also, as larger independent pharmacies gain in number relative to small independent pharmacies (because of more failures among small pharmacies and newly established pharmacies tend to be larger), there will be an increase in partnerships and corporations at the expense of proprietorships among independent pharmacies. Thus, corporations will become the more viable form of ownership of pharmacies in the future.

A similar trend is that fewer pharmacists today own the building housing the pharmacy. In fact, the notion that owning a pharmacy meant owning the building as well is long past in the scheme of things, although that option remains a possibility. The investment in the pharmacy is sufficiently large that few pharmacists would contemplate purchasing a building to house the pharmacy.

The following discussion is designed to provide the basic information for choosing the most appropriate legal form of organization for a pharmacy practice. However, it is strongly recommended that an attorney be retained to assist in that decision.

240

Sole Proprietorship

ADVANTAGES

As the sole owner of a pharmacy there are no formal requirements for establishing the business other than obtaining the facility in which it will be housed and various licenses and permits which are required for the pharmacy.

The owner has complete freedom, within the limits of the law, in determining the operating policies, methods, and controls. There is no one with whom the profits or decision must be shared. As a consequence, personal incentive is strong and the responsibility is definitely established. Regulations by governmental agencies are less than for the corporate form, resulting in fewer and simpler reports which have to be submitted. Income taxes are only those required of the pharmacy owner as an individual. This is an advantage over a corporation up to a certain income level of income because corporations must pay income taxes on earnings, and the stockholders must pay income tax on the dividends.

DISADVANTAGES

Probably the main disadvantage of the single proprietorship is the *unlimited personal liability* of the owner for the debts and legal liability of his practice. In the event of failure of the pharmacy or a lawsuit, all the owner's personal property outside of the pharmacy may be required to satisfy an indebtedness against the pharmacy. Another limitation is that the owner alone must spread his attention, time, and efforts over the many activities of his business, with none of the benefits of specialization available to a large organization. The owner is responsible for supplying all of the capital required to start and maintain the business, and often the amount of available capital is limited. Unlike a corporation, the sole proprietorship usually terminates with the death of the owner.

General Partnership

DEFINITION AND FORMATION OF PARTNERSHIPS

When a voluntary agreement between two or more persons forms an association to carry on a business together and to share in its profits or losses, they have formed a partnership. This agreement, known as articles of co-partnership, should be in writing and should specify the name and address of the partnership or firm and the names and legal addresses of the partners. It should also identify the contributors' interests, and the duties and responsibilities of each partner. If the partnership selects a trade name for the pharmacy, a certificate indicating the trade name and the articles of co-partnership should be filed with the County Court Clerk in most states. Salaries to be paid to partners should be documented as well as expenses in connection with business functions, drawing accounts, sharing of profits, and withdrawal of the firm's merchandise for personal or family use. There should be clear-cut provisions established for dissolving the partnership, partitioning the assets and dividing the profits.

ADVANTAGES

There are two or more owners, usually one of whom is a qualified pharmacist, who can combine their respective skills, capital, knowledge, time, and efforts in establishing and operating a pharmacy under the partnership form. Several partners should obviously possess among themselves *more capital, greater knowledge and competence* and *more diversified interests* than one person. This will allow for a degree of *specialization of functions*. For instance, one partner could be primarily responsible for the professional aspects of the pharmacy; another could handle the buying, selling, and inventory control, and a third could assume chiefly the financial, accounting, reporting, legal, and equipment responsibilities. Certainly all of the partners would be interested in, and legally responsible for, all phases of the operation. Like the sole proprietorship, the partnership has *less regulation* and *taxation* than the corporation and has fewer reports to make to governmental agencies.

LIMITATIONS

The partnership has a serious disadvantage in the *unlimited liability of each of the partners*. The personal property of each of the several partners is subject to be used to meet any obligations of the partnership which exceed the ability of the business to pay from its own assets and income. The personal property of a partner may be liable for the indebtedness of the partnership up to six months after assignment of his personal property to another person. Since each partner has the capacity to bind the other partners by his actions within the scope of the partnership business, any partner is at risk through foolish moves or bad judgment of another. This disadvantage is derived from the legal concept of *unlimited agency*. Because of this, it is important that formal articles of co-partnership should be drawn by a competent attorney.

As with the sole proprietorship, the partnership usually terminates in the event of death, insanity, or certain other circumstances of withdrawal by a partner. It is possible to establish a new partnership, however, and the business need not be liquidated. This is normally accomplished with a purchase agreement between the partners. Business life insurance on members of the partnerships will make funds available, so that surviving partners can purchase the interests of the survivor's heirs or his estate, thus permitting continuity of the business without interruption.

RIGHTS OF PARTNERS

A general partner *may:* (1) obligate the firm by all the transactions carried out in the apparent course of the business of the partnership; (2) make the firm responsible for all commercial paper signed or endorsed by the partner in the course of partnership business, unless restricted; (3) buy and sell goods, hire representatives, and give warranties; and (4) share in profits.

A general partner *may not,* without the consent of all partners: (1) submit a partnership claim to arbitration; (2) dispose of the good will of the partnership; (3) transfer all or a major portion of partnership property; and (4) confess judgment against the partnership.

DISSOLUTION OF PARTNERSHIP

A partnership is considered dissolved: (1) when a partner dies; (2) when the time for which the partnership was formed has expired; (3) upon notice of termination of the partnership given by a partner if the partnership was not formed for a specified time; (4) by court decree; and (5) by the bankruptcy of any partner.

A general partner may request the court that a partnership be dissolved: (1) when due to constant disagreement between the partners the business cannot be carried on profitably; (2) when one of the partners is judged legally incompetent; and (3) when any partner has persistently breached the partnership agreement.

Upon dissolution of a partnership, due notice should be given through newspapers and by the mail, to those with whom the partnership has done business, in order to protect the interests of partners, creditors, and others concerned.

Partnership assets on dissolution are applied in the following order: (1) to partnership creditors other than partners; (2) to partners for debts due them, except for capital investment; (3) to partners for capital investments; and (4) to partners for profits.

If partnership assets are not sufficient to meet all of the above, then distribution is made as follows: (1) partnership assets to partnership creditors; (2) the deficiency is contributed by the solvent partners from their personal assets in the proportion of sharing of profits.

Specialized Types of Partnership

Various safeguards toward reducing the responsibility and liability of any partner for the conduct of the other partners' financial activities may be placed in the agreement, as well as stipulations for certain limitations in the partnership related to such matters as incurring additional indebtedness, the giving of bonds or securities, and prohibition of various unilateral actions. These, of course, must be specified in the articles of partnership.

INACTIVE PARTNER

Sometimes a person is willing to furnish part of the required capital but does not wish to take an active part in the management of the pharmacy. The articles of partnership should indicate clearly all parts of the agreement including contribution of the inactive partner, percentage of profits to the inactive partner, and a provision for the active partner(s) to purchase the interest of the inactive partner in the event of his death or withdrawal. An inactive partner, often referred to as a silent partner, is *subject to unlimited liability* to the same degree as an active partner.

LIMITED PARTNERSHIP

There may be one or more limited partners and one or more general partners in an organization of this type. The *liability to creditors* by the limited partners is confined to their investment of capital, and they cannot have a part in the management of the business. There must be a formal affiliation agreement prepared indicating the limited and the regular partners, and the length of the life of the agreement. The contributions of each partner must be indicated along with specification of the distribution of profits. The other usual details of the articles of partnership, such as names and addresses, must be included. This formal agreement of partnerships must be registered with proper authorities in the county where the firm is located and published weekly for six successive weeks in two newspapers in order for the limited liability to be effected.

PARTNERSHIP BY ESTOPPEL

Partnership may exist even when parties do not intend partnership or where the agreement between them is otherwise. When persons conduct themselves in a manner from which it may reasonably be inferred that they are partners, and a third party, relying thereon, extends credit, they may be held to be partners as to such third party. This is called partnership by estoppel.

The Corporation

DEFINITION AND FORMATION

A corporation is an association of three or more individuals chartered under the laws of the state to conduct business as an entity, separate from its members. There are various kinds of corporations such as municipal, membership, and business corporations. We shall deal only with private business corporations.

When a corporation is formed, it must file articles of incorporation with the Secretary of State. The articles must state: (1) the name of the corporation, which must not be too similar to the name of another corporation or be deceptive; (2) the duration of the corporation; (3) the names and addresses of the incorporators; (4) the location of the principal office of the corporation; (5) the business or purpose of the corporation; (6) the amount of capital stock and the value assigned to each share having par value or the number of shares of stock without par value; and (7) the names and addresses of the directors for the first year or until the first meeting of the stockholders.

After the certificate of incorporation is issued, the corporation is organized. The stockholders then proceed to elect their Board of Directors and adopt bylaws to govern the corporation during its existence. However, these rules cannot contravene State or Federal law. Bylaws may be modified or amended only by the stockholders and are binding upon the directors.

The Board of Directors then meet and elect the officers of the corporation. The officers of a corporation include the president, secretary, treasurer, and chairman of the Board of Directors. A corporation, being an artificial person, can act only through its agents. The corporation is liable for all its own lawful debts and the acts of all its agents done in the performance of their duties. It must sue and be sued in its own name.

POWERS

Every corporation has the following powers: (1) to admit stockholders; (2) to elect officers and to determine their remuneration; (3) to adopt bylaws; (4) to buy and sell real property, if granted by its charter; and (5) to make such contracts and agreements as are necessary for the transaction of the business stated in the articles of incorporation and to carry on business.

BOARD OF DIRECTORS

The Board of Directors are the agents who manage the corporation. They in turn elect the officers who are removable at the pleasure of the Board. There must be at least three directors. The Board of Directors are responsible only to the stockholders, who elect them by a plurality vote of those present at a meeting called for such a purpose. If three directors are to be elected, a stockholder is voting on three questions and casts his full vote for *each* director to be elected.

The Board of Directors must act as a board and not individually. They must act by a majority vote, and any other provision of the bylaws in this respect is illegal. The directors must act faithfully in performing their duties and display a high degree of fidelity to the stockholders.

The Board of Directors, without the consent of two-thirds of the stockholders, cannot mortgage or sell real estate, dissolve the corporation, vote to merge or consolidate it, or sell its machinery or property. The Board of Directors has the sole discretion to declare dividends, including the amount per share.

STOCKHOLDERS

A stockholder is a person, partnership or another corporation that owns one or more shares of stock in a corporation. A stockholder may vote on any major question or decision affecting the corporation and he may vote in person or by proxy.

A stockholder also has the right to preemption. When a corporation increases the number of shares of authorized stock, the stockholders have a prior right to purchase the increased shares. This is called the right of preemption. The ratio of new shares, which any stockholder has the right to purchase, is proportional to the number of shares currently held.

These rights are valuable and may be sold by the stockholder, and his vendee may acquire them and all the privileges incidental to them. In cases of stock listed and sold on a security exchange, these rights are also dealt in.

Stockholders may sue directors to account for negligent acts or acts done in bad faith or for the appropriation of any assets to their individual uses, but not for errors in judgment committed in good faith.

Stockholders are only liable for the amount of the par value of their stock, if fully paid, or the amount of the purchase price of no par value stock.

If a stockholder has not paid the full par value of his stock or the purchase price of the no par value shares, he is liable to the corporation's creditors for the difference between the amount paid in and the par value or purchase price in the event of insolvency of the corporation.

STOCKS AND DIVIDENDS

Stocks are one of two classes, common or preferred. A *common stock* is the usual class issued in the formation of a corporation. The owner of a common stock has one vote for each share, and receives a dividend on the basis of the number of shares he owns. Dividends can be paid only from the surplus or earnings and to do otherwise is a crime.

A *preferred stock* has unique features. First, the owner of a preferred stock does not have the right to vote. The dividend for a preferred stock is predetermined as a percentage of its par value, and such dividends are paid before dividends may be declared for common stock—hence the term, preferred stock.

DISSOLUTION OF A CORPORATION

A corporation can be dissolved: (1) when it voluntarily applies for dissolution; (2) when it fails to abide by its charter, and the Attorney General of the State applies to the court for its dissolution; (3) when two years have elapsed and it has not conducted the business for which it was organized; (4) when it reaches the time limit for which it was organized; (5) when it fails to pay State Franchise Taxes for three years. Except in voluntary dissolution by consent of stockholders, a legal action for a dissolution must be instituted.

ADVANTAGES OF A CORPORATION

A corporation is preferred to a proprietorship or partnership for the following reasons: (1) the duration is perpetual unless the articles of incorporation specify otherwise; (2) inasmuch as the corporation is an entity separate and distinct from its members, the death of any or all of its members does not affect its existence or its operation; (3) it permits the attraction of capital in small or large amounts from innumerable sources and without regard to geographic location; and (4) liability of investors is limited to the amount of their investment and, therefore, one does not risk any more than he desires to invest, whereas in a partnership or individual form of conducting business, one's entire assets may be lost.

LIMITATIONS OF A CORPORATION

A corporation incurs considerable legal expense in connection with the procuring of its charter, issuing stock, and paying filing fees and capital stock taxes. The corporation must employ a brokerage firm if the Board of Directors decides to "go public," that is, make the stock available to the general public. It is subject to more governmental regulation than the proprietorship or partnership. It must submit more complex and detailed reports and is subject to higher tax rates up to a certain level of income. The corporation must also pay income tax on its earnings, and then the shareholder is taxed again on the corporation income he receives as dividends, thus incurring double taxation.

The Federal corporate tax rate as of 1985 was as follows: (1) up to $25,000, 16 percent, (2) the excess above $25,000 up to $50,000, 19 percent, (3) the excess above $50,000 up to $75,000, 30 percent, (4) the excess above $75,000 up to $100,000, 40 percent, and (5) the excess above $100,000, 46 percent, and 5 percent of income above $1,000,000 but not to exceed $20,250. There is a great deal of talk about revising the income tax law.

The "Subchapter S" Corporation

In 1958, Congress enacted a law giving businessmen the opportunity to do business as a corporation and allowing them the right to elect to be taxed as a partnership or sole proprietorship, thus bypassing the federal corporate income tax. This type of corporation has the following advantages: (1) it may secure tax advantages from the fringe benefits that are available to the employees of the corporation; (2) the stockholders of a young corporation have the right to deduct on their personal income tax returns the early losses incurred while the business is getting under way; and (3) the stockholders may use a corporate fiscal year different from the stockholder's tax year resulting in income deferment for the stockholder and controlling within limits the time when corporate income is counted as the stockholders income.

For the purpose of this Subchapter of the Internal Revenue Code, the term "small business corporation" means a domestic corporation that is not a member of an affiliated group according to section 1504, a financial institution, or an insurance company and that does not:

1. have more than 35 shareholders (husband and wife, and their estate, are treated as one shareholder);
2. have as a shareholder a person (other than an estate and other than a trust described in subsection (c)(2) of Subchapter S of the Internal Revenue Code) who is not an individual person;
3. have a nonresident alien as a shareholder; and
4. have more than one class of stock.
5. All shareholders must consent to the election (decision) to be exempted from corporation income tax under the provision of this Subchapter during the preceding tax year or on or before the 15th day of the 3rd month of the current taxable year.
6. If more than 80 percent of the firm's gross receipts are derived from sources outside the United States, the firm cannot elect to be exempted from corporate income tax.
7. More than 25 percent of the firm's gross receipts cannot be derived from passive investments (royalties, rents, dividends, interests, annuties, gains from the sale or exchange of stock or securities) for three consecutive taxable years, or have any corporation C earnings.
8. Small business corporation is subject to capital gains tax under certain conditions.

Stockholders can elect to become a corporation under Subchapter S regulations one year and revoke it the next provided shareholders holding more than one-half of the shares vote for revocation. But if there is a cancellation, another election cannot be held until the fifth year starting after the year of cancellation, unless the Commissioner of Internal Revenue consents to a shorter waiting period. It is not necessary to reelect Subchapter S treatment every year; it continues until revoked or cancelled for failure to follow the rules.

Summary

The choice of legal organization will depend on a number of factors: (1) the size of the pharmacy and the investment, (2) the number of principals involved, (3) anticipated growth and source of capital to finance the growth, (4) income tax statutes and regulations, and (5) the philosophy of the owner(s). Of course, the larger the pharmacy, investment and number of principals, the more advantageous the corporate form will be. Also, the corporate form of organization makes it easier to raise additional capital from several individuals via sale of stock, either common or preferred. Presently (1985), it is difficult to predict the income tax structure in the future since there are three or four tax reform proposals being discussed. Of course, the personal choice of legal organizational form is a private matter.

In any event, the aspiring pharmacist-proprietor should consult his attorney and/or accountant before making his final decision. Attorneys tend to be specialized, and therefore, not every attorney is fully knowledgable concerning legal organization. A tax-lawyer or tax-accountant can normally provide better counsel on the most advantageous legal form from a tax perspective.

REVIEW

1. Describe the formation and characteristics of a sole proprietorship.
2. List five advantages and four disadvantages of a sole proprietorship.
3. Describe four types of partnerships. Compare their formation and the different characteristics.
4. List four advantages and three limitations of a general partnership.
5. What are the five bases for dissolution of a partnership?
6. What are the three reasons a general partner may use to request a court to dissolve a partnership?
7. How are assets distributed upon the dissolution of a general partnership?
8. Explain the purpose of an inactive partner and a limited partner.
9. What is a partnership by estoppel?
10. Define a corporation and discuss the steps in the formation of a corporation.
11. What are the seven items that must appear on the articles of incorporation?
12. List four advantages and four limitations of a corporation.
13. What are the five powers of a corporation?
14. Give the distinguishing features of the two classes of corporate stock.
15. Who are the stockholders of a corporation, what are their functions, what rights and liabilities do they have?
16. How are the members of the Board of Directors of a corporation chosen and what are their functions?
17. What are five reasons for dissolving a corporation?
18. Discuss the "Subchapter S" corporation, its purpose and advantages, and the seven requirements for its legal formation.

12 | Personnel Administration

> *What we frankly give, forever is our own.*
> George Granville

Personnel administration probably is the most important aspect of pharmacy management; yet it is the most neglected phase. Today we read and hear a great deal about pharmacy becoming people-oriented or patient-oriented. Most *successful* practitioners have always been people-oriented. Furthermore, these practitioners have used this philosophy in their relationships with their employees. Just as "charity begins at home," people-orientation begins with the employees in our pharmacies.

Importance of Personnel Administration

There are *three important reasons* why good employee relations should be emphasized and practiced in every pharmacy. The *first* involves *finances*. According to the 1984 *Lilly Digest*,[1] the "average" independent pharmacy spent $89,000, or 16.8 percent of sales, for salaries and wages. The respective figures for the typical chain pharmacy reported in the 1984 *NACDS Lilly Digest*[2] were $209,000 or 10.5 percent of sales. The typical general hospital pharmacy reported an annual payroll of approximately $305,000 in the 1984 *Lilly Hospital Pharmacy Survey*.[3] The typical pharmacist-proprietor earns approximately $32,000 in salary and $15,500 in profit ($47,500 total) for a 47-hour work-week. The range of total income is $18,000 to $107,000 ($25,000 to $78,000 excluding the two extreme groups). The typical chain pharmacy manager earns $32,000 with a range of $29,000 to $40,000 for a 46-hour work-week. The typical hospital pharmacist earns approximately $14 per hour. Note that these figures were taken from 1983 calendar year data. The above figures represent the largest single expense item in the profit and loss statement. Some pharmacists may view expenditures for salaries and wages as a type of investment, but in reality, they are not. Money expended

250

for salaries and wages must be productive as it is spent, or at least in the near future; otherwise the money will not be recovered or produce a net return. Therefore, payroll inherently has an immediacy which creates an urgency in its judicious use.

Another way to view the financial importance of the payroll is to contrast it with the investment in inventory. Inventory represents an *investment* on which a net profit may be earned, while the payroll is an *expense* of doing business. A pharmacist has at least two options in the use of the inventory investment: (1) he may return the goods for credit under certain conditions, and (2) he may reduce the price and enhance the sale potential. Such options are not available in respect to the payroll expense.

There is yet another financial aspect of personnel administration, namely, the high cost of personnel turnover. Normally it requires several months of training before a new employee becomes sufficiently productive to be profitable. If a pharmacy has a high personnel turnover rate, an unprofitable situation could easily exist because of the cost associated with the constant training of new employees who, at the beginning, are not proficient enough to be productive and profitable.

The *second reason* personnel administration is important derives from the interrelationship between the behavior of the employees and the *pharmacy's public image*. To a great extent, the attitudes and behavior of the employees will create the public image of the pharmacy. Of course, their attitudes and behavior reflect the personality of the proprietor or pharmacist-manager and the type of employee relationship he maintains. This points to *one of the basic rules of* personnel relations, that is, *good employee relations begin with the proprietor or manager* himself. His attitudes toward work, people, and the profession have a tremendous influence on those in his employ. A good personnel relations program is essential to cultivate a good public image for any organization. This is especially true of a pharmacy because a successful, professional enterprise such as a pharmacy must exhibit a warm and friendly atmosphere.

The *third reason* personnel administration is important relates to the *achievements of the objectives of the pharmacy*. From a strictly economic point of view, the proprietor, in addition to his enterpreneurship, provides a managerial function, an economic input. The economic reward is reflected in the form of the proprietor's salary before the net profit is computed. The *net profit* is the economic reward for entrepreneurship, and it is one of the basic objectives of the pharmacy. Without good employees supporting the proprietor, a healthy net profit cannot be achieved.

Principles of Personnel Administration

There are several basic principles of good employee relations. These include: (1) people-orientation begins with the proprietor and the employees;

(2) good employee relations emanate from the attitudes, philosophy, and leadership of the employer-manager; he should know his true attitudes and feelings and should make desirable adjustments, while remaining open and honest with those within his relationships; (3) the "golden rule" is an excellent principle to follow, but most people need additional guidelines and principles to assist them in making personnel decisions; (4) human dignity must be maintained at all times; therefore, techniques and methods of employee relations should not be depersonalized, although objectivity and fairness must be used judiciously; (5) a good manager will delegate authority to the lowest level consistent with the capabilities of the employee; (6) adequate resources should be supplied and authority should be delegated to subordinates commensurate with the delegated responsibilities; (7) most people want to achieve and to perform at a high level, and they will, if the objectives, and procedures for achieving the objectives, are well articulated and understood; and (8) a feedback of performance results is a powerful motivating tool, especially a positive feedback of high performance.

These principles apply to all types and sizes of pharmacies; however, the scope of the application of specific techniques and methods is limited by the number of employees. In this regard, trends toward fewer smaller phamacies and more larger ones are significant considerations. (See Chapter 3).

Methods of Personnel Administration

STAFFING REQUIREMENTS

Minimum Staffing. This section is so self-evident that it may seem almost needless; however, for the inexperienced student it may serve a useful purpose. Initially in a new pharmacy, the pharmacist-manager must resist the temptation of employing a "full complement" of personnel. However, sufficient personnel to provide good service is required, which normally is one person for each major service center as determined by the size of the pharmacy and the layout design as discussed in Chapter 7. No patron who appears to want or need assistance should be allowed to wait more than a couple of minutes before a clerk offers assistance. Even so, the manager should staff personnel on the basis of personnel cost of no more than 10 percent of sales in each service center within a reasonable time, e.g., three or four months. This statistical guideline is the first-line, elementary rule for deciding staffing requirements.

Queuing Model. Since payroll is the single largest expense item and employee wages are variable expenses, pharmacists should be interested in any means of determining the appropriate level of personnel staffing. Queuing theory provides a model by which this can be done.

The queuing theory model is used to determine the optimum number of personnel for servicing any station at which people may wait to be served on a first-come/first-served basis. Barber shops, telephone switchboards, check-

out lanes, and prescription departments are examples of places where the model can be used. The model requires four factors or characteristics.
1. A pattern of probability distribution of the arrivals at the station.
2. A probability distribution associated with the time required to serve the individual.
3. The queue or waiting line (although people do not have to wait in line, only wait their turn) may be organized on a first-come/first-served or on a random basis. (If a person has to wait too long, he will go to another place for services.)
4. There may be multiple channels for service, but the model requires only one channel of service, even though several people can work simultaneously at the station. The number of arrivals cannot exceed the service rate, i.e., the number that can be served during a given period.

With certain assumptions about these factors, it is possible to apply the theory and determine the behavior of the queue at a prescription department.

First, the arrivals occur in a random pattern within a time unit and the probability of an arrival is independent of the service rate or the number of arrivals in the previous or the next unit of time. Such a distribution is known as a Poisson distribution or process. It is assumed that the number of prescriptions dispensed per unit of time is also a Poisson distribution. Therefore, the number of arrivals and the number of people served during one hour are independent and have no effect on the arrivals or service rate during any other hour. Thus, the service rate, which is the reciprocal of the average service time is also a Poisson distribution. Another assumption is that patients will accept service on a first-come/first-served basis. Finally, the assumption is made that the number of arrivals of prescriptions and the dispensing (service rate) of same are from an infinite universe. This is true in the theoretic sense.

The queuing theory model is expressed mathematically in the following formulas.

$$E_n = \frac{A^2}{S(S - A)}$$

where: E_n = The expected number in the queue
A = the average number patrons arriving per unit of time
S = the average number of prescriptions dispensed per unit of time;

then

$$E_w = \frac{E_n}{A}$$

where: E_w = the expected waiting time in the queue in hours.

A Case Study. Huffman used the queuing model to determine the optimum staffing pattern for a prescription department.[4] The study was conducted during

Table 12–1. Average Number of Prescription Arrivals by Days and Hours

Time	Mon.	Tues.	Wed.	Thurs.	Fri.	Sat.	4 wk. avg.
8–9 a.m.	4.5	5.0	3.5	3.5	5.0	5.0	4.4
9–10 a.m.	7.0	6.5	12.0	5.5	8.0	16.0	9.2
10–11 a.m.	15.0	18.5	18.0	14.0	16.5	23.0	17.5
11–12	23.0	21.5	22.0	23.5	23.0	22.0	22.5
12–1 p.m.	15.0	16.0	12.5	12.0	12.0	16.5	14.0
1–2 p.m.	11.0	8.5	9.5	5.5	9.0	5.0	8.1
2–3 p.m.	10.0	8.0	13.5	5.0	9.5	4.0	7.7
3–4 p.m.	8.0	11.5	9.0	5.0	11.0	3.0	7.9
4–5 p.m.	5.0	5.0	8.0	5.0	8.0	1.0	5.3
5–6 p.m.	2.0	4.0	2.5	1.0	3.0	1.0	2.3
6–6:30 p.m.	1.0	1.0	1.0	0.5	1.5	0.5	1.0

Adapted from Huffman, D.C.: The Feasibility of Modern Managerial Systems and Innovative Professional Services in a Community Pharmacy. A Case Study. Dissertation. University of Mississippi, University. Miss., 1970.

1969 and 1970 as a part of a doctoral research project and later published by the American College of Apothecaries.[5]

In Huffman's study, the days were segmented by hours, Monday through Saturday, and the average number of prescription arrivals for each hour was computed over a four-week period. The data are replicated in part in Table 12–1.

The average dispensing (service) time was calculated from random sampling of time periods for the existing staffing pattern. It was found that a pharmacist working by himself averaged 6 minutes to dispense a prescription and to perform all related paper and clerical work. This time also included other duties such as answering the telephone, if they interfered with the dispensing process. One pharmacist and one clerk reduced the dispensing time to 4.3 minutes; two pharmacists and one clerk, 2.7 minutes, and two pharmacists and two clerks, 2.4 minutes. The respective service rates were 10, 14, 22, and 25 prescriptions per hour, respectively.

Two cost factors enter into the calculations in the application of the model. One is the cost of service and the other is the waiting cost. The latter is based on the theory that patients will wait only so long before going to another pharmacy. If a patient waits only five minutes, there is usually little or no consequence. If the patient has to wait for one hour or more, the consequence will be substantial and the patient will probably patronize another pharmacy.

In the 1969 Huffman study, the following costs were assigned: pharmacists' service @ $5.00 per hour, clerks' service @ 1.50 per hour, and waiting cost @ $10.00 per hour. (The last figure is a rather subjective one.) However, more realistic figures for the current market would be $15.00 per hour for pharmacist(s), $5.00 per hour for clerks, and $40.00 per hour for the waiting cost. Calculations using the queuing theory model and the more current cost data indicate that one pharmacist working alone can dispense as many as six prescriptions per hour most economically. One pharmacist and one clerk can handle 7 to 12 prescriptions, two pharmacists and one clerk can handle 13 to 17 and two pharmacists and two clerks can dispense 18 or more per hour more economically.

A few calculations will illustrate how the queuing theory model operates in determining staffing patterns. Suppose 12 prescriptions arrive regularly during a given hour and the average number of arrivals for that hour is 12. "A" equals 12; with one pharmacist and one clerk "S," the service rate, is 14; with two pharmacists and one clerk, "S," is 22. Using one pharmacist and one clerk, the total costs are:

$$E_n = \frac{12^2}{14(14-12)} = \frac{144}{28} = 5.1428$$

$$E_w = \frac{5.1428}{12} = 0.4285 \text{ hour (waiting time)}$$

Service Cost + Waiting Costs = Total Costs
$15 + \$5 + [0.4285 \times \$40] = \$37.14$

Using two pharmacists and one clerk, the total costs are:

$$E_n = \frac{12^2}{22(22-12)} = \frac{144}{220} = 0.6545$$

$$E_w = \frac{0.6545}{12} = 0.0545$$

Service Cost + Waiting Costs = Total Costs

$30 + \$5 + [0.0545 \times \$40] = \$37.18$

The conclusion is not obvious in this case. Sometimes the difference in total costs is so small that the pharmacist must use judgment in deciding the number and type of personnel. The above example is a case in point. The pharmacist must decide whether to staff one pharmacist and one clerk or two pharmacists and one clerk. The respective total costs are $37.14 and $37.18–only 14 cents difference! Since the situation usually occurs near the noon hour and the pharmacist will probably favor ample time for patient consultation, he should decide to employ two pharmacists and one clerk for this time period.

A study of Table 12–1 indicates that a pharmacist alone can operate the prescription department between hours of 8 to 9 a.m. and 5 to 6:30 p.m. He can also handle the prescription department all of Thursday and Saturday afternoons. Other considerations also enter into staffing decisions such as work other than direct service to the patron. Other such work may include stocking shelves, taking inventory, rearranging merchandise and displays. These activities are usually done during "slow" periods when few patrons are being served by the prescription department. As a practical matter, a clerk or prescription assistant will normally be present most of the time from 9 a.m. to 5 p.m.

The queuing theory model is applicable during the peak period, 10 a.m. to 4 p.m. in this case, when a decision on staffing is critical. Additionally, Kitler and Lamey have reported the potential use of queuing theory in a hospital pharmacy.[6]

The queuing theory model is applicable for the decision of purchasing a computer and concomitant staffing patterns. The primary difficulty is how to determine the service rate utilizing the computer. What is needed is research on the problem designed to permit generalizations to various pharmacies within ranges of prescription volume.

JOB ANALYSIS AND SPECIFICATION

Queuing theory model is useful in determining the number of staff that is needed for a particular work station or service center with a well defined set of work elements. Job analysis is used to determine the type of work that is needed for a particular work station or function.

Job Analysis. Before a manager begins to recruit and select employees, he should perform certain analyses and describe the jobs or functions for his pharmacy. Job analysis has both a qualitative and a quantitative dimension. The qualitative dimension describes the nature of the various tasks that have to be performed. The quantitative dimension describes the time required and/ or the frequency of the several tasks (or particular components of the various tasks) to be performed. This process is aptly called job analysis, and the description written from the analysis is called job description. This process is meticulously carried out in a large organization using time and motion, work monitoring, and work sampling techniques. It may not be necessary for the usual community pharmacy; however, each job or position to be filled should be analyzed and described in sufficient detail to permit both employer and employee to know what is expected in each position. The emphasis in job analysis and job description falls upon the work elements to be performed, and by implication or explicit descriptions, the qualifications of the person who will fill the position.

Job Specification. Based on the personal qualifications extracted from the job description, a job or position specification is written. Whereas, a community pharmacist may not perform a detailed job analysis or write a detailed job description, he should write a fairly complete job specification based on the requirements of each job or position to be filled. Job specification emphasizes personal qualities, while job description emphasizes work elements to be performed. The job specification provides the basis for selecting the right employee for each position in the pharmacy.

RECRUITMENT AND SELECTION

Recruitment. A pharmacy manager can launch an intelligent employee recruitment and selection program on the basis of the job specifications for unfilled positions in the pharmacy. The sources for *recruitment* will be determined by the manager's needs at any particular time. For staff pharmacists, the colleges of pharmacy are the best source at graduation time. During the rest of the year, other pharmacies, health care institutions, government, and industry may be utilized. These sources are the only ones for experienced pharmacists for managerial positions. Another good source (and perhaps an important one for the future) consists in the married female pharmacists who want to reenter the profession after their childern have reached school age. Part-time employees, both professional and nonprofessional, may be a solution to the profit squeeze caused by rising costs on the one hand and increased competition on the other. Classified ads are the medium used most widely to locate experienced pharmacists, but employment agencies can be useful in large competitive markets.

Different means are used to recruit nonprofessional personnel. High schools and colleges offer possibilities for part-time personnel, as do married women. However, school "dropouts" usually do not make good pharmacy personnel. Newspaper ads and word-of-mouth advertising are the best media. "Help Wanted" signs in the windows have fallen into disuse for good reason. Such signs usually are not attractive or dignified, and they use valuable space that can be used better for professional displays.

Personnel Selection. The *selection process* is probably the most *critical phase* of personnel administration. Here the decision must be made. The question to be answered is, "Is he the kind of person I want in my organization?" Once an employee is hired, it is difficult to discharge him without some repercussions and considerable cost.

There are *four steps* in the selection process. The *first step* is the *initial interview* with the prospective employee and completion of a prepared *application form*. The initial interview serves as a means of appraising the applicant's apparent qualities—appearance, speech, mannerisms, and attitudes. The application form should provide essential personal, educational, experience, and health data as well as references to serve as a basis for preliminary selection. From a list of seven applicants, four might be eliminated on the basis of the application form and the initial interview.

Tests, although not widely used in community and hospital pharmacies, are the *second step* in the selection process. They are more common in chain pharmacies, industry, and government. Simple tests, properly constructed, can prove useful in personnel selection. Such a test may be written, oral, or practical, and it must be designed for the level of the position being filled. Although a proprietor may think it unnecessary to test a registered pharmacist on professional knowledge, he may want to ascertain some measure of the applicant's managerial potential.

For professionals: Written tests may cover problems, letter writing, or general knowledge about drugs. Oral questions may determine the applicant's ability to express himself and to handle a particular situation, or again, his general knowledge about drugs and patient consultation. Practical or performance tests for nonprofessionals may include making change, typing speed and accuracy and preparing a prescription label. Many such tests may be simulated; however, an actual test under real conditions is to be preferred.

Honesty and *ethics* are difficult to measure. A test can be made of an individual's basic honesty through a few questions, the answers to which can be validated. For example, the manager may ask the applicant about relationship with his previous employer(s) and then check with the employer(s). Polygraph tests are widely used in many industries, including the chain drugstores. A survey indicated that 73 percent of the responding drugstore chains use the polygraph and 80 percent stated they favor its use. The widest use of the polygraph is reserved for theft and robbery problems; however, 40 percent of those using this technique also use it for pre-employment examination.[7]

The *third step* is to employ *references* to assess the applicant's honesty and willingness to work, the quality of his work, and any personality or disciplinary problem. References may include former employers, teachers, and friends, but former employers are preferred. Oddly enough, *oral recommendations are more reliable than written ones.* People are more inclined to "tell it like it is" about a person if they do not have to put it in writing.

The *final interview* is the *last step* in the selection process. After studying the application, the results of any tests that were used, and the recommendations of former employers, the manager is ready to make a decision. On the basis of preliminary considerations, the field may have been reduced to two or three applicants. In any case, a final interview should be conducted to check on any unanswered questions and to clarify any potential problem area. The final decision will be made at this time, and the manager will want it to be the best possible.

A pitfall to be guarded against in any interview is the "halo" (positive) or "horn" (negative) effect. This is simply a lack of objectivity on the part of the interviewer by which he allows one particular characteristic to color his judgment about other characteristics or qualities. For example, the interviewer may like or dislike a certain color of hair, accent, or manner of dress so much that his judgment of other qualities is distorted. The use of two or three interviewers serves to minimize the halo or horn effect and provides for more objectivity in the interviews.

ORIENTATION AND TRAINING

Orientation. The purpose of *orientation* is to acquaint the new employee with the organization, its history, its objectives, its policies, and other employees. Personnel psychologists have demonstrated a high degree of relationship between good orientation programs and the results of subsequent training programs. It is important for each new employee to be properly indoctrinated and made to feel "at home" in the new work surroundings. Failure to orient and indoctrinate new employees properly is probably the most common failing of community pharmacy proprietors and managers.

Orientation can be made more effective by the use of concise written statement of policies and by the use of the "buddy system." Written policy statements may be compiled into a booklet that functions as an employee manual. The American College of Apothecaries has compiled a prototype policies and procedures manual for its members.[8] This manual contains a statement of objectives and general policies, employee policies and procedures, including company rules, fringe benefits, information for pharmacy personnel, such as telephone technique, consulting with patients, information for typists, and use of the patient medication record system. This manual can be easily adapted for an individual pharmacy. The large chain drugstores have seen the wisdom of writing employee's manuals and developing extensive training programs for nearly all levels of employees.

Training. Training and development of employees should be distinguished from education. Whereas education has broad objectives, training has specific objectives related to proficiency on a particular job. Training objectives are either the acquisition of skills or a change in behavior. Personnel training may be either formal or informal, but most of the training in pharmacies is considered to be informal.

The most common method of conducting training for nonprofessional personnel is *on-the-job training*. This type of training consists of four basic steps:

1. Tell the trainee what the job is, how the job is done, and why it is done.
2. Show or demonstrate how the job should be done.
3. Allow the trainee to do the job.
4. Follow up by explaining what was done correctly and what was done incorrectly. Corrections always should be made as privately as possible.

The *conference* is the next most frequently used means of training pharmacy personnel. Conferences may be either formal or informal. A formal, regularly scheduled meeting is effective in maintaining the proficiency and morale of experienced personnel if it is planned and conducted well. Each conference should have an objective (or objectives) and a planned agenda covering such subjects as sales, special promotion, public relations programs, or product knowledge. Experience has shown that combining an evening meal or breakfast with a conference is a good morale booster. Advantage should also be taken of the special schools and seminars offered by cosmetic manufacturers, surgical supply houses, veterinary drug manufacturers, vocational and pharmacy schools.

Information to be supplied in an orientation and training program should include the history, objectives, and policies of the pharmacy. Next, the pharmacy's systems and procedures, especially those for which the new employee will be responsible, should be taught. These should include the organization of the pharmacy, lines of responsibility and authority, location of departments, maintenance of inventory, handling of cash, checking registers, special controls for certain departments and products, and related restrictions. Methods of dealing with patrons, especially in unusual situations, require more time. Knowledge of new and existing products requires still more time, and teaching this is a continuous project.

The proprietor or manager of a pharmacy should realize that a personal example is a powerful teaching tool. It is especially true that poor examples have a negative effect on the learner. The principles and concepts embodied in the sections on leadership development in Chapter 10 are especially applicable to the training of personnel.

Employee orientation and training are the most neglected aspect of personnel administration. There is too little—far too little—of it done. Too frequently the training that is provided is neither well planned nor often evaluated.

SUPERVISION

Supervision is necessary even in a small pharmacy in which only two or three people are employed; it cannot be avoided if the employees are to perform satisfactorily and achieve their objectives and those of the pharmacy. There is the danger, however, of oversupervision, which reduces the self-confidence of the employees and creates a morale problem. MBO provides one of the best frameworks for good supervison. Principles and techniques for motivation and leadership in Chapter 10 are especially useful in supervision.

Supervision is simply a process of open communications between the supervisor, the manager in most small pharmacies, and the employees, and the general direction and overview of work performance by the supervisor. Communications always should be conducted on a two-way basis to be effective. Being a good listener is inherent in good communication. Understanding is important, but listening and understanding must be genuine. This is especially true in performance review and evaluation.

It is a well-known fact that there are good and bad supervisors and leaders. Since good supervision and leadership are so important to the success of any organization, there must be an explanation why there are many poor supervisors and leaders. Laurence Peter offers a plausible explanation in his book entitled *The Peter Principle*.[9] According to Peter, our modern society has the inherent tendency toward developing hierarchies in all organizations. In these structures, every person tends to rise to his first level of incompetence. The phenomenon is universal and inevitable because of the characteristics of our social system. These characteristics include: (1) social mobility which rewards competent people in a specific area of endeavor with a promotion to a higher position for which the person is not trained or qualified; (2) the tendency to preserve the hierarchy which produces conformity of action for the security it provides; and (3) the absence of a method or system of identifying and distinguishing the necessary qualities for good supervision and leadership.

The reasons for, and the methods used in, promoting people to their level of incompetency are beyond the scope of this book. However, the tendency for top management to replicate themselves is a common mistake and the organization becomes "lopsided" in its philosophy and managerial style. *The Peter Principle* and its companion, *The Peter Prescription,*[10] are recommended reading on this subject. The books not only provide a good insight into organizational hierarchy; they permit a better understanding of society in general, and, more specifically, how one can cope with the difficulties encountered in many organizations.

EVALUATION AND COMPENSATION

A manager should realize that he is evaluating himself and his personnel relations program when he evaluates employees. This procedure is even more personal than a teacher's evaluation of his students. After all, the manager selects and trains the employees, whereas the teacher normally does not select the pupils.

Principles of Personnel Evaluation. There are some general principles of employee evaluation which should be observed.

1. The manager must have a genuine desire to be fair and honest. Personal bias must be avoided if at all possible. Again, MBO provides a good method for personnel evaluation. Objectives should be explicit and realistic.
2. Allowance must be made for nonproductive (nonselling) duties. This is one of the purposes of a rating system.
3. The pay scale must be competitive within the market. Parsimony is unprofitable in personnel relations.
4. Incentive and opportunity for advancement should be incorporated into the pay scale. Insufficient incentive and opportunity for advancement are the most common faults in current pay scales for pharmacists. This may be overcome if the starting salaries are lowered and a profit-sharing plan and/or an opportunity to purchase an interest in the pharmacy is provided as a strong incentive for achievement.
5. The method of calculating wages or salary should be simple enough to be easily understood by the employee involved.
6. Clerks' wages should be approximately 10 percent of their sales, but this rule should not be applied to managers or to pharmacists.
7. Wages should be fairly uniform from week to week, especially for young married people with tight budgets.
8. Finally, compensation alone cannot replace proper supervision and good human relations.

Personnel Evaluation. Achievement measurements and rating scales are

Characteristic   *Scale*

Characteristic	
Dependability	
Loyal attitude toward the firm	
Awareness of assigned responsibilities	
Knowledge of the stock in assigned departments	
Order and cleanliness of assigned sections	
Courtesy and cooperativeness with fellow employees	
Courtesy and genuine interest in dealing with patrons	
Alertness and promptness in dealing with patrons	
Warm and pleasing personality	
Appearance	

1	2	3	4	5
Poor	Fair	Average	Good	Excellent

Figure 12–1. Rating scale for evaluating employees.

the two primary means of evaluating employees. The former are more objective, easier to devise, and easier to use. Examples of such measurements include sales per employee, number of transactions or patrons served per day, dollar value per transaction, and incidents of out-of-stock situations in an assigned department of the pharmacy.

Rating scales are more difficult to design, use, and interpret. One such instrument, the graphic rating of employees on various qualities, as illustrated in Figure 12–1, is sufficiently simple to be used by the typical pharmacy proprietor or manager. A composite score may be computed for each employee, with a low of 10 to a possible high score of 50. Also a graphic representation may be used to compare employees and to measure progress over time. However, rating of employees on a scale used alone is inferior to a system of management by objectives.

Compensation. Methods of compensation were implicit in the discussion of principles of evaluation. Although straight salary is commonly found, it offers the least in incentive. It does provide wage stability, it is simple and easily understood, and it can provide compensation for nonselling duties. Selling on commission provides a strong incentive, but it may create overly aggressive attitudes. It also lacks wage stability. Salary plus PM ("push merchandise") techniques are to be discouraged for the same reasons. In addition, PMs may divide employee loyalty between the proprietor and the manufacturer of the product. Salary plus profit sharing and/or opportunity to own an interest in the pharmacy seems to have most of the advantages and none of the disadvantages of other methods.

Employment and Wage Administration. It is beyond the scope of this text to cover in detail all of the laws and regulations governing employment and wages. However, the most common and relevant requirements are discussed briefly. First, an employer cannot discriminate on the basis of sex, race, age or religion in hiring, promoting, discharging or paying wages of anyone. Also, handicapped persons cannot be discriminated against in any employment situation that such persons could reasonably be expected to perform the work.

Second, there are regulations concerning the number of hours per day and week that minors or females may be employed, and also concerning the number of hours without a rest period. A related set of laws and regulations covers the health and safety of the work environment. These include fire hazards, stairways, toxic gases, anything that could be considered hazardous. Also, there are sanitation codes that must be considered especially if a fountain is operated within a pharmacy.

Third, any firm that employs two persons and is engaged in interstate commerce (and that includes producing or selling a product that will move or has moved in interstate commerce) is required to abide by the Federal Wage and Hour Law. Small retailers and service businesses, which include pharmacies, with annual sales less than $362,500 are exempted. The minimum wage for all other covered firms is $3.35 per hour up to 40 hours per week. The minimum wage is one and one-half times the regular hourly rate for time over the 40-hour work week. In addition, most states have a wage and hour law, which may be different from the federal law.

Fourth, the Federal Insurance Contribution Act (FICA) was designed to provide a base for retirement income. The Act levied a tax on the employee and employer at the same rate to finance the program. There are two categories: (1) the Old-Age Survivors, and Disability Insurance (OASD) and (2) Hospital Insurance (medicare). The combined tax rate for the two programs was 7.05 percent on wages up to $39,600 for 1985, 7.15 percent for 1986–1989, and 7.65 percent for 1990 and thereafter. The ceiling on which the tax is levied will increase by the cost-of-living index (CPI) each year. The employer must deduct the tax from the employee's wage and add a like amount to be forwarded to the federal government quarterly.

Fifth, pharmacies are also subject to the unemployment insurance programs that are joint programs between the federal government and the respective states. The overall program was begun by the enactment of the Federal Unemployment Tax Act, which established minimum guidelines for states and a federal unemployment fund to assist in financing the programs. Any firm that employs one or more persons for any part or a full day in each of 20 different weeks during a calendar year, or has a payroll of $1,500 or more for any quarter during a year is subject to the law. Domestic services and a few other special cases are exempted.

The program is financed entirely by employers, except for three states, by a payroll tax that is placed in a special trust fund in each state. The tax rate and wage base may vary from state to state, but the federal program levies a 3.5 percent tax on the first $7,000 of nonexempt wages for each employee (as of 1984). However, the firm will receive credit against the federal tax liability for all the tax it pays the state fund up to 2.7 percent—or up to the full federal liability if the state program conforms to the federal program. Not all firms have the same rate because each firm's rate is computed on its *experience rating,* i.e., the lower the unemployment or lay off rate, the lower the tax rate. Thus the program encourages efforts toward stable employment. Also, the firm is allowed the full 2.7 percent tax credit, if its state tax rate is less than 2.7 percent, because of a good experience rating.

The maximum benefit usually will range between 40 percent (sometimes less) and 50 percent (sometimes more) of the average weekly wage of the employee up to 26 weeks. The employee must meet four tests to qualify: established record of employment and earnings, must be willing to work, be actively seeking employment, and not have voluntarily stopped working.

The pharmacist-manager can establish a good experience rating by: (1) not hiring people on temporary basis unless absolutely necessary, (2) establishing a permanent but fexible work group in terms of trade-offs in work schedules, jobs and a "helping spirit,"(3) assisting a former employee to find a job before or soon after a layoff, (4) maintaining good records of performance evaluation, grievances, absenteeism and similar events, (5) projecting ahead for labor needs, and (6) vigorously protesting unwarranted unemployment claims.

Sixth, pharmacies are subject to workman's compensation laws. This program generally parallels the unemployment insurance program, but with less federal involvement. In most states the state program is compulsory, but in those states where participation in the state program is voluntary, the firm must carry insurance for disability that is work related. The latter approach is unwise because the firm is not automatically protected from damage suits as is the case with the state program. The state program is based on the assumption that the injury was unintentional; employers pay the entire cost and receives limited liability. The tax for any given firm is based on his injury record. Again, this program encourages safety and accident prevention programs.

Although the program varies from state to state, all programs cover five major categories of costs:

1. *Medical expenses* (hospital, surgical, physician's services, drugs and related costs).
2. For *permanent and total disability,* weekly income for life (or at least an extended period of 300 to 500 weeks) that generally will range between 50 to 75 percent of prior weekly earnings with a minimum and maximum income.
3. For *temporary but total disability,* same as above for a period of 208 to 500 weeks.
4. For *permanent but partial disability,* provides a lump sum of money according to a schedule for loss of a limb or other body member.
5. *Survivors benefit,* provides a weekly income for the surviving spouse and children up to a prescribed age plus a lump sum to cover burial expenses.

Some six states have a similar mandatory program to cover disabilities caused by off-the-job injuries or illnesses that are not covered by workman's compensation.

Recently, Congress passed the Employee Retirement Income Security Act (ERISA) to provide standards for retirement and pension programs.

Summary

The importance of good personnel cannot be overemphasized. Although purchases represent the largest expenditure, they are an investment that can be recovered if the purchases have been restricted to salable goods. Payroll is the second largest expenditure and the largest single expense item in a typical pharmacy. In contrast to inventory investment, money spent on payroll is gone forever once the checks are written. Only through efficient and effective employees can one hope to reap a return from the money spent on other expenditures and to achieve business and professional objectives. All phases of employee administration are important, including selection, pleasant working conditions, supervision, compensation, and motivation. A wise proprietor or manager will do well to practice good personnel management.

REFERENCES

1. Deiner, C.H.: *The Lilly Digest 1984, Community Pharmacy Operations for 1983.* Indianapolis: Eli Lilly and Co.
2. Deiner, C.H.: *1984 NACDS-Lilly Digest for 1983.* Indianapolis: Eli Lilly and Co.
3. Deiner, C.H.: *Lilly Hospital Pharmacy Survey 1984.* Indianapolis: Eli Lilly and Co.
4. Huffman, D.C., Jr.: The feasibility of modern managerial systems and innovative profes-

sional services in a community pharmacy: a case study. Doctoral Dissertation, The University of Mississippi, January, 1971.

5. Huffman, D.C., Jr. and Smith, H.A.: *Building a Successful Pharmacy Practice: A Case Study.* Memphis: American College of Apothecaries, 1972.

6. Kitler, M., and Lamey, P.: Statistics in hospital pharmacy. *Hosp. Pharm.* 4:17–21, 1969.

7. NACDS *Executive Newsletter,* July 16, 1973.

8. Eiler, L.E., et al: *Policies and Operational Procedures for Community Pharmacy Managers.* Memphis: American College of Apothecaries, 1972.

9. Peter, L.J.: *The Peter Principle.* New York: William Morrow & Co., 1969.

10. Peter, L.J.: *The Peter Prescription.* New York: William Morrow & Co., 1972.

REVIEW

1. Discuss the three reasons for emphasizing the importance of personnel administration.

2. Discuss the application of management by objectives to personnel relations, especially supervision, by relating the benefits accruing to both employees and the organization.

3. What are the six principles of good personnel administration?

4. Discuss the six major aspects of personnel administration procedures.

5. Discuss the theory and the rationale underlying the queuing theory model.

6. For various average prescription arrivals—5, 7, 11, 14, 18 and 20—calculate the total cost of service and waiting and select the most economic staffing pattern.

7. Define and differentiate between job analysis, job description, and job specification.

8. Describe the four steps in the employee selecting process.

9. Explain why the selection process is so critical.

10. Explain the "halo" and "horn" effects and how these influence the selection process.

11. Explain the purpose, importance and basic objectives of orientation of a new employee in a pharmacy.

12. Distinguish between training and educating as it relates to employees in a pharmacy.

13. Distinguish between the two types of training methods.

14. Outline the steps of on-the-job training.

15. Discuss the purpose and use of the conference in employee training and development.

16. Discuss the importance and the role of supervision.

17. Explain the importance of motivation and why motivation is the most difficult aspect of employee relations.

18. Name the primary methods of evaluating employees, and contrast the two in terms of objectivity, value, and difficulty of implementation.

19. Which of the above means of employee evaluation is better adapted to a system of management by objectives?

20. What are the eight principles of employee evaluation?

21. What are the four methods of employee compensation and the relative merits and disadvantages of each?

22. Discuss the relationship between MBO and good personnel administration.

23. Discuss the basis for the antidiscrimination and safety and health law.

24. Discuss the purpose and requirements of the Wage and Hour Law, the FICA and the Workman's Compensation Law.

25. Discuss the philosophy, purpose, requirements and financing of the Unemployment Insurance Act.

DIRECTING

Directing is the one managerial function that most closely approximates the term managing. As used in the management context, directing is the function of management that is a continuous process. In contrast, planning or organizing are more of a continuing process with greater emphasis given to each of the functions at various stages, especially the early stages of a firm. This is not meant to indicate or imply that either planning or organizing is not performed throughout the life of the firm. The influence of planning and organizing is continuous, but the effort given to these functions is intermittent. Based on these definitions, we have included chapters on purchasing, inventory control, pricing, pharmaceutical services and patronage, and promotion/merchandising within this section. As indicated in the introduction to the organizing section, personnel administration has various components that are directing in nature, but we chose to include the chapter on personnel in the previous section. There is some functional overlapping between this section and the control section, which will be considered in the introduction to that section.

13 | Purchasing

Good purchasing policies and inventory control are closely interrelated because one cannot be effective without the other. Without the information provided by some type of inventory control system, it is difficult to buy the correct quantities. Conversely, inventory control procedures are of little value unless the information generated is used to determine appropriate quantities to buy. The best policy is to reinforce good purchasing policies and procedures with a good inventory control system, the subject of Chapter 14.

There is an old saying among retailers, including pharmacists, "goods well bought are half sold." Certainly there is much validity in this saying, and pharmacists who neglect the buying function operate under a severe handicap. An extension of this saying is that goods not well purchased cannot be profitably sold. There is another old saying among retailers and pharmacists as well that says "you buy yourself poor and sell yourself rich." Certainly a balance between these two points of view is the best policy.

The *specific functions of purchasing* are: (1) formulating effective buying policies; (2) determining the demands or desires of the patrons; (3) selecting the best sources of supply; (4) determining and negotiating the terms of purchase; (5) receiving, marking, and stocking merchandise; and (6) transferring the title of the goods, including payment in time to receive maximum discounts.

Formulating Effective Buying Policies

There are *three basic considerations* in formulating buying policies.

1. Buying policies should be *compatible with the general objectives of the pharmacy,* which, in turn, are determined largely by the type of pharmacy and location. For example, a pharmaceutical center stocks fewer merchandise lines, and probably a lesser assortment of merchandise in each line, than a traditional pharmacy. Similarly a traditional pharmacy carries fewer merchandise lines, and a lesser assortment within each line, than a super drugstore. Pharmaceutical companies normally close their books a few days before the end of the month, and the efficient manager places monthly orders just in

time for them to arrive at the manufacturer's office on the first day or so of each new discount period.

2. *Needs and desires of the patrons* must be recognized. Obviously, there is an interrelationship between these two basic considerations. The type of pharmacy practice has a substantial influence on the patrons it attracts. The needs and desires of the patrons in a particular market should be the basis for establishing a particular type of pharmacy. The buying policies should reflect basic changes in demographic factors such as age distribution, young families with children, and purchase preference and buying habits caused by both demographic and economic factors.

3. The manager should select, based on experience and research, one primary drug wholesaler as the *primary source of supply.* This will provide efficiency and lower merchandise cost by concentrating the bulk of the purchases from one source. One other drug wholesaler, two in some situations, should be utilized to provide another source whenever the primary source is out-of-stock or does not carry the item. Sufficient trade should be given to the secondary source to keep him interested in your business. The primary source should not be selected on price alone, although that should be the single most important criterion. Other criteria should include promptness in delivery, frequency of delivery (although this can be overdone for optimum efficiency and total costs, which is discussed in the next chapter), return goods policy, frequency of out-of-stock situations, breadth of merchandise lines and assortment, and all around good service relations. The utilization of direct accounts with manufacturers should be carefully scrutinized to be sure each such account is more profitable than the primary source. Again, price alone (discounts) is not the only criterion; order quantity and turnover must be considered within the parameters of good inventory control system.

Determining the Needs and Desires of Patrons

The needs and demands of patrons of a pharmaceutical center or apothecary shop are determined primarily by the prescriber's preferences, which in turn are determined by the prevalence of disease entities, the drugs available to treat these diseases, and the promotional efforts of the producers of these drugs. However, it remains for the proprietor or manager to determine whether certain needs, such as home health care aids and surgical appliances, are to be met. The latter consideration has more relevancy for the traditional pharmacy that stocks rather wide assortments and lines of merchandise, and is even more significant to the super merchandising pharmacy.

Where does the proprietor or manager of a pharmacy find the information on kinds, types, and prices of goods his patrons and potential patrons want? The primary sources are outlined below:[1]

A. Inside sources (in the pharmacy)
    1. Past sale trends by departments and/or lines

2. Returned goods and adjustment data
3. Patrons' inquiries—want slip or want book
4. Suggestions of employees
B. Outside sources
   1. Salesmen's offerings and suggestions
   2. Trade journals and magazines
   3. Survey of patrons' desires and needs
   4. National and local advertisements of manufacturers
   5. Offerings of other pharmacies
   6. Visits to large merchandise marts

Selecting the Sources of Supply

There are basically two kinds of sources of supply, *direct* and *indirect* through either a wholesaler or jobber. A jobber is a wholesaler with limited services and usually limited lines. Before discussing the obvious advantages and disadvantages of each source of supply, we should consider certain similarities and basic marketing functions. These similarities can best be described within the framework of the basic *marketing functions,* which are outlined below.
A. Exchange function
   1. Buying
   2. Selling
B. Physical supply function
   1. Storage
   2. Transportation
C. Facilitating or Ancillary functions
   1. Standardization and grading of products
   2. Financing
   3. Risk-bearing
   4. Market information and research, and related service

UNIVERSALITY OF MARKETING FUNCTIONS

Careful consideration of the above functions points to the fact that all of these functions must be performed, if not by the wholesaler, then by either the manufacturer or the pharmacy. This concept is known as the universality of marketing functions. For example, if a manufacturer decides to do all of its marketing, including functions normally performed by the wholesaler, either the manufacturer or the pharmacy must provide additional storage space and pay for the transportation, and the manufacturer must provide a salesman who, in turn, provides the information about the goods offered for sale. Either the manufacturer or the pharmacy must absorb the cost of these functions. Unless there are economies of scale or other economic efficiencies, the only marketing cost that can always be avoided by direct selling is the pure net profit, or risk cost of the middleman or wholesaler.

In contrast, the wholesaler provides the intrinsic role of a middleman by which inherent economies accrue to society. The middleman role encompasses three related concepts: minimum total transactions, sorting, and market proximity.

MINIMUM TOTAL TRANSACTIONS

This term is used to describe the reduction of the actual number of transactions involving many sellers (manufacturers) and many buyers (pharmacies). This concept can be explained best by an illustration: If each of 1,000 manufacturers were to process one order for each of 50,000 pharmacies each month—a situation that would not be conducive to best inventory management because of out-of-stock situations and possible overstocking—the total number of annual transactions would be 600,000,000.[2]

$$\underset{\text{(pharmacies)}}{50,000} \times \underset{\text{(manufacturers)}}{1,000} \times \underset{\text{(months)}}{12} = \underset{\text{(no. of annual transactions)}}{600,000,000}$$

If, on the other hand, we assume there were 250 drug wholesalers who ordered weekly from the 1,000 manufacturers and who, in turn, made daily sales to their "share" of pharmacy customers for 255 working days a year, the total number of transactions would be 25,750,000.

$$\underset{\text{(wholesalers)}}{250} \times \underset{\text{(manufacturers)}}{1,000} \times \underset{\text{(weeks)}}{52} = 13,000,000$$

$$\underset{\text{(wholesalers)}}{250} \times \underset{\text{(pharmacies per wholesaler)}}{200} \times \underset{\text{(days)}}{255} = +12,750,000$$

$$\text{Total annual transactions} = 25,750,000$$

The number of annual transactions can be reduced to almost 4 percent of the original number with the use of the pharmaceutical wholesalers. If we assume that on the average each of the 200 pharmacies will order from two drug wholesalers (255 days/year) and from 15 manufacturers monthly—a more realistic assumption—the total number of annual transactions would be approximately 60,500,000, or approximately 10 percent of the number of annual transactions without the use of wholesalers. This means a reduction in the cost of billing, bookkeeping and freight, and in the number of errors in billing.

SORTING

Sorting is a marketing term composed of two elements or activities, *concentration* and *dispersion*. This is basically what the wholesaler does. He buys from thousands of suppliers in relatively large quantities. He may buy from several to many gross of a product at much lower distribution cost than could an individual pharmacy. The wholesaler, in turn, may sell only one or a few units of a product to a pharmacy at a given time, but he combines this order with other items, perhaps one to several dozen products, and again economizes in the distribution process. The distribution cost would be tremendous if each pharmacy had to purchase all of its products directly from the manufacturers.

MARKET PROXIMITY

This marketing concept simply means being near to the final market. Market proximity is certainly true of drug wholesalers, and has obvious advantages in providing product and market information faster, more frequent deliveries, and an all-around closer working relationship with customers.

All three of these concepts—minimum number of total annual transactions, sorting, and proximity—are interrelated, and together they permit the wholesaler-middleman to perform his unique role.

To better understand the role of the wholesaler-middleman, the marketing concept, *utility,* which largely is the result of the market proximity, will be briefly described. There are four types of utility, viz, *time, place, possession,* and *form utility.* The latter is the result of production or manufacturing, which does not concern us here. The first three types are the result of marketing activities. Simply stated, time, place, and possession utility is defined as providing the right good at the right time to the right person at the right place. Dispensing prescriptions is a special, professional case of marketing utility. Of course, the proper dispensing of a prescription includes much more—the correct directions, checking for appropriate dosages and possible drug interactions, and consultation with the patient. Even these activities fall within the marketing function of market information and related services. Thus, the pharmacist assumes a unique professional as well as marketing role.

SERVICES OF DRUG WHOLESALERS

According to Fay,[3] the pharmaceutical wholesaler provides 13 specific services to pharmacies. Unlike the 15 traditional services enumerated by Smith[4] in 1975, the services described by Fay[3] are related to management information systems and are derived from computerized data systems. In addition to the 13 management services, drug wholesalers still provide the following four basic, traditional services:

Assembly of Goods. The wholesaler has at his disposal trained and experienced buyers who can, and do, purchase and maintain extensive inventories in knowledgeable anticipation of the pharmacist's needs.

Delivery. Not only is regular delivery service available, but traditionally the members of the NWDA maintained separate, more frequent delivery schedules for prescription drugs.[5]

Credit. The value of credit to retailers has already been explored in a

Table 13–1.   Factors Related to Sources of Supply

	Purchased From	
Item	*Manufacturer*	*Wholesaler*
Inventory size	Larger	Smaller
Turnover rate	Less	Greater
Delivery	Slower; less frequent	Faster; more frequent
Return of goods	More difficult	Less difficult
Availability of goods	Only source for certain lines	Only source for certain lines theoretically
Time involved in ordering	More overall	Less overall
Product information	More complete; possible bias	Less complete; less bias
Available credit	Readily in most cases	Readily if not in default
Cost of handling	More	Less
Cost of product	Lower in some cases	Higher in some cases

previous chapter. This simply means an expansion of working capital for the pharmacist.

Special Services. The pharmaceutical wholesaler has historically provided, free of charge, a number of services to the community pharmacist which are only indirectly related to the product itself. Past and present services of this type include: prescription drug information services, store layout and design, store modernization, location analysis, and traffic-flow analysis in addition to the 13 computerized management services.

DIRECT VERSUS INDIRECT PURCHASING

Table 13–1 compares the advantages and disadvantages of purchasing from the pharmaceutical wholesaler or directly from the manufacturer under normal conditions.

To select the best source of supply one needs to assess all the advantages and disadvantages. If the saving in extra discounts warrants direct purchasing, it is wise to buy in this way. This decision can be made with greater accuracy after studying the economic order quantity phase of inventory control. In general, the typical pharmacy can purchase advantageously from about 10 prescription drug manufacturers and about the same number of "out front" manufacturers, including the franchise lines. The remainder of the products should be purchased from one wholesaler primarily, using a second "back-up" wholesaler in servicing your pharmacy as needed.

Because of the competitive resilience of drug wholesalers, there has been a remarkable turnabout in the market position of the wholesale drug industry. Beginning in 1974, a long-term decline in the market share of prescription drugs was reversed with an average annual increase of 1.4 percent in market share. Between 1973 and 1980, sales increased 103 percent. During this period, gross margin percent decreased from 13.67 percent to 11.22 percent, but operating costs were decreased even more, from 11.84 percent to 8.60 percent. The net result was an increase in net profit from 1.83 percent of sales to 2.62 percent, a 43 percent increase.[3] Drug wholesalers lowered the prices of drugs while increasing their net profits by utilizing new technology, primarily the computer.

Because of these shifts, there is less need, and less effort being expended in developing purchasing coops. However, there is still a real need for independents to combine their resources, as discussed in Chapter 8, in order to be competitive with the chains and remain a viable institution. Because of these shifts, there is less need to form coops for the purpose of purchasing only; therefore, the following section on cooperative buying groups should be viewed with this reservation in mind. There is a *real need* for a better *integrated financial structure for independent pharmacies* even more than an integrated marketing structure via wholesale relationships or buying co-ops.

COOPERATIVE BUYING GROUPS

Another source of supply, which was popular in the recent past, is the cooperative buying group. Competition and the profit squeeze have caused pharmacists to forego some of their independence and form buying groups to survive. Some of these groups have been initiated by drug wholesalers, others by pharmacists. Some restrict their cooperative efforts to buying whereas others include promotion and advertising.

The increasing importance of cooperative buying groups in pharmacy, and even the greater potential they offer the independent practice of pharmacy, warrant more than a passing view of this development. The following discussion of cooperative buying groups is based, in part, on a paper by George Grider.[6]

For several decades the drug trade literature and drug wholesale houses have been discussing the problems and dark future of the independent pharmacist. For several years the National Wholesale Druggists Association (NWDA) has told the drug wholesaler to develop voluntary chains for the community pharmacist.

In 1978, McKesson purchased a small coop of 20 pharmacies with the trade name, VALU-RITE and has expanded the coop to over 2,000 participating pharmacies in 1982 with a projected number of 4,000 by 1986. In 1981, Bergen Brunswig and 10 other independent drug wholesalers started another coop with the designation Family Value Drug Centers. There were 20 participating pharmacies initially. The Foxmeyer Co. has established a coop that is a hybrid between a wholesale sponsored coop and a franchise system with the name, Health Mart. The program has the following four basic functions: (1) purchases at competitive prices, (2) cooperative advertising, (3) pricing of merchandising that is competitive in the respective market, and (4) financial analyses. Foxmeyer emphasizes the latter two functions in the context of management support service. They serviced about 300 members in 1985. These types of programs are a big boost to independent pharmacies, but they fall short of the potential "financial muscle" that is available in a fully integrated financial and market plan described in Chapter 8.

The independent retail grocery co-op chain and the wholesaler-directed voluntary chain of independent grocery stores realize a large 50 percent of the retail food dollar volume today, whereas 30 years ago they were selling only 30 percent of the retail food volume in this country. They are providing their members with lower prices through group buying and furnishing them an advertising program. Thirty years ago the independent grocery stores were at a crossroad similar to that of community pharmacies today; food chains were rapidly forcing the independent grocery stores out of business, just as the chain drugstores are making it difficult for the community pharmacy to compete in the marketplace today.

Today drug wholesalers are merging, computerizing, offering recordkeeping and inventory control service, push-button and scanning ordering service, line extension discounts, and across-the-board special discounts to some pharmacies. If the number of community pharmacies continues to decline at the present rate, the drug wholesaler's computer service, push-button ordering service, bookkeeping and inventory control service, and line extension discounts may be of little use.

Some say the pharmacist is too independent and will not join with his fellow pharmacist to form a buying group or voluntary chain. However, there are hundreds of community pharmacies that are members of buying groups and advertising groups, including McKesson and Robbins Economost, a computerized accounting and inventory service as well as a buying and advertising group; Rite-Way Discount System, a Chicago-based advertising and marketing firm; Leader Advertising Group in the Cleveland area; and Kentucky Drug Stores, a buying and advertising group in Kentucky.

The purpose of a pharmacy buying group is to promote the economic welfare of independent community pharmacies by utilizing their united efforts for efficient and economical distribution through buying and advertising of products sold in the members' pharmacies. In plain language, it is a large number of pharmacies combining their purchases in order to buy merchandise at the lowest possible price for each member. This is accomplished through a membership organization that may be either a stock corporation or a nonprofit corporation.

The next logical question is: how can pharmacists organize a buying group? Following is a brief discussion of how the Kentucky Drug Stores buying group was organized. Originally, five pharmacy owners formed a nonprofit corporation and this corporation contracted with Kentucky Food Stores, a Lexington-based grocery buying group of 105 members, to purchase, warehouse, and deliver merchandise to their pharmacies. Next, a manager was selected who had several years of experience as a salesman for a major drug wholesale company and five years of experience in pharmacy layout and design. His job was to help the group to increase its membership and set up the warehouse operation. He was paid a good salary, absolutely necessary if the buying group is going to be successful. The manager for the Drug Store Division was placed in charge of the buying and warehouse operation of the Drug Division and fixture installation for both the drug and grocery divisions. The Kentucky Food Stores' warehouse stocked all types of drugstore merchandise except prescription legend drugs. A contract was negotiated with a full-line drug wholesaler to supply the member pharmacies with prescription legend drugs and other merchandise that was not stocked in the Kentucky Food Stores. A full-service drug wholesaler could do it as well or better.

The price of merchandise is the same to each member and is calculated by using actual cost of the merchandise, plus 5 percent operational and warehouse cost, plus 3 percent for transportation. To reduce the net cost of merchandise and operational cost, Kentucky Drug Stores and Kentucky Food Stores buy merchandise and warehouse and deliver it on an integrated basis. Pharmacy members order once a week and pay for the merchandise the following week. A computer system of purchasing, invoicing, and billing is used for both divisions. An advertising specialist serves both groups on a combined contractual basis for developing advertising, printing of handbills, and painting of purchase and window signs.

To finance the pharmacy buying group, each member bought $3,000.00 in Kentucky Drug Stores stock. There are no monthly dues or initiation fees. If a member sells his pharmacy or desires to leave the buying group, Kentucky Drug Stores will buy his stock in the corporation and pay him the original purchase price.

Economics was the basic reason the Kentucky Drug Stores co-op group joined the Kentucky Food Stores. Since Kentucky Food Stores already had an organization, a warehouse, delivery trucks, a computer, and expertise in cooperative group buying, it was patently uneconomical to duplicate these facilities. The Kentucky Food Stores group was happy to have the Kentucky Drug Stores group join them, because this increased their efficiency and productivity simply through economy of scale. The joint venture reduced the initial investment and risk for Kentucky Drug Stores.

Mr. Goodwin Rosen, managing director of National Drug Cooperatives Associated, an organization of drug cooperatives, franchises, voluntary chains, and wholesalers from coast to coast, states that the only way for the independent community pharmacy to compete with the chain drugstores is to belong to a buying group or a wholesaler sponsored co-op. Mr. Rosen's organization is composed of 13 cooperative groups in various parts of the country, representing 1,650 independently owned pharmacies.

According to Mr. Rosen, some of the advantages of buying groups are as follows: (1) maximum discounts available through quantity buying; (2) advertising and promotional programs at a much lower cost; (3) special merchandise shows provided for members; (4) the remodeling and installation of pharmacies at savings from 40 to 50 percent; (5) exchange of ideas among members; (6) consulting service providing new methods and techniques of pharmacy operation, in such areas as inventory control, management, financing, individual advertising and promotions, and sales schools for clerks; (7) computer service provided for individual members; and (8) development of a group logo for advertising and pharmacy identification, while the individual member retains his individual pharmacy name.

Because of the essential role of drug wholesalers, I feel that pharmacists and drug wholesalers must work closely with one another in the future when establishing any type of coop arrangement, in order for both groups to survive. Chain pharmacies now do 60 percent or more of the total drug and "other drugstore" sales, and the trend is increasing rapidly. Bold action is required to reduce this trend or to reverse it.

Members of the American College of Apothecaries (ACA) have established a private label program of high quality generic prescription drugs and selective O-T-C drugs. Members of the American Society of Consultant Pharmacists have organized a purchasing coop group for selected high volume prescription drugs. These are other measures to attempt to be competitive.

SPECIALTY WHOLESALERS

There are other sources of supply that nearly all pharmacists use, depending on the scope of the operation. These are the speciality wholesalers, usually relatively small wholesalers dealing in a limited line of merchandise, but with wide assortments within these lines. Sometimes special services, especially assistance in inventory control, are provided. Examples include veterinary drug wholesalers, tobacco or tobacco and confectionary wholesalers, costume jewelry and gift merchandise wholesalers, suppliers of photography equipment, and leather goods wholesalers. These specialty wholesalers can be of tremendous assistance in the development of special skills departments within a pharmacy.

Determining the Terms of Purchase

The terms of purchase include several important items that are not as generally known as they should be. The significance of the terms is too frequently taken for granted until some misunderstanding develops. The major points in terms of sale include discounts of various kinds, the date payment is due, policy on credit extension, and return of goods policy.

Manufacturers' catalogues contain this information, usually in the front portion of the catalogue. Pharmaceutical wholesalers make this information readily available on request. Invoices contain a large portion of this information as a formal part of the sales contract. In this respect, each transaction, whether a $500 drug order or the sale of a ten cent bar of candy, is a sales contract, and every written, spoken, or *implied* bit of information that has any bearing on the consummation of the sale is a part of a binding contract. Specifications for generic drugs are a part of the terms of the purchase.

DISCOUNTS

Discounts are probably the most frequently discussed aspect of the terms of a sale. Buyers are constantly wanting larger discounts. This is natural and commendable; however, buying the right merchandise that will sell, or the proper quantity of merchandise, can be much more important than a large discount or lower price.

Trade Discounts. There are several kinds of discounts, and each should be understood in terms of its intended purpose. The *trade* (or *functional*) *discount* is given to a firm for performing a level or set of marketing activities. Wholesaling and retailing are examples of marketing levels. The trade discount is not well understood because it is not used directly as frequently as the other types. The trade discount is based on a base line figure known as the *list price,* which is falling into disuse. Some firms use a list price that corresponds to the "suggested" retail or consumer price, while others use what is called a wholesale list price, which confuses the matter. The choice of the type of list price used depends partly on the custom of a particular company and the policy of favoring direct buying by the pharmacist or selling through the wholesaler. A trade discount for a drug wholesaler normally ranges from 15 to 20 percent; for a pharmacy it ranges from 30 to 50 percent. An illustration will explain the two approaches:

Company A sells only through a wholesaler. The catalogue for a drug in a bottle of 100 tablets shows a "retail list" price of $10.00. The pharmacy is given a trade discount of 40 percent and the wholesaler a trade discount of 20 percent. The pharmacist pays the wholesaler $6.00 per hundred [$10.00 − (.40 × $10.00)]. The wholesaler pays the manufacturer $4.80 [$6.00 − (.20 × $6.00)].

In contrast, Company B has a direct selling policy. For a similar drug, costing about the same to manufacture and to market, the company's catalogue shows a "wholesale list" price of $7.00, with a "direct purchase" discount of 15 percent. The pharmacist can buy the drug for $5.95 per hundred [$7.00 − (.15 × $7.00)]. The wholesaler can buy the same drug at a 20 percent "wholesaler's" discount for $5.60 [$7.00 − (.20 × $7.00)]. The wholesaler has to sell the drug to the pharmacist for $6.10 just to break even or make a very small profit. The operational cost of a full-line drug wholesaler ranges from eight to ten percent of sales. The economic pressure for the pharmacist to buy direct from Company B is obvious. Trade discounts generally are exclusive of other types of discounts.

Quantity Discounts. Quantity discounts are given when a designated quantity is purchased at one time or when a cumulative dollar volume is purchased over a specified period of time, usually one year. The discount normally ranges from 5 to 20 percent of a base line or quoted "list" price. These discounts are offered to both wholesalers and retailers and are based on economies of larger purchases. Sometimes the discount is given in the form of "free" goods. Often the discounts that include "free" goods and "deals" are misleading. A few examples of the various kinds of quantity discounts will illustrate and explain how they differ and are used in practice.

The most frequent type of quantity discount is a percentage discount from the regular price extended for the purchase of a larger single order. For example, a product that normally sells wholesale at $6.00 a dozen may be offered at $6.00 per dozen less 10 percent in quantities of five dozen. Thus the unit cost is $.45 rather than the usual $.50. Again, the cash discount is not considered here, and often the quantity discount will be inclusive of the usual cash discount. If this were the case in the foregoing example, the actual quantity discount would be less than 10 percent, approximately 8 percent. Sometimes the quantity discount is offered if a designated dollar amount is ordered for an assortment of different products from the same manufacturer. For example, a 5 percent quantity discount on a $50.00 order or a 10 percent discount on a $125.00 order is typical.

Some direct-selling pharmaceutical manufacturers provide a quantity discount during an ensuing year provided a quota was met the previous year. The discount may be 5 to 10 percent in addition to the usual 15 percent "trade" discount for direct accounts. As with all discounts in a series, one does not add the 5 percent to the 15 percent to arrive at an overall 20 percent discount. The basic 15 percent discount is first deducted, then the 5 percent discount is deducted. For example, on a $100 order the pharmacist first deducts $15 ($100 × .15) from the $100 and obtains the difference, $85. Next, the pharmacist subtracts $4.25 ($85 × .05) from $85.00 to obtain the net cost of $80.75, if there is no additional cash discount. The terms of sale indicate whether the 5 percent quantity discount includes the cash discount.

A variation of the above example is sometimes used by companies with a wide variety of drugs—some that are not profitable, such as biologicals, some that are very popular with a high turnover rate, and some that are fairly popular, but with a slower turnover rate. These types of products would be classified at A, B, and C with quantity discounts of 5, 10, and 15 percent, respectively.

The "free" goods or "deal" discount can be misleading, as stated previously. A typical example is a 10 percent quantity discount, including the cash discount, plus four "free" bottles of a four-ounce size of cough syrup with the purchase of one dozen of the four-ounce size and one-half dozen of the eight-ounce size. The eight-ounce size sells for $1.69 each and normally costs $1.13 each. The four-ounce size sells for $.98 and normally costs $.65 each. The regular cost of the dozen four-ounce size is $7.80 and the half dozen eight-ounce costs $6.78 for a total of $14.58. The quantity discount is $1.46, giving a net cost of $13.12. The total sales for the entire deal, provided all units are sold, are $25.82, providing a gross margin of $12.70 or 49.2 percent.

Too frequently the advertisement of the "deal" indicates a discount of $1.46 plus $3.92, the retail value of the four free bottles. The total quantity discount is stated as $5.38, or 36.9 percent, off the regular cost of $14.58 for the dozen of the four-ounce size and the half dozen of the eight-ounce size. This is misleading on two accounts. First, the free goods should be valued at the regular wholesale cost and not at the retail value. Second, the free goods should not be considered a discount until they have been sold. If, for example, two of the four free bottles are never sold, the effective extra discount would be $1.30, and the total *effective* quantity discount would be $2.76, or 18.9 percent, off the regular wholesale price.

Cash Discounts. The cash discount is the smallest discount of all, but it is the most important one. A cash discount is given to a buyer for payment within a time period specified on the invoice or statement. The discount is normally 1 or 2 percent of the regular or *net* amount of the invoice or statement. Note that *net* refers to the amount paid after the designated time period before calculating the cash discount.

The importance of the cash discount can be explained best by an illustration. Suppose a pharmacist finds himself in a financial position in which he is unable to pay his statements for merchandise in time to earn the cash discount. Further assume that the pharmacist purchases $10,000 worth of goods each month. The cash discount rate is 2 percent. Under these conditions, he will lose $2,400 over the entire year. This loss can be prevented by borrowing $10,000 from the bank at 10 percent interest. The $1,000 interest, subtracted from the $2,400 gained in cash discounts, yields $1,400 additional profit. If the pharmacy is being managed appropriately in other respects, it should yield approximately $10,000 normal net profit on an annual sales volume of $225,000. The $1,400 additional profit from cash discounts represents a 14 percent increase in the normal net profit of the pharmacy.

The pharmacist can fare even better than this, provided he has both the financial status and expertise to utilize the financial or money market to its fullest extent. Of course, he would have to have an excellent credit rating and be known as a "prime risk debtor" among financial institutions, a reputation he is not likely to enjoy since he is unable to pay his bills. However, for the sake of students' and practitioners' edification, let us assume these possibilities and determine their net effect. Since the pharmacist normally has until the tenth of the month following the month the goods were purchased to earn the cash discount, he could borrow the $10,000 for 20 days at 10 percent. The interest charges would be only $55.55 for the 20-day period ($10,000 × .10 ÷ 360 days × 20 days = $55.55). If the pharmacist astutely generates sufficient cash from cash sales, collecting accounts receivable, and perhaps reducing inventory levels to pay the $55.55 interest charge and 10 percent of the principal, he possibly could have this note renewed on a 20-day basis. This would result in the liquidation of the debt in ten months at a cost of only $555.55 interest charge.

Let us hasten to warn that the typical pharmacist who has gotten behind in paying his invoices is not likely to receive such favorable treatment in the money market. However, a successful pharmacy, a solvent cooperative buying group, or a chain of drugstores that found itself in a temporary, nonrecurring position of not being able to take the cash discounts could well take advantage of a short-term 20-day loan and yield a handsome return for its effort. Students should also realize that the interest rate has varied between 8 and 20 percent over the past several years.

Serial Discounts. The term "serial discounts" is used occasionally in explicit language and frequently in an implicit manner. Students and practitioners should know the manner in which such discounts are computed. Some trades use the term as such and state them as 50, 20, and 5. More often in pharmacy, the series is implied and typically will be 40 percent (trade discount), 10 percent (quantity discount), and 2 percent (cash discount). In *neither* case are the discounts *added* and then multiplied by the amount of the invoice. Rather they are multiplied and subtracted in steps, beginning with the largest discount, which is usually listed first. An illustration will explain how serial discounts are computed.

Step 1. $500.00—Net amount of invoice at retail list
           × .40—Trade discount as decimal
           $200.00—Allowance for trade function

Step 2. $500.00
           − 200.00
           $300.00
           × .10—Quantity discount
           $ 30.00—Allowance for quantity purchased

Step 3. $300.00
           − 30.00
           $270.00
           × .02—Cash discount
           $ 5.40—Allowance for paying invoice by specified time

Step 4. $270.00
           − 5.40
           $264.60—The amount the pharmacist pays

DATINGS AND CREDIT TERMS

There are a number of terms and notations that pertain to the delivery of goods, date of payment and cash discounts. Collectively, these are usually referred to as "datings." Following are the more common terms with definitions. The last definition is the most common set of cash and dating terms encountered in pharmacy.

AOG or ROG   Arrival of goods or receipt of goods
COD   Collect on delivery

EOM	End of the month
FOB; FOB (city)	Free on board; free on board at designated city
N	Pay the net or full amount
N/30	Pay net 30 days from date of invoice
N/10 EOM	Pay net within 10 days after the end of the month
2/10, N/30	Deduct 2 percent within 10 days after invoice date; otherwise pay net within 30 days after the invoice date
2/10 ROG, N/30	Deduct 2 percent within 10 days after receipt of goods; otherwise pay net within 30 days after receipt of goods
2/10 EOM c̄ 60 extra	Deduct 2 percent within 70 days after the end of the month in which the goods were purchased
2/10 EOM, N/30	Deduct 2 percent cash discount if paid within 10 days after the end of the month; otherwise pay net within 30 days after the end of the month.

RETURN GOODS POLICY

Another important sales term is the return goods policy. The pharmaceutical industry is generous in this respect. Most company catalogues contain a statement on the return of goods in front of the catalogue as a part of the general statement on policies, credit terms, and the like. There are limitations placed on the return of goods, the most common being broken packages (i.e., a part of the contents has been used); mishandling of stored goods, and a time limitation for credit, usually five years, but this varies with the company. Each pharmacy should have a new product section in the prescription department, and this should be checked weekly. If a new product has not been used in three or four months, it should be returned for credit. To maintain an orderly and efficient goods return system, each pharmacy should build a series of small bins in the stock room with each labeled for the respective manufacturer and wholesaler from whom the goods were purchased. All return goods—wrong merchandise, wrong size, damaged, or nonsalable—should be placed in the appropriate bin, and a list maintained of these items.

Receiving, Marking, and Stocking Goods

This aspect of purchasing may seem to be ordinary and not too important, but this is not the case at all. Each invoice should be checked for the appropriateness, both quality and quantity of the merchandise, the terms of the sale, and the accuracy of the extension of the cost (number of units multiplied by the unit cost). Then goods should be marked appropriately. The latter should include the cost per unit (in code), the source, the date, and quantity received. Then the merchandise is placed on the shelf or display with new, fresher products placed behind the older products.

There are hundreds of *cost codes*. Only two will be indicated, one a letter code, the other a simple system of straight lines in two directions. The first, the best known of all cost codes, is an aberration of the spelling of pharmacist.

P H A R M O C I S T
1 2 3 4 5 6 7 8 9 0

(It should be noted that this code is not, and probably never was, the official code of the NARD.)

The second code uses a vertical line for zero, a horizontal line attached but extending to the right to represent one (L), and extending to the left to represent two (⌐), and so on as follows:

L ⌐ ⌐ ⌐ ⌐ ⊥ ∃ ∃ ∃ |
1 2 3 4 5 6 7 8 9 0

Letters are usually used to designate the source, for example, A, B, and C represent three wholesalers that the pharmacist frequently utilizes, and D is used when merchandise is purchased direct. Most pharmacists also indicate the date the merchandise was received, either by number (1/4/74), letter (A-Jan.) or different colors of stickers to indicate the year of purchase. Some use five or six colors and change the color of the sticker every quarter. The quantity frequently is indicated by an arabic numeral preceded by a dash (-). All of these codes may be put together as a composite such as (PAM)D 1/4/84-12, meaning that twelve units of a product were purchased directly from the manufacturer at a cost of $1.35 per unit and were received the fourth of January, 1984.

A final word of advice on marking the cost of merchandise. It is the best policy, in most instances, to mark the exact cost per unit to the nearest whole cent after allowing for all discounts, including free goods. The exception would be when the accounting system included an account for discounts and rebates, which is not a common practice. Also, the cost of freight and postage should be evenly distributed over the order unless, again, a separate account is maintained for freight and postage. In this regard, most mechandise is shipped to the pharmacy with the freight prepaid.

Title to Goods

As a general rule, the intention of the parties determines when the title passes. Difficulty arises in that the parties may not express any intention on this point. When the parties fail to do so, the law, with the aid of certain assumptions, must decide this question for them. There are about a dozen such assumptions under the law, but discussion will be limited to only those instances most applicable to pharmacy.

If the goods are to be shipped to the pharmacy with freight prepaid, the title passes to the pharmacist when the goods arrive in *good condition*. If there is any damage or shortage, a notation to that effect must be made on either the bill of lading or freight bill (even if it is a prepaid freight bill) before signing for the receipt of the merchandise in order to protect the interest of the purchaser.

If the goods are sold without reference to delivery or prepaid freight and they are in a deliverable state, title passes immediately. If, on the other hand, the terms of sale include a statement that the merchandise will be delivered FOB at the railroad depot in Chicago, title passes when the goods arrive in Chicago in good condition.

When goods are delivered on *consignment,* they remain the property of the supplier, and the pharmacist is required to pay for only the amount he sells. Unfortunately, this includes merchandise that may be stolen, because the pharmacist is the legal custodian of the goods.

REFERENCES

1. Duncan, D.J., and Phillips, C.F.: *Retailing Principles and Methods,* 6th ed., Homewood, Ill.: Richard D. Irwin, 1963, p. 266.
2. Fay, J.T. (Jr.): "The Wholesaler" in Smith, M.C. (ed). *Principles of Pharmaceutical Marketing,* 3rd ed. Philadelphia: Lea & Febiger, 1983, p. 251.
3. *Ibid.,* pp. 248–270, especially Table 12–3.
4. Smith, M.C.: *Principles of Pharmaceutical Marketing,* 2nd ed., Philadelphia: Lea & Febiger, 1975, p. 227.
5. *Pharmaceutical Distribution Plus.* New York: National Wholesale Druggist Association, 1962, p. 9.
6. Grider, G.W.: Advantages of a Buying Group. A paper presented in a seminar at the University of Kentucky College of Pharmacy, September 24, 1971.

REVIEW

1. Discuss the two points of view or philosophies of purchasing.

2. Name and discuss in detail the six purchasing functions.

3. Discuss the three basic considerations in formulating purchasing policies.

4. Outline the sources of information for determining the kinds and types of goods patrons want.

5. Outline the various marketing functions and relate each to purchasing activities in a pharmacy.

6. Discuss the advantages and disadvantages of purchasing from a wholesaler and directly from a manufacturer.

7. Explain the concept of the universality of marketing functions.

8. Explain and give an illustration of the concept of minimum total transactions.

9. Define and explain the significance of the following terms: sorting, market proximity, and time, place, possession, and form utility.

10. Name and describe four services the full-service drug wholesaler provides to a pharmacy.

11. Discuss cooperative buying groups, including the two basic types (or manner they are initiated), the advantages of a cooperative buying group, and especially the economics of joining an existing cooperative group in another trade.

12. Describe and give examples of specialty wholesalers.

13. Define and be able to work problems relative to the following kinds of discounts: trade, quantity, cash, ''deals'' with free goods, and serial discounts.

14. Define or explain the following dating and credit terms: AOG; ROG; COD; EOM; FOB; N; N/30; N/10 EOM; 2/10, n/30; 2/10 ROG, N/30; 2/10 EOM c̄ 60 extra; and 2/10 EOM, N/30.

15. Explain the value of a new product section and special return goods bins in a pharmacy.

16. Discuss and be able to describe the procedure of receiving, checking, marking, and stocking an order of merchandise.

17. Explain the conditions that determine when the title of goods transfers to the buyer.

18. Explain the term consignment.

19. What are the names and features of the three wholesaler initiated co-ops?

20. Discuss the two cooperative iniatives by two professional organizations, including the purpose and scope of each.

14 | Inventory Control

Among the many problems facing pharmacy today, the challenge of maintaining the appropriate inventory investment and providing superior pharmaceutical services at a competitive price is perhaps the most critical. Inefficient use of capital in general, and inventory specifically, is the cause of many of the problems in pharmacy. Utilizing capital more effectively, especially better control of the inventory investment through more efficient control techniques, can provide the necessary funds to offer *new* and traditional pharmaceutical services at a competitive price.

In one reported study, a majority of the 5,000 pharmacists surveyed indicated they did not consider inventory to be a major problem.[1] Surely these pharmacists were not fully aware of the significance of inventory control or the magnitude of the investment in inventory. According to *The Lilly Digest* inventory investment exceeds the investment in any other single asset by nearly fourfold.[2] The average investment for the 1,547 pharmacies reporting for 1983 in *The Lilly Digest* was $78,946.[3] Proper inventory control can reduce the inventory investment from 10 to 25 percent, depending on the degree of overstocking. In one research project,[4] the inventory was reduced by 22 percent over a nine-month period.

A simple example will illustrate the significance of an inventory control system by reducing the inventory investment from $50,000 to $40,000, a 20 percent reduction. If we assume a sales volume of $300,000 and a net profit of $12,500, both of which are typical, the significance of inventory reduction on both the return on investment, and the length of time to liquidate a debt that may have been incurred in purchasing the inventory, can be readily demonstrated. Assuming all other factors remained constant, the reduction in inventory would have increased the return on the inventory investment from 25 percent to 31 percent. Also, disregarding the interest charge, the debt incurred by financing the inventory on credit could have been liquidated with the net profit in 3.2 years instead of four. Another aspect of the savings resulting from inventory control is the interest that could have been earned if the inventory had been financed with cash (or equity funds) by the pharmacist-proprietor. In the example above, the $10,000 inventory reduction would earn $1,200 per year at 12 percent simple interest. The $10,000 would have more than doubled if the 12 percent interest charge were compounded annually for seven years.

Methods of Inventory Control

There are at least six methods of inventory control, ranging from the elementary and ineffective to sophisticated and effective methods.

INTUITIVE METHOD

The first method is designated as the intuitive method, aided by the well-known *wantbook*. This is the most common method in practice today and surely the least effective. Items are recorded in the wantbook when the number of units in stock reaches one to three, and the amount ordered is the best estimate of the pharmacist-manager or proprietor.

SYSTEMATIC WANTBOOK METHOD

The second method is a set of systemic wantbooks. In this case, there is a wantbook for each direct account and each major wholesaler. Items are recorded in the appropriate wantbook based on the need as indicated by an order card located with each product, or a strip of cardboard on the edge of the shelf. The information on the card or strip simply indicates the minimum/maximum quantities—the number at which the item is ordered and the quantity to order to bring the inventory to the maximum level. The selling price and sometimes the cost, in code, are also included. The items are ordered at the appropriate time, at which point the quantities and date of the order are recorded in the wantbook. When the order is received, notation is made of shortages and related information. Reviewing the data in the wantbooks periodically aids greatly in the establishment and refinement of the minimum and maximum quantities.

OPEN-TO-BUY BUDGET SYSTEM

One of the simplest and easiest inventory control systems to implement is the open-to-buy (O-T-B) budget method. The rationale underlying this method is simply to adjust each month's purchases based on the increases or decreases in the sales of the previous month in comparison to the corresponding monthly sales a year ago, and to make adjustments of any overbuying or underbuying during the previous month. Based on this principle, a purchase budget is established for each month.

When a purchase is made, it is subtracted from the balance of the purchase budget maintained in a separate purchase journal or register. In this manner, the pharmacist-manager can determine whether he is buying too much or too little by referring to his budget balance in his purchase journal during the month. This part is easy to do, but establishing the purchase budget for each month requires more skill. To assist students and practitioners in developing a monthly purchase budget for the prescription department, Table 14–1 was constructed to explain each step in the process.

As illustrated in the table, the pharmacist-manager implemented his O-T-B budget in January. Note that no adjustment was made for January's purchase budget because the sales for the month were not known until January 31, and the purchase adjustments necessarily are based on the events of the prior year and month. To illustrate the system, we will follow each step taken to establish the adjusted purchase budget for February:

First, the sales for January this year were $500 more than for January of last year. This figure was multiplied by .50, the decimal form of the 50 percent cost of goods sold, to transform the increased sales figure to a purchase figure of $250. Second, we note that purchases were $500 less during January than had been budgeted. This means that there was a balance in the adjusted purchase budget, and an additional amount of $500 should be included in February's adjusted budget to bring the inventory up to the proper level. Third, the $250 ($500 multiplied by .50) should be added to the $500 budget balance to arrive at the $750 adjustment, as shown in the adjustment column. Finally, we note that February sales for last year amounted to $10,500, which when multiplied by .50 provided an unadjusted purchase budget of $5,250, to which the $750 adjustment was added to obtain the final adjusted purchase budget for February of $6,000.

The O-T-B budget system may be applied in several ways. It may be used for one or more departments or the entire pharmacy, or for the slower moving drugs in the prescription department when the inventory of the faster moving prescription drugs is controlled by a more sophisticated system, for example, the stock record card system.

To implement the O-T-B budget method, a pharmacist should set up a format similar to the one illustrated in Table 14–1 and obtain the following information: (1) sales for each month for the unit being controlled, and (2) the percent cost of goods sold or at least a fairly accurate estimate.

For the latter estimate, a sample of 480 prescriptions can be drawn by taking the first 40 of each month over the year for the prescription department. It would be preferable to take the first 40 prescriptions dispensed on Monday in January, the first 40 prescriptions on Tuesday in February, and continuing this rotation through June, but skipping Sunday, and repeating the days of the week beginning with July. The total cost of ingredients (drugs) for the 480 prescriptions is divided by the total sales for the same prescriptions to estimate the percent cost of goods sold. In addition, the sales and purchases for the current year have to be recorded each month and the adjustments calculated as outlined above. This procedure requires little additional time or information for most pharmacies.

Table 14–1. Open-to-Buy Budget Method for Inventory Control

Month	Sales Past Year	Sales This Year	Unadj.* Purchase Budget	Adjustments Sales† + Purchases‡ = Adj.	Adj. Purch. Budget	Actual Purchases	Monthly Balance in Budg.§
January	$ 10,000	$ 10,500	$ 5,000	NA** + NA = NA	$ 5,000	$ 4,500	$ +500
February	10,500	10,500	5,250	(+500 × .5) + 500 = 750	6,000	5,500	+500
March	11,000	10,500	5,500	(0 × .5) + 500 = 500	6,000	5,750	+250
April	10,500	11,000	5,250	(−500 × .5) + 250 = 0	5,250	5,250	0
May	9,500	10,000	4,750	(500 × .5) + 0 = 250	5,000	5,250	−250
June	10,000	10,500	5,000	(500 × .5) − 250 = 0	5,000	4,750	+250
July	9,000	10,000	4,500	(500 × .5) + 250 = 500	5,000	5,000	0
August	8,500	9,000	4,250	(1000 × .5) + 0 = 500	4,750	5,000	−250
September	8,500	9,500	4,250	(500 × .5) − 250 = 0	4,250	4,500	−250
October	9,500	10,000	4,750	(1000 × .5) − 250 = 250	5,000	5,000	0
November	10,500	11,000	5,250	(500 × .5) + 0 = 250	5,500	5,000	+500
December	11,000	12,000	5,500	(500 × .5) + 500 = 750	6,250	6,250	0
TOTAL	$118,500	$124,500	$59,250	— — — —	$63,000	$61,750	$ 1,250

*Based on a 50 percent cost of goods sold for the same month one year before.
†The difference in sales between the previous month and the same month a year ago.
‡The difference between the adjusted purchase budget and the actual purchase of the previous month.
§A positive monthly balance in the purchase budget indicates an inventory depletion of the same magnitude, and vice versa.
**No adjustment is made the first month the method is implemented.

Name: Manufacturer A
Address: 1428 W. 22nd St., New York, N.Y. (Use Self-Addressed Order Form when available)
Discount Terms: 2% 10 days E.O.M., Net 30. Books are closed on 28th each month.

Item	*Cost*	*Size*	*Inventory minimum/ maximum*	*Inventory and Purchases by Date*								
				1/25	2/25	3/25	4/25	5/25	6/25	7/25	8/25	9/25
Tetracycline Syrup	3.42	Pt.	1 / 2	1 /	<1 / 1	.5 / 2	.5 / 2	1 / 2	1+ / 1	1.5 / 1	0.5 / 0	1 / 2 / 1
Tetracycline 250 mg. Cap.	6.17	1000	1 / 3	2 / 1	1 / 2	1 / 2	2 / 1	1 / 2	2 / 1	2.5 / 0	1.1 / 2	1.5 / 2
Meprobamate 400 mg. Tab.	18.50	500	1 / 3	2 / 1	1.5 / 2	1 / 2	.5 / 2	1 / 2	2 / 1	1.5 / 1	1 / 2	1 / 2

Figure 14–1. Typical stock record card.

The real value of the O-T-B budget system is that it is much easier to make twelve small adjustments, one each month, than to try to make one large adjustment at the end of the year when the physical inventory is taken. To illustrate further, let us assume a pharmacy had an inventory of $41,000 and a turnover rate of 3.4 per year with a cost of goods sold of $140,000. The pharmacist-manager decided that his inventory was too high and should be reduced to at least $35,000 during the following year to provide a turnover rate of 4. The $6,000 reduction in inventory represented 14.6 percent of his current inventory. Each month after the pharmacist calculated his adjusted monthly purchase budget as outlined above, he deliberately reduced this adjusted budget by an additional 14.6 percent. On the average the reduction was $500 each month.

STOCK RECORD CARD SYSTEM

Even though one can control the inventory investment for major departments by means of the open-to-buy budget, he cannot use this system to determine the optimum number of individual units of a product to be ordered. To determine the optimum number of individual units for each product in each major department, a more formal control, such as the stock record card system, must be utilized. A stock record card system, as illustrated in Figure 14–1, has proved to be effective. Ideally, the stock record card should have at least 12 columns to record data for each month. The heading of the stock record card normally shows the supplier's name and address, the discount, and other sale terms, such as the date the company closes its books.

After the general information has been recorded for a company, the name, size, cost per unit, and the minimum and maximum quantity of the product to be stocked are recorded as indicated by the column headings. Figure 14–1 demonstrates that the pharmacist in our example stocks tetracycline syrup in pints, tetracycline 250 mg. capsules in 1000s, and meprobamate 400 mg. tablets in 500s.

This stock record card system was begun in January and the first inventory taken was on Janury 25. On January 25, the pharmacist had one pint of tetracycline syrup, and the pharmacist recorded the value 1.0 in the upper part of the block under the date, January 25. On this date he also had 2 units of tetracycline 250 mg. capsules and 2 units of meprobamate 400 mg. tablets, plus various other products. Based on the minimum and maximum quantities the pharmacist had previously established from experience, he decided to purchase one pint of tetracycline syrup and the number of units of other products as indicated. This information was recorded in the lower part of the block. Upon completing the order, the manager can ascertain whether he has purchased the minimum amount necessary to receive the maximum discounts available. This can be easily determined by multiplying the units ordered times the cost per unit, totaling the costs, and comparing the total with the supplier's minimum order requirement. On February 25 and each month thereafter, the pharmacist again recorded the quantity of items in inventory and repeated the process.

Some product lines do not warrant the additional time required to maintain the inventory on stock record cards because of their small investment and slow turnover rate. The pharmacist must decide which products warrant stock record cards and which should be controlled with the open-to-buy budget. As a starting point for setting up the stock record card system, it is suggested that the system include all prescription products purchased directly from the top 10 to 20 major pharmaceutical manufacturers and all other prescription drugs with a high turnover rate pruchased from wholesalers, especially if the product appears in the top 200 products listed in the National Prescription Audit.[5] Stock record card inventory control of the top 200 prescription drugs will include the investment of about two-thirds of the prescription sales volume. Another consideration is that most of these drugs are routinely inventoried and ordered monthly by a majority of community pharmacists. The stock record card system should be restricted to prescription drugs in the beginning because the average investment in major lines of prescription drugs is usually greater than the average investment per line of nonlegend drugs or other merchandise.

By maintaining stock record cards on prescription drugs with high turnover rates, the pharmacist is in a position to place a larger order at the end of the month and thus have the suppliers finance the inventory investment for as long as 40 to 45 days. The system also ensures the earning of cash discounts on the products controlled by the system and provides more cash for other investments. The extra cash can be invested in other products with a high gross margin and/or high turnover rate or can be invested in securities or other property. Also, the additional money may be used to improve services for patients, for example, a patient medication record system.

THE ECONOMIC ORDER QUANTITY

The basic problem of inventory management is having the right amount of stock on hand, neither too much nor too little. Fundamentally, inventory control is deciding how much to buy and when. The economic order quantity (EOQ) deals with both *how much* to purchase and the appropriate reorder point, or *when* to buy. Also, the EOQ is the amount to buy that will keep total costs at a minimum.

There are two sets of costs involved in purchasing, *procurement* costs and *carrying* costs. Procurement costs vary with the number of orders and may be reduced for any given item by placing fewer and larger orders. However, the result is an increase in inventory and consequently in the other set of costs, the carrying costs. Procurement costs vary directly with the number of orders and inversely with the amount of investment. On the other hand, the carrying costs may be reduced for any given item if smaller orders are placed. However, the result will be an increase in the number of orders and consequently an increase in the first set of costs, the procurement costs. Carrying costs vary directly with inventory investment and inversely with the number of orders.

The various individual expenses of the two sets of costs are:

PROCUREMENT COSTS	CARRYING COSTS
Checking inventory	Interest, imputed and/or real
Purchasing	Obsolescence
Receiving and checking the merchandise	Loss through theft
Marking and stocking the merchandise	Deterioration or damage
Paying for the merchandise	Storage (insurance and property tax)

The EOQ model provides a level of inventory at which the combined costs of procuring and carrying inventory are at a minimum. For example, Table 14–2 shows how total costs are affected by the size of the order with a procurement cost of $4.00 per order and a carrying cost of 10 percent of the average inventory investment, on a product with annual cost of goods sold at $720.

First, if an order for $720 is placed only once each year, the total cost of procurement is $4. Since the average value of the stock will be $360, or one-half of the value of the order, the carrying costs will be 10 percent of $360, or $36. The sum of the two costs will be $40.

If two orders are made each year, the value of each order will be $360. This will double the procurement costs and reduce the carrying costs to one-half. Total costs will be $26 instead of $40. However, by placing 3 orders of $240 each, the total cost will be the least of all. Beyond this point the increase in procurement costs will always be greater than the decrease in carrying costs, as can be seen in the table. The total cost is at a minimum

Table 14–2. How the Value of Orders Determines Total Costs

Value of Order	No. Orders Per Year	Procurement Costs	Average Active Inventory	Carrying Costs	Total Cost
$720	1	$ 4	$360	$36	$40
360	2	8	180	18	26
240	3	12	120	12	24
180	4	16	90	9	25
144	5	20	72	7	27
120	6	24	60	6	30

when the procurement costs and carrying costs are equal. For practical considerations, the two sets of costs may be only approximately equal.

For any one item, a reduction in *one* set of costs causes an increase in the other set. This is also true for a group of items under ordinary purchasing practices. The application of EOQ to any group of stock items will cause the sum of the two sets of costs to be lower than under any other system of purchasing. This will happen in one of the following ways: (1) by balancing or equating the two sets of costs; or (2) by reducing one set of costs without increasing the other. (This latter possibility is not a likely event under normal purchasing practices.)

Any other order quantities may: (1) produce a certain stock turn, but at unnecessarily high costs; (2) reduce procurement costs by increasing carrying costs; or (3) reduce carrying costs by increasing procurement costs.

Under many replenishment systems, items are ordered at regular intervals. Such systems result in maintaining on the average a constant level of supply for all items in the group. Under other systems, the number of orders may vary according to demand. For items with a high dollar demand, orders may be placed more frequently than for low dollar demand items, in which case, fewer and larger orders, relative to demand, are placed. In addition, under some of these systems, consideration is properly given to special characteristics such as limited shelf life, space requirements, and seasonal demand. But after all these characteristics are considered, the questions still remain, how many orders per year are the right amount for any given item? How much should be ordered at a time? How much stock should be maintained?

The economic order quantity (EOQ) equation is difficult to derive but not difficult to use. The model is expressed by the following equation:

$$Q = \sqrt{\frac{(2)(C_p(D))}{C_h}}$$

where Q = the economic order quantity;
C_p = procurement cost;
D = the demand for the product expressed either in dollars or physical units; and
C_h = the holding or carrying cost of the investment.

Table 14–3. Table of Square Roots

Number	Square Root	Number	Square Root	Number	Square Root	Number	Square Root
1.0	1.0	10	3.2	100	10	1,000	32
1.2	1.1	12	3.5	120	11	1,200	35
1.4	1.2	14	3.7	140	12	1,400	37
1.5	1.2	15	3.9	150	12	1,500	39
1.6	1.3	16	4.0	160	13	1,600	40
1.8	1.3	18	4.2	180	13	1,800	42
2.0	1.4	20	4.5	200	14	2,000	45
2.5	1.6	25	5.0	250	16	2,500	50
3.0	1.7	30	5.5	300	17	3,000	55
3.5	1.9	35	5.9	350	19	3,500	59
4.0	2.0	40	6.3	400	20	4,000	63
4.5	2.1	45	6.7	450	21	4,500	67
5.0	2.2	50	7.1	500	22	5,000	71
6.0	2.4	60	7.7	600	24	6,000	77
7.0	2.6	70	8.4	700	26	7,000	84
8.0	2.8	80	8.9	800	28	8,000	89
9.0	3.0	90	9.5	900	30	9,000	95

To find the square root of a number larger than 9,000, simply drop the last two numbers. Find the square root of this resulting number and add a zero to it.

Suppose the value of the yearly demand of an item is $29,750. Rounding to 30,000 and dropping the last two numbers, you get 300. You will find in the table that the square root of 300 is 17. Adding a zero, you get 170. This is approximately the square root of 30,000.

To find the square root of a number less than 9,000 not in the table, take the square root of the nearest number or one in between. For example, use 25 for the square root of 640, which is between 600 and 700. The approximate square roots you will get will be accurate enough for determining EOQ.

Table 14–3 is a modified table of square roots, and contains instructions for its use in determining the EOQ.

One important consideration in using the EOQ equation is that both D and C_h must be expressed in comparable terms with respect to time and quantity. For example, if D is expressed as the amount in dollars that will be purchased in one year, the C_h must be expressed as the annual percent in decimal form which represents the holding (carrying) cost. Currently, this cost will range from 20 to 30 percent in most pharmacies. However, if D is expressed as the number of physical units that will be purchased in a period, for example one month, C_h must be expressed as the holding cost for the average cost per unit purchased each month. The following examples explain how to calculate the EOQ using monthly and annual data.

Assume that a pharmacy purchased $3,000 worth of goods from one company in a year, with an average of 50 physical units of the various products each month. It was determined with the aid of a stop watch that, on an average, 12 minutes were required to inventory and place an order from this company. If this were done by a pharmacist with a salary of $15.00 per hour, the procurement cost (C_p) would be $3.00 ($15 × 12/60 minutes). It was determined that the average cost per physical unit of the product mix ordered during the year was $5.00 and C_h is 30 percent per annum. The carrying cost per unit per month (C_h) can be calculated as follows: $5.00 × 0.30 ÷ 12 = $0.125. Substituting in the equation, we solve for Q as follows:

$$Q = \sqrt{\frac{(2)(C_p)(D)}{C_h}}$$

$$Q = \sqrt{\frac{2 \times \$3.00 \times 50}{\$0.125}}$$

$$Q = \sqrt{\frac{300}{0.125}}$$

$$Q = \sqrt{2400}$$
$$Q = 48.99 \text{ or } 49 \text{ units in round figures}$$

When the number of units is converted to dollars, the EOQ is $245, in round figures. The idealized average investment is one-half the EOQ value or $122.50. The optimum turnover rate is approximately 24 ($3,000 ÷ 122.50) or 12 orders per year.

The economic order quantity may be calculated by use of annual data—the total amount purchased per year, the same procurement cost per order, and the 30 percent carrying cost for the year. The calculations are as follows:

$$Q = \sqrt{\frac{2 (C_p)(D)}{C_h}}$$

$$Q = \sqrt{\frac{2 \times \$3.00 \times \$3,000}{.30}}$$

$$Q = \sqrt{\frac{\$18,000}{.30}}$$

$$Q = \sqrt{\$60,000}$$
$$Q = \$245$$

Now let us calculate the EOQ, using the yearly demand in dollars for the same company but under a different set of conditions. Instead of having the pharmacist take the inventory and place the order, the pharmacist-manager hired a stock clerk for $4.00 per hour to do the job. (He found the clerk could do this chore just as efficiently after two months of training.) Procurement cost (C_p) was $0.80 ($4.00 × 12/60 minutes). The holding cost remained the same. The yearly demand (D) remained $3,000. Substituting into the equation:

$$Q = \sqrt{\frac{(2)(C_p)(D)}{CV_h}}$$

$$Q = \sqrt{\frac{2 \times \$0.80 \times \$3,000}{.30}}$$

$$Q = \sqrt{\frac{4800}{0.30}}$$

$$Q = \sqrt{16,000}$$
$$Q = \$126.50—24 \text{ orders per year, twice per month.}$$

Under these conditions, the idealized average inventory investment is $63.25 (1/2 × $126.50). The optimum turnover rate is now approximately 48. This latter set of conditions represents a "money-saving" approach to the problem. It is readily apparent that the inventory investment has been reduced to one-half, and if other cost factors remain the same, the percentage return on the investment in inventory would increase significantly.

The economic order quantity model will determine the optimum quantity to order, in terms of either dollars or physical units, and the optimum turnover rate. This can be applied to a line of merchandise or to an individual product. Since the actual number of units of each product that a pharmacist can expect to dispense during a given month can be rather closely estimated by inspection of the stock record card, it is more feasible to apply the model to the monthly order of the entire manufacturer's line. This, of course, requires that the pharmacist use the stock record cards or a computerized counterpart along with the EOQ.

Once the EOQ for the line has been calculated, quantity adjustments among the various products may be necessary to obtain the most economic product mix for each order. In any case, the company's minimum direct order quantity must be considered, especially if the minimum direct order quantity exceeds the EOQ by a considerable amount. This could be a good indication that this company's line of products may be purchased more economically through the wholesaler. Of course, the discount for direct buying should enter into the decision.

A simple example illustrates a way to approach such a decision. Assume a pharmacy has a low sales volume of $200 per year for a small manufacturer's line. Also, assume a 50 percent cost of goods sold (CGS) and gross margin (GM) and a net profit of 10 percent of sales. The manufacturer requires a $100 order for direct purchases with a 10 percent quantity discount. Under these conditions, the CGS is $100, the average investment in inventory is $50.00 (1/2 × $100 CGS) and the net profit (NP) is $20.00. The return on the investment in inventory is 60 percent ($20.00 NP + $10.00 in discount divided by the $50.00 average investment).

However, the EOQ is calculated to be $33.33 purchased every four months. The average investment is now $16.67 (1/2 × $33.33 CGS), but the net profit is only $20.00 since the pharmacist-manager must forgo the discount. His return on investment is now 120 percent ($20.00 ÷ $16.67); he has doubled his percentage return on the inventory investment. It should be noted, however, that his actual net profit declined by $10.00, and the real issue is whether the pharmacist could have invested the difference in the average inventories ($33.33) in some other venture and earned more than the $10.00. This could have been achieved by investing the $33.33 in a product with a 40 percent gross margin, with four turnovers per year and a net profit potential of 5 percent of sales. This investment would yield $11.11 in net profit.

PERPETUAL INVENTORY METHOD

Perpetual inventory method is the most efficient method of inventory control provided the pharmacist has the necessary technology for this method, which is a computer. The software is more important than the hardware in providing such a sophisticated system. Perpetual inventory system simply means the system can tell you precisely the amount of inventory on hand for any product in the system at any time, and the system is programmed to provide a list and quantities of products (actually it normally will execute a purchase order) to be ordered to maintain the inventory at a designated level.

There are two algorithms for achieving the perpetual inventory optimum or target quantity. One is the EOQ model, which is really the better of the two simply because it includes more variables, C_h and C_p. The second method is the "usage pattern" method. At the beginning, the pharmacist has to specify the minimum and maximum quantities for each product based on historic data from either a stock-record-card system or a systematic wantbook system. The usage pattern algorithm must specify the time period for each product, e.g., week, month, two or three months. Also, the program should revise the minimum and maximum quantities based on the usage pattern. For example, if the minimum quantity was one and the maximum was four for a one-month period, and the usage quantity (number dispensed) was four at the end of three weeks, the maximum quantity would be revised to five. Also, that product would be flagged in the next printing of an order list or purchase order. The pharmacist would then order the quantity to hold the inventory level until the next order cycle at which time the automatic order quantity would be printed or executed. An alternate program could automatically order five units and start a new order cycle beginning that day.

Some computer inventory control systems are less sophisticated and provide only a list of products with the quantity dispensed during a specified period.

Based on this historic data, the pharmacist then decides the quantity to be ordered. It is obvious that this is only a sophisticated record keeping system similar to the systematic wantbook system with speed and accuracy being the only advantage of the computerized system.

There are a couple of important points concerning the computerized EOQ mode. First, once the investment cost of the computer has been amortized, the procurement cost becomes very low, probably about $1.00 per order, unless the order is very large with many items. In this case, it is the cost of checking the order and stocking the merchandise that determines most of the cost. However, when that cost is prorated over several lines or many products, the procurement cost per line or product remains small.

Second, the carrying cost now becomes the primary consideration, which favors smaller, more frequent orders. If the supplier submits a statement weekly with remittance specified within a few days, then a weekly order cycle becomes very feasible. With automatic purchase orders, billing and check writing via computer for both parties, a weekly order cycle is very efficient and feasible. Note that if remittance is required monthly, there is little, if any, economy in a weekly purchase cycle. The pharmacist can purchase a montly supply early in the month and sell a large portion (possibly 85 to 90 percent) of the order before paying for it. Thus, carrying cost would not be optimized by weekly orders, and the traditional monthly purchase cycle would remain the most economical option.

Selection of the Optimum Method(s)

No one method of inventory control is the most appropriate for every pharmacy. The least any pharmacist-manager should do is to maintain a systematic set of wantbooks to assist him in ordering more nearly the appropriate quantities of merchandise. This will only approximate the desired results, but it is an improvement over the usual use of wantbooks.

Pharmacies with annual sales over $150,000 can use the more sophisticated methods profitably. Any pharmacy can use the open-to-buy budget method for the prescription department, or any of its other major departments. This method, however, only provides control of the dollar amount of the inventory. Together with a system of wantbooks, with appropriate entries in them, the O-T-B method will be fairly effective for small pharmacies with sales volumes of $150,000 or less.

The stock record card system should be used for those products or lines of goods on which the economic order quantity model indicates the feasibility of the system. Under most conditions, the carrying cost will range between 20 and 30 percent. With interest and inflation rates so high, it is essential that pharmacist-managers use every means possible to reduce inventory investment. Small pharmacies will have an inventory of $20,000 to $25,000 at an effective annual interest cost of $3,300 to $4,200. Never has there been such economic pressure for good management of assets.

The following example illustrates the way to determine the feasibility of using the S-R-C system and the EOQ model. A pharmacy purchases $500 worth of drugs annually from Company A. The minimum order is $100, providing a 15 percent discount. Judicious purchasing from a local drug wholesaler provides a 10 percent quantity discount on line extension of $10 per product, a 5 percent difference. If a trained clerk checks the inventory and does the ordering, procurement cost is $1.33 per order. If a pharmacist does the job, the cost is $3.00. Carrying cost is 30 percent.

When the clerk is used, the EOQ is $66.58, rounded to $62.50 for eight orders per year. The total cost is $20.02 [(1/2 × 62.50 × .30) + (8 × 1.33)]. To earn the 15 percent quantity discount, $100 in goods must be ordered each time. The total cost under these conditions is $21.65 [(1/2 × 100 × .3) + (5 × 1.33)]. It appears that taking the $25 extra quantity discount is economically feasible, since the total purchasing cost is increased by only $1.65 when making orders of $100 each time. However, this is not the full picture; the appropriate comparison is between pruchasing directly from the manufacturer and from the wholesaler.

If the demand is evenly distributed over the 12 months, then approximately $42 in goods would be ordered each month from the wholesaler. The carrying cost is $6.30 (1/2 × $42 × .30). Assuming that the procurement cost is reduced to $1 per order, then the total procurement cost is $12 for a total purchasing cost of $18.30. This $3.35 savings in total purchasing cost should be compared with the additional extra quantity discount of $25 for the year. Even if the pharmacist performs all the purchasing and inventory functions, the total purchasing cost is $30, which is $11.70 more than the purchasing cost through the wholesaler. This additional cost ($11.70) is $13.30 less than the additional quantity discount of $25.

If a pharmacist installs an efficient S-R-C system with a well-trained stock clerk, or a combination of a stock clerk and a prescription aide, annual purchases of as little as $300 from one source can be profitable using the S-R-C + EOQ system. Only with stock record cards or a computerized inventory control and the EOQ model is the pharmacist able to determine with a high degree of accuracy the most advantageous quantity and frequency per order.

An inventory control system maintained with a computer, together with the EOQ model, can be profitably used to control the inventory for individual products and the entire inventory. This situation will be found in most pharmacies dispensing 65 prescriptions or more per day. Unit control is feasible under these conditions and an example will illustrate this.

A hospital pharmacy uses 1,200 units annually at a cost of $2.00 per unit for a total dollar volume of $2,400. The procurement cost is $1.35 and the carrying cost is 16 percent annually. The EOQ is $200 or 100 units.

$$Q = \sqrt{\frac{2 \times \$1.35 \times \$2,400}{0.16}}$$
$$Q = \sqrt{40,500}$$
$$Q = \$201 \text{ or } 100 \text{ units for } 12 \text{ orders per year.}$$

The same result is obtained by substituting the demand in units per month for annual dollar demand and $0.0267 for 16 percent as the carrying cost per month per unit cost.

Effect of Inventory Control: A Mini-Case Study

A professional pharmacy was located in a medical building in a city of approximately 40,000 population.[4] Fifteen physicians and an oral surgeon practiced in the building. About 65 percent of the $245,000 sales volume was derived from prescriptions and physicians' supplies. The pharmacy was heavily overstocked with prescription drugs. The inventory for the prescription department was $34,866 before a program of purchasing and inventory control was implemented. The turnover rate for the previous year was 1.6 for the prescription department.

During the initial preparatory stage of the project, 51 percent of the inventory was returned to the suppliers or written off as nonsalable and nonreturnable merchandise. The balance of the inventory of $16,970 was considered to be usable and constituted a well-balanced prescription drug inventory for this pharmacy.

At this stage of the project, two inventory control methods were implemented, the stock record card system and open-to-buy budget system. Product lines of eleven manufacturers were selected for stock record card control based on the observed utilization rate during the preparatory stage and the policy of direct selling to pharmacies. It had been observed that at least the minimum order quantity was purchased monthly from each of the companies during the preparatory stage. The EOQ was used to determine the optimum order quantity.

The inventory controlled by the stock record card system was reduced by an additional 17 percent during the six months' test period. The turnover rate increased to 6.1, on an annual basis for the first three months, and 8.0 on an annual basis for the second three months. The inventory controlled by the open-to-buy budget method was reduced by 4 percent. The turnover rate for this group of drugs increased to 2.4 on an annual basis. Overall, the turnover rate for the prescription department increased from 1.6 to 3.22, a two-fold increase.

It was determined that, on an average, only 24 seconds were required to inventory and place an order for a single product among all the products of the eleven manufacturers controlled by the stock record card system. An additional 36 seconds were required to check, mark, and stock a product on receipt of the order—for a total of 60 seconds. The out-of-stock rate was almost exactly the same for each method and averaged 1.2 prescriptions per day.

REFERENCES

1. Cullman, W.A.: What pharmacists think. *NARDJ, 88*:24–34, 1966.
2. Deiner, C.H.: *The Lilly Digest, 1984*. Indianapolis: Eli Lilly and Company, 1984, Table 22.
3. *Ibid.,* p. 5.
4. Huffman, D.C., Jr.: The Feasibility of Modern Managerial Systems and Innovative Professional Services in a Community Pharmacy: A Case Study. Dissertation, University of Mississippi, January, 1971.
5. *National Prescription Audit General Information Report*. Ambler, Pa. IMS America, Ltd. This information is published in several pharmaceutical journals each year.

REVIEW

1. According to the latest *Lilly Digest,* what was the average investment in inventory, and how did this investment compare with other items of assets?

2. Describe the six methods of inventory control.

3. Given the necessary data, complete a table of open-to-buy budget inventory control including the adjustments, adjusted purchase budget, and the monthly balance in the adjusted purchase budget.

4. Discuss the procedures and be able to devise and complete a system of stock record card inventory control.

5. Explain the concept of the economic order quantity (EOQ) including the terms of the formula and the specific information it provides the pharmacist.

6. Given the appropriate data, calculate the EOQ in either units per order or dollar value per order, the reorder point, and the optimum turnover rate for a given line of products or for a company. Table 14–3 has been included to assist in determining square roots.

7. Given the necessary data, including quantity discount rates, determine when a minimum direct order, example $100, is feasible using the EOQ model.

8. Discuss the various situations (sizes of pharmacy, sales volume) under which each method of inventory is most feasible, especially a computerized perpetual inventory system.

9. Discuss how the turnover rate is indicative of a good inventory control method.

10. Discuss the relationship between the return on investment in inventory and the efficiency of an inventory control method.

15 | Pricing and Professional Fees

General Pricing Considerations

BASIC FACTORS

When a pharmacist makes a determination of the pricing philosophy, policy and method(s) for his pharmacy, he must consider at least five basic factors that affect his decisions.

Philosophy. The philosophy of the pharmacist is a primary consideration. This philosophy is a product of the pharmacist's socioeconomic background, the market in which he practices, and his education and experience. In the final analysis, however, the philosophy is determined by the pharmacist's volition.

Competition. This factor is certainly a major consideration. Since it has already been discussed in some detail, the point of emphasis here is that the pharmacist can deal effectively with various forms of price and non-price competition through a well-designed strategy of market segmentation. The application of the principles of economics and marketing is the principal tool in this case.

Merchandise Cost. The cost of merchandise is a necessary factor that must be considered in determining methods of pricing and the pricing of individual merchandise or services. The cost of the merchandise forms the fundamental base line for determining prices. Cooperative buying groups and other buying methods are important in determining prices and profits. Again, the application of economic and marketing principles is necessary to purchase merchandise in a manner to be competitive.

Expenses. The control of expenses is another essential element in price determination. Control of expenses, especially variable expenses, provides one of the bases for more competitive pricing. In the long run, prices must

305

cover all expenses, and more, to yield a profit. The application of accounting and economics can assist the pharmacist in reducing unnecessary expenses, and thereby to price competitively.

Legal and Social Constraints. These combined forces make up the fifth basic factor in price determination. There are franchise agreements that prohibit the pharmacist from charging less than the stipulated or suggested price. Certain lines of cosmetics are sold exclusively through franchise agreements. Fair trade laws are largely inoperative now, but may still be in effect for certain lines in certain jurisdictions. These operate more in the nature of a franchise, through individual contractual agreement, than through the general operation of statutory law, with the exception of the sale of alcoholic beverages. In addition, certain goods sell for a certain price because of long-standing custom. Although inflation has largely displaced these ''customary prices,'' there still may be some residual constraint to sell some items at a customary price. This latter socioeconomic factor is included here more for a historic purpose and to apprise the reader of the necessity to consider this factor, especially franchise agreements, in price determination.

There are many factors, policies, and strategies which must be considered in the making of pricing decisions. These considerations vary with the market, the type of pharmacy practice, and the pharmacist himself.

COMPETITIVE RANGE

As discussed in Chapter 1, competition has been a problem in American pharmacy from the beginning. The report of a recent study by the Dichter Institute for Motivational Research, Inc.,[1] commissioned by the American Pharmaceutical Association, may provide the pharmacist with some useful insight into the design of a competitive posture for his pharmacy. The research revealed that in purchasing prescriptions, the public is not so much *pulled* toward discounters by their price advertising as it is being *pushed* away from the regular community pharmacy by a sense of alienation. The community pharmacists are not communicating and consulting with their patrons and showing a genuine concern for their welfare, which the public so desperately desires. The public perceives prescription and comprehensive pharmaceutical services as a vital part of their health care and have very deep-seated feelings about the services provided and concern shown in providing these services.

Types of Competition. The two major types of competition are *price* and *nonprice*. Nonprice competition takes several forms of promotion in which price is not a primary factor. These include advertising, displays, broad lines and assortments of merchandise, extra services (both professional and nonprofessional), and, probably the most important form of all, a vast number of competing units vying for the consumers' dollars for the same or similar products and services. This latter form of competition may be divided into nondrug firms and the various types of pharmacies and drugstores. The large discount emporium with a prescription department and a drug counter can be classified in either category, but traditionally it is not considered to be a "regular" pharmacy or drugstore and, therefore, is placed in the nondrug class. This type of firm is found in the larger cities where competition, both price and nonprice, is the severest.

Market Segmentation. Nonprice competition, in many ways, is associated with the concept of market segmentation. Market segmentation is the strategy of identifying a segment of the market who are desirous to purchase a particular, and frequently unique, line of goods and/or services. The pharmacist attempts to measure the extent of the demand for the special line of goods and/or services and offers the line and/or services if the demand seems to warrant it.

Market segmentation can range from stocking a single product, such as a very expensive imported perfume, to the design, decor, stock and services of an entire pharmacy, such as the pharmaceutical center. In the first instance, the pharmacist is appealing to a small number of wealthy female patrons. In the latter instance, the pharmacist is appealing to a much larger number of people of both sexes who prefer a highly personalized, professional service. Other market segments include a complete home health care, convalescent, and orthopedic department; hypoallergenic cosmetics; complete veterinary drug and pet department; a complete baby department supervised by a licensed nurse; a professionally operated medication record system; and a clinical laboratory—just to mention the more common lines and services that appeal to particular segments of the market. The stocking or implementation and promotion of these special lines and/or services are viable examples of nonprice competition.

Quasi-Price Competition. In addition to direct price competition, there exists a technique known as quasi-price competition. The trading stamp is a classic example of quasi-price competition. Another example of this technique is the inclusion of a product "free" with the purchase of another product. This is more frequently done at the manufacturer's level and passed on to the customer. Another example is providing coupons in a newspaper ad or circular that permit a person who tenders the coupon to purchase an item at a reduced price *provided* he or she purchases other goods costing a designated amount, for example, $5.00. There are many variations of this, but they are not used in pharmacy to the extent that they are used in supermarkets. Although quasi-price reduction is not a true, direct price reduction on a product, it is similar in some respects to price competition.

Direct Price Reduction. Direct price reduction on a particular product is the most obvious mode of price competition. Direct price reduction may take several forms also. The broadest form is the *across-the-board* reduction of prices below normal or average market price on all the merchandise. At least two chain drugstore firms have adopted this approach.

A second form of direct price reduction is the *loss leader.* In this case, the management selects a group of products and reduces the prices below the market norm by a significant amount. This practice was once restricted to "out front" merchandise, but now it is used extensively by "discounters" and some other pharmacies on *popular* or *maintenance* prescription drugs.

Another approach is to use *weekend "specials,"* offering a significant discount on selected products from Thursday evening through Saturday or Sunday. The group of products is selected each week from a larger, master list of popular shoppers' items. This also gives the impression that the drugstore or pharmacy offers substantial discounts over a wide range of products, while in fact, the range of products discounted is less than the image created— at least that is the objective of the promotional method. This method of competition has been designated "shadow boxing."

A fourth method of price competition is to have *sales* or *"special events"* coinciding with holidays (e.g., Washington's birthday), anniversaries, seasons, and the so-called close-out sales. Usually there are discounts on the prices of selected merchandise, but sometimes the "sales" are at the regular price. Some firms even buy special sale merchandise, usually not a regular line of goods, and sell them at the usual or regular margin, but marked to indicate a discount price. This is practiced more frequently in the dry goods trade. Needless to say, this practice is unethical, if not fraudulent. Any false close-out sale also comes under this indictment.

Last, there is the famous annual or semiannual *one cent sale*. This type of sale was introduced by Rexall many years ago, and it later was used by Walgreen drugstores. The original concept was that the purchaser could buy a second unit of a product for one cent provided the first unit was purchased at the regular price. The Federal Trade Commission stopped the use of the phrase "one cent sale" and a somewhat different title is used today. However, older consumers still associate the sale with the "old-time one cent sale."

The foregoing discussion covers competitive practices ranging from selective nonprice, service-oriented programs to "hard-hitting" across-the-board discounting, as well as the once traditional "one cent sales." The pharmacist should select the competitive posture that is best for him. The choice, of course, will depend on the individual, the type of pharmacy, and the market.

PRICING POLICIES AND STRATEGIES

The pharmacist's pricing policies should correspond to the competitive strategy of his pharmacy. He may choose from among the following approaches to pricing merchandise or use a combination of these approaches for various departments or product lines: (1) traditional or regular pricing, (2) competitive pricing, (3) price leadership, (4) pricing based on an estimation of what the market will bear, (5) odd pricing, and (6) professional discount.

Traditional Pricing. Traditional or regular pricing simply means that, for a particular product or merchandise line, the pharmacist uses a markup that has become the general custom or practice over the years. The markup varies with the nature of the product and its turnover rate. (The markup percentages are always based on the selling price equaling 100 percent.) These range from approximately 10 percent on tobacco products up to 50 percent on products with high service requirements and relatively slow turnover rates. These various percentages are estimated on the basis of the turnover rate, the service costs, the carrying costs, and the procurement costs. These intuitive estimates, derived through may years of experience, parallel the marketing theories of Professor Aspinwall.[2] Pharmacists who practice this approach are not considered either to be very competitive or to have extremely high prices. Many pharmacists who have good locations and provide superior professional pharmaceutical services and use market segmentation strategy have been successful with traditional pricing. In contrast, pharmacists with an inferior location or who provided inferior professional pharmaceutical service have faced bankruptcy as a result of this pricing policy in a highly competitive market.

Competitive Pricing. Competitive pricing approximates fairly well what has come to be known as the game plan by sophisticated managers. Game theory, a mathematical and statistical model, is designed to guide managers in decision-making. However, experts in game theory admit the impossibility of encompassing all of the varieties of economic behavior in their model. The theory presumes that people pursue their own interests, whatever they may be, and each individual has a preference pattern among the available options and follows the pattern rather consistently.[3] Statistically, this theory is sound, but in practice it is subjective individuals who make the decisions, and their choices are subjective, isolated acts that often cannot be treated as aggregates. Thus, the game plan is a rather tenuous method of long-range planning. However, the game plan works well in the area of competitive pricing. The following cases illustrate the application of the game plan on a scale that is practical.

One drug company tabulates the advertisements of its competition, most of which are the weekend specials variety. A chart is constructed to show what products, by classes of categories, are advertised with the quoted price by firm and week. These charts are updated continuously, and the general, composite pattern of advertising behavior of the competition is easily discernible. The management of this company simply selects the product mix and the price of each product to convey a competitive image and not a deep-cut discount image. The company provides many services not offered by the larger competitors. This game plan is successful because it is directed toward a specific objective; it is based on data that provide a fairly high degree of predictability of the behavior of the competition; and finally, it is flexible enough to permit desired changes in the plan. This game plan is in sharp contrast to a long-term game plan based on data providing less predictability and designed to achieve broad and general objectives.

Two other mini-cases illustrate the concept on a much smaller scale. In a small town of approximately 6,000 with four pharmacies, one of the pharmacists was rather aggressive from a professional viewpoint (or progressive from a business viewpoint) and ran "weekend specials" advertisements in the weekly newspaper. One of his colleagues, or competitors if you prefer, consistently cut out the advertisement and taped it on the front door of his pharmacy with the notice that he would match all of the prices advertised for the items that he also stocked.

The other case is a little more subtle in the game plan used. A pharmacist who operated a traditional pharmacy with a professional orientation and atmosphere and a large prescription volume suddenly found himself in a highly competitive market. He designed an attractive poster that indicated that he offered competitive prices consistent with the services he provided on those products he stocked. The notice indicated the average cost for charge service, delivery service, patient medication record system, and personal professional consultation. It also indicated that for those who did not want these services, a cash and carry price would be quoted. Since most of his patrons wanted these services, he had few inquiries about the cash and carry price. The pharmacist was able to satisfy those few patrons in his trade area who were especially price oriented without loss of patronage or profit.

Price Leadership. This is the most aggressive approach to pricing policies and strategy. As the term implies, the management of the pharmacy or firm attempts to have the lowest prices in the market. This is characteristic of the discounters and at one time some well-known department stores such as R.H. Macy and Company of New York. Some chain drugstore companies practice this policy.

Most of these firms have several characteristics in common: (1) they buy in large volume and search out the lowest possible price; (2) they cut their expenses as much as possible, both by carefully controlling necessary expenses and by not offering many services such as credit, delivery, and personalized attention or selling; (3) many use the least expensive fixtures and furnishings; (4) many carry only the fast turnover products or sizes and styles. Most of these firms practice price leadership on all merchandise, while some use price leadership on a large portion of their stock, but not necessarily on a majority of the items.

People other than pharmacists condemn this "cut throat" type of practice. Mr. J.C. Penney, founder of the company that bears his name, had this to say about the practice: "The item we sell at 79 cents is a 79 cent item. We neither expect nor want customers of ours to think either that we are such poor business people as to believe we can sell them a dollar item for 79 cents, or we think them of such poor intelligence that they would actually think we could do so."[4]

What the Market Will Bear. Pricing based on what the market will bear is the worst of all approaches to pricing. First, it is the most inconsistent pricing policy of all. Second, it shows a lack of social responsibility and sensitivity *unless* the practitioner makes allowances for the indigent, which would require great astuteness and a sense of fair play. Third, the policy is undemocratic in that the practitioner takes advantage of both the ignorant and the rich—if he can get away with it—without adequate information to determine a just price.

Unfortunately, some pharmacists have been practicing on the fringe of this policy with respect to prescription charges because they did not have a logical method of prescription pricing, but priced them in a haphazard manner. Although the prescription pricing surveys that have appeared in several newspapers and *Consumer Reports* were poorly designed with faulty analysis and conclusions, the wide divergence in prices for the same prescription in different pharmacies is cause for some apprehension in the minds of thinking pharmacists as well as the public. When these discrepancies in prices appeared for the same prescription dispensed from the same pharmacy, there was indeed cause for alarm![5] This latter inconsistency, together with severe competition on popular and maintenance drugs from discounting pharmacies in a nearby city, caused one independent pharmacist to adopt the professional fee for prescriptions.[6] For these reasons, the policy of "what the market will bear" should be discouraged.

Odd Pricing. This is an old gimmick that has been used for so long that it has lost most of its potency in accomplishing its intended purpose. Odd pricing is simply using an odd figure, for example 49 cents, instead of the round figure of 50 cents, in the belief that the public would think the price difference was more than one cent. The basis of this theory is that 49 cents is associated with the decimal class of 40s in contrast to the decimal class of 50s, a 10 cent difference. In other words, 49 cents carries the connotation of being less in price than the one cent difference it really is. Also, it is supposed that the public thinks the merchant is pricing the item as low as possible by reducing the price a penny to its lowest possible level.

Odd pricing probably was first used by price leaders and later by those who priced competitively. Odd pricing became so common that it became a characteristic of traditional or regular pricing. Although odd prices are still prevalent for many products sold in pharmacies, at least one chain drugstore company has discontinued its use for clerical reasons. The company found that fewer errors and greater efficiency were achieved at the cash registers when rounded prices were used.

Some pharmacists and other retailers have installed computerized cash registers that read the price from a bar code on the product with an electronic wand. There are few cashiering errors with this system, and therefore, no advantage with round-figure pricing when utilizing the automatic bar-code registers.

Professional Discounts. Most pharmacies generally adhere to a one-price policy except for special or professional discounts. Professional discounts have been a problem for pharmacists for many years. Most pharmacists, if not all, will agree that professional discounts are good if used on a reciprocal basis. The crux of the problem is that prescribers in general, and physicians in particular, expect discounts on drugs and other pharmaceutical products, but they do not reciprocate for their services in many instances. Furthermore, professional discounts do not stop with the prescribers but are extended to nurses, receptionists, and others, either by request or voluntarily. The question is where the professional discount should stop. Many pharmacists gladly extend these discounts when requested in the hopes of enhancing their professional relations with the prescribers and those associated with them. The ultimate goal, however, is the increase in the number of prescriptions from these sources. Other pharmacists actively seek the opportunity to offer professional discounts to prescribers and their associates.

It is the abuse of the professional discount that demeans pharmacy, and some logical and fair guidelines or policy should be established in every pharmacy. In addition, pharmacists in each market should establish a uniform policy or guideline and abide by it. Since the discount is based on professional courtesy, I do not see such an agreement as a violation of the Anti-trust Laws; however, such activity should be reviewed by an attorney in each case.

Sometimes, special discounts are offered to ministers, policemen, and others. In my opinion, there is no rational basis for these discounts.

Pricing Methods

Having discussed the competitive range and various competitive strategies to deal with the market situations, let us turn our attention to pricing methods. The competitive strategy and pricing policy of a pharmacist provide the theoretic and philosophic framework for price determination. However, the actual mathematic or nonmathematic methods of pricing constitute the final step of price determination.

NONMATHEMATIC METHODS

These methods of pricing are used under various circumstances described in the discussion of competitive strategy and pricing policies. They include the suggested selling price for products sold under a franchise agreement, fair trade laws where they are operative, and certain circumstances of competitive pricing in which the competitor's price is simply emulated. The haphazard pricing used in an attempt to get the price the market will bear is determined without the benefit of rational arithmetic calculation.

MATHEMATIC METHODS

The use of mathematics is a rational approach to price determination. The mathematic calculations should be based on a thorough understanding of management's objectives and policies, operational costs, and financial analysis of the financial statements. The *mechanics* of mathematic methods of pricing is based on the equation representing the relationship found in the profit and loss statement. The equation is expressed as follows:

$$SP - CGS - Exp = NP$$

where: SP = the selling price
    CGS = the cost of goods sold
    Exp = the expenses
    NP = the net profit

The basic equation may be broken down into two other equations:

$$SP - CGS = GM$$
$$GM - Exp = NP$$

where: GM = the gross margin.

In pharmacy, contrary to many other industries, the selling price always equals 100 percent, unless otherwise specified, just as net sales volume equals 100 percent in the profit and loss statement. The combined equations may be illustrated by percentages and dollars as follows:

SP − CGS = GM	and	GM − Exp = NP
100% − 65% = 35%	and	35% − 31% = 4%
$5.00 − $3.25 = $1.75	and	$1.75 − $1.55 = $0.20

The relationships illustrated are such that the desired selling price may be calculated if any one of the other terms of the equation and its corresponding percent are known. The dollar value is divided by the percent, expressed as a decimal, for example, $3.25 ÷ .65 = $5.00. The selling price in the above example may be calculated algebraically as follows:

Let X equal the selling price: then

$$(X)\,(.65) = \$3.25$$
$$.65X = \$3.25$$
$$X = \$5.00$$

Pharmacists have devised short cuts or easy methods for arriving at the selling price, given the unit cost, to provide a desired percent gross margin. An overview of the more commonly used short cuts should be valuable to the reader. To yield a 50 percent gross margin, double the cost; for a 40 percent gross margin, take two-thirds of the cost and add this figure to the cost, or divide the cost by 6 and multiply the quotient by 10; for a 33⅓ percent gross margin, take one-half of the cost and add this value to the cost; for a 25 percent gross margin, take one-third of the cost and add this figure to the cost; and for a 20 percent gross margin, take one-fourth of the cost and add this value to the cost. In each instance, the resulting selling price will yield the specified or desired percent gross margin.

PRICING OBJECTIVES

The mathematic method of pricing will permit the pharmacist to mark up a product or product line to accomplish specific objectives and to adjust the percent gross margin to compensate for turnover rates and other variables.

Return the Usual Net Profit. One pricing objective is to cover average expenses and usual net profit. The *Lilly Digest* percentage total expenses was 30.2 for 1983, and the estimated percentage for nonprescription sales was approximately 28 percent. The NACDS *Lilly Digest* average percentage for total expenses was 23.5 for 1983, and the estimated percentage expenses for nonprescription sales was approximately 20 percent. The percentages net profit were 2.9 and 5.1 and for gross margin, 33.1 and 28.6 for independent and chain pharmacies, respectively. Thus, the independent pharmacist sets his percentage gross margin for the bulk of nonprescription products at 28 to 33 percent, whereas the management of the chain drug firms targets the percentage markup of the bulk of nonprescription products at 22 to 26 percent.

Promotional Image. Another pricing objective is to cover variable expenses only for selected products and occasionally some net profit. If the objective is to cover variable expenses only, then the general purpose is to project a promotional or low price image. If the objective is to include some net profit, then the purpose is to maintain profits while projecting a promotional or low price image. For the purpose of this discussion, the following expense items are classified as *strict variable expenses,* even though they may be fixed to an extent for a given pharmacy: accounting and legal fees, advertising, bad debts, employees' wages, and miscellaneous expenses. Employee wages and miscellaneous expenses are semivariable, but they are classified as variable expenses for the purpose of delineating all expenses into two categories. Variable expenses for independent pharmacies were estimated at 15 percent from *Lilly Digest* data for 1983. For nonprescription sales, the variable expenses were estimated at 16 percent. If a pharmacist wishes to cover variable expenses only, he can take one-fifth of the unit cost and add this figure to the unit cost. If he wishes to make about 3 percent net profit on sales, he can add one-fourth of the unit cost to the unit cost. This method of pricing is used mostly for promotional, nonstaple merchandise.

It should be understood that pricing merchandise to cover variable expenses is *not* pricing at the marginal cost. The two are somewhat similar concepts, but the economics as well as the method of arriving at the marginal cost are quite different.

This type of pricing is *not* the true "loss leader" type of pricing whereby a product is priced at or near cost and sometimes below cost. The *objective* of the *loss leader* strategy of pricing is to create a definite low price image. Both special and staple goods are used for loss leaders.

Turnover Rate Variations. The percent gross margin should vary inversely with the turnover rate of a product. Turnover rate is determined by dividing the cost of goods sold by the average inventory investment. Table 15–1,

Table 15–1.   Relationship Between Gross Margin and Turnover Rate

Turnover Rate Per Unit	1.5		3		6	
Selling price	$1.00	100%	$1.00	100%	$1.00	100%
Cost	.50	50%	.60	60%	.65	65%
Gross margin	$ .50	50%	$ .40	40%	$ .35	35%
Expenses	.30	30%	.30	30%	.30	30%
Net profit	$ .20	20%	$ .10	10%	$ .05	5%
Annual NP	$ .30	—	$ .30	—	$ .30	—

composed of hypothetical data, illustrates how gross margin and turnover are inversely related while achieving the same annual net profit.

The same principle can be illustrated by actual data derived from the *Lilly Digest*. The pharmacies were divided into two groups for comparison—those with low turnover rates and those with high turnover rates. The gross margin, total expenses, proprietor's total income, and inventory were related to the respective turnover rates as shown in Table 15–2.

The data in Table 15–2 clearly indicate the relationship between increased turnover rate and proprietor's total income. This is achieved with a smaller percent gross margin and a smaller investment in inventory. The percentage of total income to sales is increased by 1.7 percent of sales, or $8,500 on $500,000 sales, as the turnover rate is increased 3-fold. With a good inventory control system, the turnover rate can be increased and the pharmacist will be in a good position to price wisely, be competitive as necessary, and still maintain good profits.

Table 15–2.   Relationship Between Turnover Rate and Other Operating Data

	Fast Turnover Pharmacies N = 228	Slow Turnover Pharmacies N = 337
Inventory turnover rate	8.9	3.0
Total sales	100.0%	100.0%
Cost of goods sold	68.4%	65.3%
Gross margin	31.6%	34.7%
Employees' wages	9.3%	11.4%
Rent and other expenses	12.2%	15.0%
Total expenses (less proprietor's salary)	21.5%	26.4%
Total income (proprietor's salary plus net profit)	10.0%	8.3%
Total Inventory	7.7%	21.4%

Source: Adapted from Deiner, C.H.: *The Lilly Digest 1984,* Indianapolis: Eli Lilly & Co., 1984, p. 36.

Prescription Pricing

The pharmacist should not be misled into believing that prescription prices are of little or no concern to the public. In fact, there is a relationship between trusting the pharmacist as a professional person to provide the necessary advice and the correct drug (including avoiding drug interactions and allergies), and trusting him to charge a reasonable price. If the trust is not fulfilled with respect to price, the pharmacist will lose the professional trust, and *vice versa*.[7] Since only a few popular maintenance prescription drugs, some 15 to 20, are discounted in most instances, this is one of the best arguments for using a reasonable professional or dispensing fee, a method that will yield a prescription price that is both competitive and defensible.

HISTORY OF PRICING

Attempts to establish fair and adequate dispensing or professional fees go back into the antiquity of pharmacy. These efforts have been both private and public. As discussed in Chapter 1, one of the earliest public attempts to regulate prescription prices was the edict of Frederick II.[8] Griffenhagen traced the early private attempts to promote "Fair Trade" in prescription pricing.[9] He described the *Catalogue of the Materia Medica and of Pharmaceutical Preparation with Uniform Prices of the Massachusetts College of Pharmacy* published in 1828. It included 40 pages and 700 items. It was the first such American catalogue with printed prices. A unique feature was a compounding pricing schedule, which included the following example: Pills: 2 to 4, 12 cents; 6 to 8, 19 cents; 10 to 18, 25 cents; and 1 cent each over 30. There was a schedule for powders, liquids, ointments, and plasters. Clearly, this schedule was a type of compounding or professional fee. Griffenhagen noted earlier catalogues, but he emphasized the uniform pricing and pricing schedule aspects of the Massachusetts catalogue.[10]

No doubt interest in prescription pricing has occupied the thinking and deliberations of pharmacists over the years since 1828. McEvilla reviewed briefly some of the early history of the changing attitudes toward prescription pricing between World War II and the 1950s.[11] Myers provided a more extensive review of the changing attitudes and approaches toward the professional fee in an article entitled, "Professional Fee: Renaissance or Innovation?"[12] Nitardy made one of the earlier contributions to rational prescription pricing when he developed the "Prescription Pricing Schedule" for the National Association of Retail Druggists (NARD) in 1908.[13] The schedule was based on the cost of ingredient(s), doubling this, and adding a compounding charge as a reward for professional skills and knowledge. Almost every pricing schedule developed since the Nitardy schedule contained a dispensing or professional fee, which included either a nominal or a substantial amount, for the professional function.

Myers briefly described two other prescription pricing schedules devised by Cutts and the Minnesota Pharmaceutical Association in 1893 and 1903, respectively.[12] The proliferation of prescription pricing methods was beginning to take place. Chase also noted that chaos and diversity of prescription prices existed from the use of the many different schedules and rules.[14] In 1915, he found that some pharmacists were "getting whatever they think the customer will stand for. . ."

Until World War I, the cost of ingredients generally was not the major factor in pricing prescriptions. The labor cost and professional skills involved were major considerations. Therefore, most of the various pricing schedules and rules contained a significant professional fee component. This began to change with the high cost of drugs and chemicals during World War I. These higher costs resulted from the fact that most drugs and chemicals were imported and Germany was the world's largest producer. The price of acetophenetidin increased as much as 2,000 to 3,000 percent.[12] As a result, "a flat-rate system of pricing was no longer feasible."

In 1915 the APhA appointed a committee to investigate the matter and suggest a proper manner of pricing prescriptions. The Committee, under the chairmanship of Harry B. Mason, made its report, and the House of Delegates adopted Evans' rule as the preferred method of prescription pricing. Evans' rule was rather simple and did not confuse the issue greatly. It simply stated that a pharmacist should double the cost of the ingredient(s) in the prescription and add $1.00 per hour for the time consumed in compounding the prescription. Ironically, one of the two papers presented by title only at the same session was written by Nitardy, who had devised the NARD Schedule, and who advocated that a fee for the professional services of the pharmacist be incorporated into the formula or schedule.[12]

From this historic moment until the present day, at least *five* major developments have increased the emphasis on the cost of the drug and the percent markup, with de-emphasis on the professional component of prescription services. First, the industrial revolution in the pharmaceutical industry brought about a reduction in the number of compounded prescriptions, with a corresponding reduction in the utilization of the manipulative skills of the pharmacist. Second, the revolution brought about a proliferation of potent, prefabricated pharmaceuticals with a "high" ingredient cost to the pharmacist. Third, with the gradual expansion of the merchandising function of the pharmacist, there was a gradual carry-over tendency to apply the markup concept more directly in the prescription department. Fourth, the enactment of the fair trade laws in the 1930s and their application to prescription legend drugs had a most profound and direct influence on the philosophy of prescription pricing. The minimum fair trade price was based on a percentage markup. Last, the various prescription pricing schedules, devised during the 1950s as a timesaving convenience, emphasized the markup aspect, but retained a substantial or nominal professional fee as a part of the final prescription price.

ANALYSIS OF PRICING SCHEDULES

Many prescription pricing schedules were devised during the years between World War II and the 1960s. Although these schedules claimed a rationale, they generally were short on sound logic. Kendall and Lee attempted to correct this deficiency by analyzing various schedules and developing an improved formula.[15] They found that most schedules used one of the following formulas:

1. *Computation type—*

$$M + C + CF = SP$$

where: M = the material cost plus a markup;
C = the container cost with or without a markup;
CF = the compounding fee, determined by multiplying the compounding time by $1 to $3, depending on the pharmacist's hourly salary;
SP = the selling price.

2. *Computation plus a flat rate—*

$$C + S + M = SP$$

where: C = the compounding fee;
S = a flat service charge;
M = the material cost plus a markup;
SP = the selling price.

The markup varied from 33⅓ to 50 percent of the cost, depending on the value of the ingredients. The improved formula of Kendall and Lee varied little from previous formulas except that an average service fee, SF, was established, based on the average time for experienced pharmacists to compound a given number of units of a dosage form. For prefabricated prescriptions, one-half of the service fee was used. The revised formula was:

$$M + C + SF = SP$$

where: M = the cost of materials plus a markup of 33⅓ to 50 percent;
C = the cost of the container, which was doubled;
SF = a flat rate based on the number of units dispensed;
SP = the selling price.

There are basically four methods of computing prescription charges.

> Percent gross margin (GM)
> Sliding scale gross margin
> Professional fee
> A combination of these

Analysis of several prescription pricing schedules revealed the following variations and combinations of the four basic methods. One schedule used a fixed percent GM and a fixed dispensing fee to determine the total prescription price. Another schedule applied a decreasing percent GM with increments of cost of the quantity dispensed without a dispensing fee. A third schedule used a decreasing percent GM with increments of the cost of the quantity dispensed plus a variable fee which increased with the increments of quantity dispensed. Four schedules utilized a decreasing percent GM based on the quantity dispensed, without respect to cost of the drug, plus a percentage dispensing fee added to the GM. Three other schedules utilized some form of professional fee concept. None of the other possible combinations of the basic pricing methods was observed.

All of the schedules examined made provision for a professional fee for compounded prescriptions. One schedule provided a fixed professional fee of $2.00 added to the cost of ingredients. The same device provided six variable percent gross margin schedules for a wide range of choices. The variable percentage markups decreased at a decreasing rate with increasing number of units dispensed. It supposedly followed a ''curve'' rather than a step-wise progression.* One other schedule also utilized a ''curve'' in establishing the gross margin to which a fee could be added, but all the other schedules were based on a decrease in percent gross margin, ranging from a minimum of two to ten steps. Some had a fee built into the selling price as shown in the schedule, while others suggested a fixed or variable fee to be added to the ''commodity'' value of the prescription drug as shown in the schedule.

There are *several objections* to most of the existing pricing schedules:

1. The price of small quantities of inexpensive prescriptions frequently is not sufficient to cover the amount of fixed costs of dispensing. This ''deficit'' is made up on larger quantities and expensive prescriptions which causes a hardship on the patrons affected.

2. The use of some of the schedules requires interpolation, especially for the more expensive drugs.

3. Some schedules vary the percent gross margin in a manner that causes inequities in prescription charges among patrons. For example, 50 tablets that cost $2.00 per 100 sell for $2.35, while 10 tablets costing $10.00 per 100 sell for $2.85. This is a 50 cent difference in price for a $1.00 ingredient cost in each instance, but fewer doses are provided in the more expensive prescription.

Professional Fees

REVIVAL OF PROFESSIONAL FEES

A serious attempt to determine the cost of dispensing prescriptions was made by Jeffries.[16] He established norms for dispensing prefabricated prescriptions using time and motion studies. An average overhead or expense per prescription was computed, which was applicable to most pharmacies. The study further indicated three levels of labor cost (5, 6, and 7 cents per minute, respectively) depending on the market. He devised three sliding charts

---

*The publisher of the schedule stated the selling price was calculated ''on a curve.'' The ingredient cost varied by a fraction of a cent in the low cost range, but the ingredient cost varied by discrete intervals (in excess of one cent) in the higher cost range and by one cent intervals in the mid-range.

corresponding to the three different labor costs per minute which, when set at the combined cost of the ingredient and container, would indicate the breakeven cost over eleven different time intervals required to dispense the prescription. To the breakeven cost, the pharmacist could add a flat or percentage fee, respresenting the net profit for each prescription dispensed. This chart was made available to pharmacists by Becton, Dickinson and Company.

Evanson's economic analysis of prescription departments provided basic operational data that gave further insight into the economics of prescription pricing.[17] In 1952, Apple published another method of calculating prescription charges.[18] His method included both a significant professional fee and a commodity value. In 1957, a student of Professor Fuller first advocated a simple, all inclusive single professional fee for all prescriptions filled in a particular pharmacy.[19,20] Since then, much has been written for, and against, the professional fee concept.[21] It generally is believed by those who have made a serious study of the fee concept that a professional fee *is* possible. It can be simple to use and is easy to adjust to meet competitive conditions or to maintain a desired profit structure.

PHILOSOPHY

Before one can really appreciate and understand or use the professional fee concept, one must examine the three basic tenets of its philosophy. They are:

1. A prescription drug is not an ordinary article of trade that the public may buy or sell at their pleasure. Prescription drugs are developed and produced to alleviate human suffering. They are potent compounds and are subject to misuse and abuse in unskilled hands. Therefore, laymen may possess these drugs only through competent professional people, including the pharmacist, after diagnosis of the illness, prescribing and proper dispensing of the indicated drug.

2. Neither the dispensing cost nor the benefit dervied from such prescription is a function of the cost of the ingredient(s) in a prescription.

3. Neither the professional and legal responsibility nor the time incurred in dispensing a prescription is a function of the cost of the ingredient(s) in a prescription.

Having accepted these three tenents, one can proceed to examine the pros and cons of the fee concept.

PROS AND CONS OF PROFESSIONAL FEES

Advantages. First, there are several economic advantges to the professional fee:

1. The fee concept tends to stabilize prescription prices, protecting the pharmacist from a profit squeeze due to prescriptions of less expensive brands or generic drugs, and protecting the public from high prescription charges resulting from a markup on expensive new drugs.

2. The pharmacist is able to recover all expense and a fair return on *each* prescription dispensed on a fee basis.

3. The professional fee permits a competitive charge for expensive, maintenance prescriptions.

4. The fee, being fixed, saves time and prevents miscalculations and errors.

5. The fee may be used to improve professional relations. Physicians have been enthusiastic in accepting the fee concept.

6. Since most patients accept the fee concept wholeheartedly, it will, when properly used, promote good public relations and image.

7. The fee could have legal advantages in negotiations with third-party payers, since it more nearly defines the professional services of the pharmacist than does the markup method. History has not proved this particular advantage to be the case.

Potential Problems. Some of the potential problems, and their resolutions, which a pharmacist may encounter with the fee are:

1. How does one price refills of prescriptions already on file? The answer to this question lies in not raising the price on any refill, but rather, adjusting downwardly the price of expensive refills.

2. What does one do about requests for refills of multiple or fractional amounts? The fee remains the same unless a certain defined upper limit is exceeded. This will discourage refills for one-half or one-fourth amounts, which are seldom economic. Such requests have been eliminated largely by third-party payment programs. Exceptions are made in the case in which only a few doses are needed until the next appointment with the physician. The fee is retained for all larger quantities up to the size of the regular stock bottle of 100 or less. An adjustment of the fee is added for the second or fraction of each additional stock bottle quantity dispensed. This rule is designed solely to protect the pharmacist economically from someone deliberately prescribing or requesting unusually large quantities.

3. What about new prescriptions for large quantities? The answer is the same as discussed above.

4. How does one compute the fee for a compounded prescription? Simply add to the regular price the appropriate rate for the pharmacist's time spent in compounding. This occurs in less than one percent of the prescription.

5. How does the fixed fee cover the cost plus a return on the investment in inventory? The answer is that only about 15 percent of the variable overhead expense can be related directly to inventory investment. Also, only about 40 to 50 percent of the inventory-related expenses is attributable to prescription inventory. The average variable cost directly associated with the investment in prescription inventory (other than *imputed* interest) is only $0.20 per prescription based on 1984 *Lilly Digest* data. Most expenses are fixed on an annual basis. Average return on the inventory investment can be calculated for each prescription, and this will ensure the proper return on inventory investments. Based on 1984 *Lilly Digest* data and a 10 percent interest rate, $0.12 per prescription will cover the average interest cost. If one uses the

full 20 percent estimated inventory carrying cost, the average cost is $0.23 per prescription. Since the professional fee uses the cost of dispensing concept and includes all allocated overhead expenses, only the interest charge is a legitimate consideration, and this cost should be included in the overall net profit component.

6. Isn't the fee unrealistic for prescription ingredients costing $15.00 or more? The answer is that a fairly small percentage of the prescriptions cost $15.00. The supposed deficit on expensive prescriptions can be adequately compensated by the increased revenue from the less expensive prescriptions.

BASIS OF FEE COMPUTATION

Regardless of the method used to determine the prescription charge, consideration must be given to three basic factors: (1) the cost of the ingredient and the container; (2) the cost incurred in dispensing the prescription; (3) the profit necessary to sustain the practice and to permit its growth.

The first of these is always computed in the same manner, regardless of the pricing method used. The second and third factors may be combined and an average value per prescription is computed to arrive at the professional fee. The markup method is based on the theory that the sum of factors two and three is a function or percentage of factor one. Since this is not true, the markup is not a logical method. The major difficulty lies in how much the professional fee should be, but this difficulty also exists with the markup method. Several methods of determining the professional fee have been proposed.

OLDER METHODS

Fuller's Formula.[22] Fuller offered the following formula:

$$\frac{(AE - PS)\,(R_xS \div TS)}{TR_x} + LC + NP = PF$$

where: AE = All expenses
PS = Proprietor's salary
R_xS = Prescription sales
TS = Total sales
TR_x = Total number of prescriptions dispensed
LC = Direct labor cost ($0.50 in the original formula; $2.00 now)
NP = Desired net profit
PF = Professional fee

Applying this formula to 1984 *Lilly Digest* data, the average professional fee for all the pharmacies is $3.14 plus desired net profit of $0.56 = 3.70 fee.

Abrams's Formula.[23] Abrams has suggested the following formula:

$$\frac{(AE - PS)(R_xS \div TS) + PS}{TR_x} + NP = PF$$

If this formula is applied to the same *Lilly Digest* pharmacies, the professional fee is $3.75 plus desired net profit of $0.55 = $4.30 fee.

Jacoff's Method. Jacoff and Evanson computed an average burden rate of $1.39 per prescription for 1960 *Lilly Digest* pharmacies.[24] The burden rate was 43.5 percent of the average prescription charge. If this percentage is applied to the average prescription charge reported in the 1984 *Lilly Digest,* the burden rate would be $4.74. To this figure the desired net profit must be added. It should be noted that $4.74 may not be the burden rate per prescription for 1984 *Lilly Digest* pharmacies, if the burden rate is recalculated by means of the technique of Jacoff and Evanson.

Jacoff and Evanson applied the cost accounting technique to 1958 data derived from a prescription-oriented pharmacy.[25] Their burden rate was $1.00. Again, extrapolating the percentage of the burden rate to the average prescription charge for pharmacies in 1984 Lilly Digest data, the estimated 1984 burden rate would be $3.55.

Knox's Method.[26] A trial and error method of computing a professional fee was suggested by Knox. This method requires the use of a representative sample of prescriptions—both new and renewals—dispensed during the previous year. From the sample, an average prescription charge is computed. A professional fee is selected and added to the ingredient cost of each prescription. The average of the prescription charges using the fee is computed and compared with the average of the original prices. The fee is adjusted so that the same average charge, gross margin, and net profit potential are realized. A simpler approach would be to compute the average gross margin for a representative sample of original prices and round to the nearest five cents or quarter. This gives a professional fee that ensures approximately the same net profit.

An average cost of dispensing a prescription of $1.69 was reported in 1968.[27] This study, sponsored by the NARD, was based on 1,638 usable questionnaires, which were purported to represent the U.S. pharmacies. This figure projected to 1984 based on CPI prescription subcomponent would be approximately $3.90.

Smith's Method.[28] Smith applied cost accounting principles to 1964 *Lilly Digest* data and computed a burden rate per prescription ranging from $.85 to $1.75 when the data were classified by sales volume and number of prescriptions dispensed per day. The Kansas Department of Social Welfare modified and refined the cost allocation method published by Smith and others, and the modified method is applied to each pharmacy that wishes to participate in the Kansas Title XIX Program.[29] The modifications in the Kansas Form require that: (1) any direct expense that can be identified as a direct prescription department expense is allocated directly to that department, for example, prescription bags; and (2) insurance premiums and property taxes are allocated to the prescription department on the basis of prescription inventory divided by total inventory and prescription fixtures and equipment divided by total fixtures and equipment, respectively. A further refinement of the Kansas Form was published in *The Kentucky Pharmacist*.[30]

REVISED METHODOLOGY

More recently, Smith modified his method to make it sensitive to inflationary pressures, the effects of high interest rate and the notion that any pricing method should integrate the cost of the capital investment.[31] The various costs associated with the dispensing process may be divided into five categories: professional labor cost, direct prescription cost, fixed cost, semivariable and variable cost. These are discussed in turn.

Professional Labor Cost. It is easy to conceptualize professional labor cost but it is more difficult to determine. The question is: what percentages of time at work is/are the pharmacist(s), technician(s) and clerk(s) engaged in prescription related activities? Most cost-of-dispensing (COD) methods require the pharmacist (proprietor or manager) to estimate these percentages. Of course, this is not a very accurate method.

There are methodologies for determining these percentages that are much more accurate than estimations: time and motion, and work sampling studies. The former method is better suited for compact, less varied work in which the time to perform each segment of the total work component is important. The latter method is better suited for flexible, more varied work such as prescription processing/dispensing with all that entails. In this latter case, the proportion of time spent in the various, diverse segments of the work is the significant concern.

Work sampling requires considerable time and expense because a large sample of time units across, weeks, days, hours and minutes must be scientifically delineated for observation to determine what proportion of time is devoted to each segment of activity of interest. For our problem, the proportion spent on prescription related work vis-a-vis all other activity is the objective of the study. The reader may conclude at this point that this is not a viable alternative, but he/she would be wrong. Even a modified, reduced version of work sampling is far better than the current method of estimation (guessimation). Since only two relatively large proportions or percentages are the dependent variables of interest, fewer observations are required for accuracy.

For example, if one accepts a 95 percent confidence level (i.e., correct 95 percent of the time) and a margin of error of 6.6 percent, then only 900 observations are required. To reduce the error rate to 5 percent, 700 more observations would be required. Assume a pharmacy is open 10 hours a day, six days a week and observations are made on a fixed time interval of every two minutes. Also, assume observations are made for one hour, then rest for one hour to prevent fatigue related errors, then 150 observations are made per day (30 × 5 hrs). Begin making observations the first hour the pharmacy is open on Monday, the second hour the pharmacy is open on Tuesday, return to the first for Wednesday, and so forth, then 900 observations will be made in one week during 30 hours of observation. A packet of instructions with indicators of prescription and nonprescription related activity and an observation schedule and form should be developed.

A pharmacy student with considerable experience in a prescription department can be trained in two 5-hour sessions to make the observations accurately for one pharmacist and one assistant on an every other minute basis. At a wage of $5 per hour for the student, a work sampling study for one pharmacist and one assistant can be completed for $200. If there is little overlap in the work schedules of two pharmacists and their assistants, then the above schedule would suffice for the entire pharmacy; otherwise two weeks of observations may be required—at a maximum cost of $400. A member of the family could perform the study without any out-of-pocket cost.

For small pharmacies with prescription volume of less than 15,000 Rx's per year, a rule-of-thumb approach may be sufficiently accurate, as follows: Allow 8 mintues per prescription for all the work associated with the dispensing function. This includes receiving the prescription and clarifying any required information, processing the prescription, delivering the prescription with consultation to the patient, filing the prescription and performing any third-party paperwork, and allowing at least two minutes per prescription for all of the associated work of talking with company representatives and prescribers, ordering, checking and stocking drugs and keeping required records. Then multiply the pharmacist's gross hourly salary by 0.133 (8 min. ÷ 60 min.). For example, if the gross hourly salary is $15, then $15 × 0.133 = $2.00, the professional labor cost.

Direct Prescription Costs. These costs are easy to conceptualize and to determine provided there are good accounting records. These expenses are allocated 100 percent to the prescription department. They include prescription containers, labels, patient profile, special forms, and bags; pharmacy permit and DEA license; pharmacist's license renewal, continuing education expense, professional organizational dues and subscriptions; laundry cost for professional attire and towels; premiums for professional and product liability insurance; direct telephone and exclusive prescription telephone expense; and any other expense of operating or promoting the prescription department exclusively.

There are few categories of expense that may or may not be exclusively prescription costs such as delivery and computer costs. In the case of delivery, if the pharmacy's policy is that only prescriptions or orders containing a prescription are delivered, then all delivery related costs are allocated 100 percent to the prescription department. If this is not the policy, the log of deliveries made (time out and in, dollar amount, name and address) should have a place to check whether the delivery contained a prescription. The daily, weekly and yearly tally of prescription and nonprescription deliveries will provide the basis for allocating delivery expenses. If deliveries are made only occasionally, then a record of these in a small notebook can be used to determine the yearly cost on the basis of the minimum cost charged by a commercial delivery service.

In the case of the computer, if it is used exclusively for prescription related work, then this cost should be allocated 100 percent to the prescription department. If the only nonprescription computer processing is accounts receivable, then 80 to 90 percent, depending on the number of accounts receivable, should be allocated to the department. If the pharmacy is fully computerized (accounts receivable and payable, general ledger and some "front" activity), then computer expenses should be allocated as variable costs to be discussed later.

Local business permit or license, chamber of commerce, better business, credit bureau, NARD dues or fees should *not* be allocated 100 percent to the prescription department; rather these expenses should be allocated as a variable cost.

Fixed Costs. Fixed costs are those expenses that do not vary with the level of sales; rather they remain fixed irrespective of sales at least in the near-term of one year. Fixed expenses include rent, (unless the rent is paid as a percentage of sales in which case the rent, or that part paid as a percentage, is allocated as a variable expense), utilities (electric, gas, water, not telephone), repairs and depreciation. If accounting records will permit, repairs and/or depreciation may be allocated on the basis of the value of fixtures and equipment in the prescription department to the total value of fixtures and equipment. Even a more precise method would be to allocate the exact cost for either repairs or depreciation of fixtures and equipment within the prescription department, if records indicate this. The depreciation of the delivery vehicle, as well as insurance, taxes and other expenses related to it should be treated as indicated under direct prescription costs. If the pharmacist owns the building, he should impute rent at the market rate.

These expenses are related to the space occupied, and often referred to as occupancy costs, and are allocated on the basis of the ratio of sq. ft. of prescription space to the sq. ft. of total space. In calculating this ratio, the following allowances should be made: (1) Be sure to include the sq. ft. in the stockroom devoted to prescription goods (containers and the like) in the prescription department. (2) Include in the prescription space the sq. ft. "out front" that are used for patient waiting and consultation, using a minimum of 60 sq. ft. (3) For each of the main traffic aisles, i.e., those aisles that run front to back only and carry most of the traffic, subtract the sum of the sq. ft. equal to 2.5 or 33 ft. × length of the aisle for all such aisles from the total sq. ft. of space. The inner space of the traffic aisles is used primarily as a traffic conduit and not as "shopping space." If the traffic aisle is 3 ft. or less, use the 2.5 ft. value; if it is more than 3 ft., use the 3 ft. value.

Semivariable Costs. Semivariable costs are of a mixed nature. For example, delivery expense has elements that vary with sales, viz. gasoline and oil, and elements that do not vary with sales, viz., auto insurance. As sales increase, deliveries will increase and so will the amount of gasoline consumed. Also other expenses, e.g., fire insurance on property, vary indirectly with sales with a time lag sometimes involved. As sales increase, the amount of inventory does not directly and immediately increase, but it will eventually. Thus the insurance premium will increase for the following period. However, it is further complicated by the fixtures and equipment portion of the insurance premium against fire. Its value decreases each year due to depreciation. This may or may not offset the increase premium on inventory of products.

Semivariable expenses include insurance, property taxes, interest paid, accounting and legal fees, and possibly imputed interest of the investment. The first three of these have a special relationship to the investment in inventory, fixtures and equipment. Thus, they are allocated on the basis of the ratio of the value of prescription inventory, fixtures and equipment to the total investment in these items. The other two items are treated as variable expenses for the present analysis.

The reader is reminded that if the professional and product liability insurance premium, pharmacy permit and DEA license, and direct telephone costs have already been allocated as direct costs, then these should be subtracted and not counted again in this category or as variable expenses.

Variable Costs. Variable costs are expenses that vary with sales. They include employee wages, accounting and legal fees, advertising, bad debts and miscellaneous expenses. Employee wages do not figure in calculating the professional fee except as a part of professional labor cost. Since these expenses vary with sales, they are allocated to the prescription department on the basis of ratio of prescription sales to total sales. That part of the proprietor's salary not allocated as professional labor is considered to be in this category for the purpose of calculating COD because he spends the remainder of his time managing the pharmacy. If delivery and telephone expenses have not already been allocated directly to the prescription department or on some other basis, then these two expenses are included here. Care should be taken not to count any portion of an expense twice.

STEPS IN COMPUTING PROFESSIONAL FEE

Step 1. PROFESSIONAL LABOR. Calculate the professional labor on the basis of percentage of time devoted to prescription related activities determined preferably by work sampling methodology. This cost is applied as an average cost per prescription.

Step 2. DIRECT PRESCRIPTION COST. These costs are identified, summed and applied as an average cost per prescription.

Step 3. FIXED/OCCUPANCY COST. These costs are allocated on the

	Dollars	%
Total Net Sales		$508,000	100
Net Prescription Sales	$330,000		65
Net Other Sales	178,000		35
Cost of Goods Sold		335,300	66
Gross Margin		$172,700	34
Expenses:			
Proprietor's Salary	$ 30,000		6.0
Employee Wages	55,000	(85,000)	10.8
Rent	12,000		2.4
Heat, Light & Power	4,800		0.9
Repairs	2,000	(18,800)	0.4
Depreciation	5,000	(5,000)	1.0
Taxes (except bldg & income)	7,000		1.4
Insurance (except building)	5,000		1.0
Interest Paid	2,200	(14,000)	0.4
Direct Expenses*	7,500	(7,500)	1.5
Accounting & Legal Fees	2,000		0.4
Advertising	7,200		1.4
Bad Debts Charged	500		0.1
Telephone	1,000		0.2
Miscellaneous Expenses	11,400	(22,100)	2.2
Total Expenses		152,400	30.0
Net Profit		20,300	4.0

*Direct Expenses include prescription containers, labels and bags; computer supplies and amortization; delivery; professional licenses, permits, dues, subscriptions, CE and insurance, exclusive prescription telephone, and laundry.

Figure 15–1. Classified income and expense statement.

basis of percentage of prescription space to total space and applied as an average cost per prescription.

Step 4. SEMIVARIABLE COST. These costs are semivariable and investment related. They are allocated on the basis of the percentage of prescription investment to total investment in inventory, fixtures and equipment. It may be applied either as an average per prescription or as a percentage of the cost of ingredients or goods sold (CGS). This is illustrated in the case to follow.

Step 5. VARIABLE COST. These costs are allocated on the basis of the percentage of prescription sales to total sales. This cost also may be applied as an average per prescription or as a percentage of CGS.

Step 6. SUM OF THE VARIOUS COMPONENTS. This is the COD or breakeven figure.

COD AUXILLARY DATA

Item	Prescription	Other	Total
Inventory	$36,000	$32,000	$68,000
Inventory Per Prescription	1.31		
Fixtures and Equipment	10,000*	12,000	22,000*
Total	$46,000	$44,000	$90,000
Percentage	51	49	100
Space, Sq. Ft.	500	2,500	3,000
Percentage	16.7	83.3	100
No. of Prescriptions Disp.	27,400	(51% new; 49%, refills)	
Average Prescription Charge	$ 12.05		
Hours per week pharmacy is open			60
Hours per week employee pharmacist works			40
Hours per week proprietor-pharmacist works			46
Employee pharmacist gross salary (incl. FICA, etc.)			$32,000
Employee pharmacist 90 percent in prescription department			
Proprietor works 65 percent in the prescription department			
Technician/Clerk works 80 percent (32 hrs.) in the prescription dept.			
Technician's gross hourly wage is $6.50 per hour.			

Figure 15–2.   Auxiliary pharmacy COD data.

Step 7. FINAL FEE. Determine the average amount of desired net profit and add this to the above COD for the final fee. Alternatively, the net profit may be applied as a percentage of CGS.

Case Study

The data for the case study are found in Figures 15–1 and 15–2. This is a typical pharmacy and is similar to the *Lilly Digest* average. A work sampling study indicated the employee pharmacist worked 90 percent, proprietor worked 65 percent, and a technician/clerk worked 80 percent in prescription related duties. Note when allocating the proprietor's salary to the prescription department, an hourly rate equivalent to the employee pharmacist's gross salary rate is used. The remainder of the proprietor's gross salary is transferred to the variable cost category for the purpose of calculating the COD.

Calculations:

1. Employee Pharmacist: $32,000 × 0.90   = $28,800
2. Proprietor: 46 hrs/wk × 0.65 × 52 wks × $15.40 hr. = 23,944
      Technician: 40 hrs/wk × 0.80 × 52 wks × $6.50/hr = 10,816

      Subtotal $63,560
      Professional Labor per Prescription   = 2.32
3. Direct Prescription cost: = 7,500
      Per Prescription   = 0.27
4. Fixed Costs: $18,800 × 0.167   = 3,140
      Depreciation: $5,000 × 0.45*   = 2,250

      Subtotal   = 5,390
      Per Prescription   = 0.20
5. Semivariable Cost: $14,000 × 0.51   = 7,140
      Per Prescription   = 0.26
6. Variable Cost: $22,000 × 0.65   = 14,365
      Per Prescription   = 0.52

7. Sum, COD   = $97,955
      Per Prescription, COD   3.58
8. Professional Fee: COD + NP
      Est. 75% of NP in Rx Dept.: $20,300 × 0.75 = 15,225
      Per Prescription NP   = 0.56
      Professional Fee   = 4.18
      (Rounded)   (4.20)

A modification of the flat dispensing fee is recommended to keep prescription prices abreast of inflation during inflationary periods. The recommended formula is as follows:

$$PF = PL + DC + FC + SC\% + VC\% + NP\%$$

Where:
    PF = Professional Fee
    PL = Professional Labor Cost Average
    DC = Direct Cost Average
    FC = Fixed Cost Average
   SC% = Semivariable Cost as a % of Selling Price (SP)
   VC% = Variable Cost as a % of SP
   NP% = Net Profit as a % of SP
We now calculate the percentages of sales for SC, VC and NP.
   SC% = $ 7,140 ÷ $330,000 = 2.2%
   VC% = $14,365 ÷ $330,000 = 4.4%
   NP% = $15,225 ÷ $330,000 = 4.6%
Consolidating the data in the formula:
   PF = $2.32 + $0.27 + $0.20 + 0.022 SP + 0.044 SP + 0.046 SP
   PF = $2.79 + 0.112 SP ; SP = CGS + $2. 79 × 0.112 SP

Apply formula to an example, cost of drug = \$7.90:

$$SP = \$7.90 + \$2.79 + 0.112\ SP$$
$$SP = \$10.69 + 0.112\ SP$$
$$0.888\ SP = \$10.69$$
$$SP = \$10.69 \div 0.888$$
$$SP = \$12.04, \$12.05\ \text{rounded}$$
$$NP = \$12.05 - [\$7.90 + \$2.79 + (12.05 \times 0.066)] = \$0.56$$

Meeting Competition

If a pharmacy practice faces severe competition in prescription prices, especially with selected popular drugs used as "loss leaders," the pharmacist-manager should develop a strategy to meet this challenge. For the professional minded pharmacist, superior service, both conventional and clinical, would be the best "offensive" weapon. In addition, he may wish to lower the price on a selected group of drugs. If he does this, it may be necessary to adjust the price on other prescriptions to offset the decreased revenue, using the following technique.

1. Determine the list of drugs on which the price will be reduced.
2. Conduct a survey of your prescription files by selecting 100 prescriptions each month beginning with the first Monday, then the second Tuesday and so forth for the past 12 months.
3. Determine the percent for each drug on the list.
4. Adjust the price on each drug to be competitive.
5. Project the number of prescriptions per year for each drug on the list.
6. Multiply the amount of price reduction for each drug on the list by the projected number of prescriptions per year.
7. Sum these amounts for all drugs on the list.
8. Subtract the total number of projected prescriptions on the list from the total number of prescriptions dispensed the previous year.
9. Divide the number (the remainder) into the total dollar amount of reduced revenue from price reductions.
10. This is the amount that you will need to add to each prescription to offset the reduced revenue.

This may be added as a flat fee or converted to a percentage, e.g., \$0.48 (loss/Rx) ÷ \$12.00 (Average SP) = 0.04 or 4%.

Summary

The methodology described in this chapter is somewhat involved but comprehensible. Any pharmacist can perform the analyses and apply the methodology with little effort. Conducting such a case study for your pharmacy at least once each year will provide much insight into the economics of your pharmacy practice. The pharmacist-manager who does not conduct such a study, using this or a similar methodology, may very well face a business loss and possibly failure during the contemporary competitive market climate.

REFERENCES

1. *Communicating the Value of Comprehensive Pharmaceutical Services to the Consumer.* Washington: American Pharmaceutical Association, 1973, p. 14.
2. Aspinwall, L.V.: *Four Marketing Theories.* Boulder, Colo.: Bureau of Business Research, University of Colorado, 1959.
3. Odiorne, G.S.: *Management Decisions by Objectives.* Englewood Cliffs: Prentice-Hall, 1969, p. 170.
4. *Supermarket Merchandising,* Nov., 1960, p. 83.
5. The same prescription means two or more prescriptions for the same quantity, the same drug, and the same strength.
6. Anon. by request, personal communications.
7. *Communicating the Value of Comprehensive Pharmaceutical Services to the Consumer.* Washington: Amer. Pharm. Assoc., 1973, p. 28.
8. Sonnedecker, G.: *Kremers and Urdang's History of Pharmacy,* 3rd ed. Philadelphia: J.B. Lippincott Co.,1963, p. 39.
9. Griffenhagen, G.: Fair Trade in 1828. *J. Am. Pharm. Assoc., Pract. Pharm. Ed. 20*:156, 1959.
10. *Ibid.*
11. McEvilla, J.D.: Pharmacy and the professional fee in theory and practice. *J. Am. Pharm. Assoc., NS 2*:520, 1962.
12. Myers, M.J.: Professional fee: renaissance or innovation? *J. Am. Pharm. Assoc., NS 8*:628–631, 1968.
13. Nitardy, F.W: Prescription pricing schedule. *NARD Notes 6*:17, 1968.
14. Chase, W.M.: Prescription prices in Detroit. *J. Am. Pharm. Assoc., 4*:1357, 1915.
15. Kendall, H.L., and Lee, C.O.: Rapid method for determination of prescription fees. *J. Am. Pharm. Assoc., Pract. Pharm. Ed., 5*:130–135, 1944.
16. Jeffries, S.B.: *The Universal Prescription Costing and Pricing Calculator.* Rutherford, N.J.: Becton, Dickinson & Co., 1953.
17. Evanson, R.V.: An Economical Study of Prescription Departments in Indiana Pharmacies. Dissertation, Purdue University, 1953.
18. Apple, W.S.: Prescription pricing. *Wisconsin Commerce Reports, 3,* No. 3 (Aug., 1952).
19. Fuller, H.J.: *Bull. Ont. Coll. Pharm., 6*:43, 1957.
20. Fuller, H.J.: *Can. Pharm. J. 90*:418, 1957.
21. For a comprehensive review of the professional fee see *J. Am. Pharm. Assoc. NS 2,* No. 9, 1962; *J. Am. Pharm. Assoc., NS 8,* No. 12, 1968; *Am. J. Hosp. Pharm., 23,* No. 9, 1966; and *Hosp. Pharm., 2*:11–20, 1967.
22. Fuller, H.J.: *Bull. Ont. Coll. Pharm., 13*:80, 1964.
23. Abrams, R.E.: *Focus on Pharmacy, 1962.* Detroit: Wayne State University College of Pharmacy, March, 1962.
24. Jacoff, M.D., and Evanson, R.V.: An expense-cost analysis for professional fee planning. *J. Am. Pharm. Assoc., NS 2*:525–528, 1962.
25. Jacoff, M.D., and Evanson, R.V.: An application of cost accounting to prescription pricing. Paper presented to the Section on Pharmaceutical Economics, APhA Annual Meeting, Washington, D.C. (Aug. 1960).
26. Knox, H.: Procedure for setting professional fee. *J. Amer. Pharm. Assoc., NS 2*:530, 1962.
27. Anon.: NARD prescription cost study. *NARDJ, 90*:17, 1968.
28. Smith, H.A.: Determining the professional fee. *J. Amer. Pharm. Assoc., NS 8*:646–649, 1968.
29. Several investigators and I have contributed to the development of present cost of dispensing formulas. Professor Hugh Cotton was one of the first persons to design a satisfactory cost of dispensing formula. He also contributed greatly to the Kansas Medicaid program.
30. Smith, H.A., and Billups, N.F.: Survey form to determine the cost of dispensing a prescription. *Kentucky Pharmacist, 36*:20, 1973.
31. Smith, H.A.: Prescription pricing: A contemporary method to account for inflation. *Current Concepts in Retail Pharm. Mngt., 3*(3):2–7, July, 1985.

REVIEW

1. Discuss and differentiate between price and nonprice competition and give examples of each in the practice of pharmacy.

2. Explain market segmentation strategy and give several examples in the practice of pharmacy.

3. Define and give several examples of quasi-price competition in a pharmacy.

4. Discuss and give examples of five types or levels of price competition.

5. Explain the push-pull effect on the public of prescription price advertising.

6. Explain each of the five basic factors that enter into pricing decisions. Include the underlying principles and concepts of each.

7. Discuss each of the six pricing policies and describe how they differ.

8. Explain and give examples of the application of the game plan to competitive pricing.

9. What is wrong with pricing according to what the market will bear?

10. Why has odd pricing lost the potency it had originally?

11. Given the appropriate data, calculate the selling price, cost of goods sold, gross margin, expenses, and net profit, in terms of both dollars and percentages.

12. Given appropriate data, calculate the selling price required to achieve the following pricing objectives: (a) average expenses and net profit, (b) variable expenses and usual net profit, and (c) variable expenses.

13. Explain the usual relationship between turnover rate and percent gross margin and given appropriate data, calculate the effect of turnover rate on total annual net profit.

14. Discuss the history of prescription pricing and the professional fee. Include: (a) the action of the APhA House of Delegates in 1917, (b) Nitardy's NARD "Prescription Pricing Schedule," (c) Evans's "Simple Rule of Determining Prescription Prices," and (d) the Kendall and Lee formulas of prescription pricing.

15. Describe five reasons the percentage markup became the usual method of prescription pricing after World War I.

16. Outline the variations and modifications of the percentage markup, with or without a fee, used in the many prescription pricing schedules.

17. Discuss the three tenets of the professional fee philosophy.

18. Given the various formula for prescription pricing and the appropriate data, determine the prescription price by each method and explain the essential difference between the formulas.

19. Calculate the breakeven cost of dispensing a prescription using the revised methodology.

20. Describe the basic differences between the flat fee and the combination fee of the revised methodology.

16 | Pharmacy Services and Patronage

Pharmacy patronage is a complex subject. Many types of motives are involved in any specific purchase or patronage decision. There is no simple explanation of motivation; it is a complex of many economic, social, and psychologic forces, both rational and emotional. This is true of both purchasing and patronage motivations.

Among the many studies on motivation, relatively few have dealt with pharmacy purchases and patronage. A study by the Dichter Institute for Motivational Research, Incorporated, provided some interesting and nontraditional insights into the deepseated, underlying motives of consumers with respect to their image and patronage of pharmacies.[1] The research utilized depth interviews, psychologic tests, and projective techniques. The depth interviews, phase I of the research, were conducted in two waves of 27 interviews each. Wave I was performed to test some hypotheses and to construct new ones through a comprehensive analysis of the findings. Wave II was performed to validate the hypotheses and to quantify them to a degree. The psychologic tests and projective techniques were performed with 447 respondents in 33 geographically diverse locations to provide further data and insight into the public's image of pharmacy. Another study by Benson and Benson provided additional, but more traditional, information and insight into pharmacy patronage.[2] There are two regularly conducted surveys of pharmacy's image and patronage attitudes held by pharmacy patrons sponsored by The Upjohn Company and Schering-Plough Corporation.[3,4]

Pharmacy's Public Image

A *key concept* emerged from the Dichter study—namely, the pharmacist has lost contact with his patients. It was found that the patients expect, and deeply desire, personal contact and attention, and genuine professional services from the pharmacist. It is a feeling of isolation and alienation that prompts

334

patients to be *pushed* away from the independent pharmacist rather than *pulled* by lower prices to the mass merchandisers. The American consumer has an uneasy feeling that permeates the entire shopping situation.

The researchers probed the respondents to determine how this feeling developed. The respondents felt that they had been abandoned by the new breed of pharmacists. This parallels the changes that have taken place in medicine, and apparently these changes are symptomatic of the cool, aloof, and scientific manner of dealing with patients today. It appears that while developing sound scientific curricula for our health practitioners, we have neglected the socioeconomic and behavioral aspects of the health professions. The famous medical historian and sociologist, Henry Sigerist, was keenly aware of this deficiency.[5] Sigerist labeled medicine a social profession; surely pharmacy is none the less a social profession. An awareness and a commitment to pharmacy as a socioeconomic institution is incumbent on both educators and practitioners if change is to be made in the orientation and behavior of pharmacists, who in turn will be able to alter the perception their patients have of them.

LOSS OF PUBLIC CONTACT

The Dichter researchers associated the alienation that patients feel toward their pharmacists with a basic instinct, the instinct for survival as represented by their health needs. Where alienation has occurred, the perception of loss is felt deeply, whether consciously or not.

The results of the motivational research revealed that the pharmacy is in a unique and complex shopping category.[1] It provides products and services that affect the well-being, even the very life, of its patrons, while offering a wide range of nonhealth products for the convenience of patrons. This peculiar mixture of professional service and commercialism produces a degree of confusion in the minds of the public. It is difficult to perceive the pharmacist as a professional on the same plane as the physician or attorney. The latter serve their patients or clients in an office type of environment, whereas the pharmacist performs his professional service in a commercial context. However, the "ideal pharmacist," as perceived by the respondents, closely resembles the "doc" of the past decades, especially when the pharmacist is friendly, approachable, and concerned about his patrons.

The depth probes revealed that the public wants more than the old-fashioned, friendly "doc;" they want a proficient pharmacist who will protect their health with medication profiles and one who strives to prevent allergic reactions and drug conflicts of all types. The key to the latter, more sophisticated role is to fill the first role—that of the friendly pharmacist who has personal contact with the patient and calls him by name. Although the physical environment and the diverse merchandise in the pharmacy can have a negative effect on the attitude of the public toward the pharmacist, it is the *attitude* and *behavior* of the pharmacist himself that exert the greatest influence with the public. When the friendly druggists of the thirties were considered the family doctor substitute, or simply "doc," the typical pharmacy realized only about 10 to 20 percent of its income from prescriptions and sold a wide assortment of nonhealth products, and the soda fountain, the antithesis of professionalism, was an integral part of most pharmacies.

An understanding of behavioral and sociologic phenomena, such as the sick role, is a necessary prerequisite to the development of expertise in the expanding new roles of the pharmacist. A better and deeper understanding of the profession as a unique social institution is also a prerequisite to assuming these new roles. A pharmacist with internal role conflicts of his own can hardly instill confidence and trust in the patient he serves. He must understand the profession-business complex in which he works and his role within it, if he is to contribute to the public confidence in the profession. "Surely no one would deny that the role of the pharmacist is crucial to the success of the pharmacy enterprise because it is he, more than any other employee, who can effectively build patron loyalty."[1] He should not be providing professional services one moment and "pushing" household goods the next, especially for the same person.

"It is also clear from the research that, for the most part, the pharmacist has not properly communicated with the public. As a result, the public is almost completely in the dark with regard to what the pharmacist really does. One of the public's most *prevalent perceptions* is that the pharmacist hides behind a specialized counter in a corner of the establishment, makes a little bit of noise, and comes up with a small bottle and a large bill."[1] This image must be reversed if pharmacy is to regain its credibility.

Although Jang and Knapp found that the provision of information by pharmacists to patrons failed to make a strong attitudinal impact on the patrons,[6] Yellin and Norwood found the opposite.[7] The latter researchers concluded that "an improvement in public attitude may be realized more through increased pharmacist-patient contact than any other means, especially when this leads to increased communication regarding health matters."

One aspect of the pharmacist's image, honesty and ethical standards, is positive. According to the Gallup Poll, pharmacists rank second only to clergymen in perceived honesty and ethical standards: clergymen very high or high—63 percent, average—28 percent, low or very low—6 percent; pharmacist very high or high—59 percent, average—33 percent, low or very low—5 percent; no opinion—3 percent for both groups. Dentists ranked third; physicians, fourth; engineers, fifth; college teachers, sixth; and policemen, seventh.[8]

There are some interesting comparisons between the findings of the Dichter motivational research and the earlier study by Benson and Benson.[2] There are points of agreement and disagreement, which can be attributed largely to the changes in the public's attitudes and pharmacy itself during the eleven intervening years. Part of this is due to the differences in methodology used in the two studies. The Benson and Benson study used both structured and nonstructured depth interviews with a sample of consumers located from coast

Table 16–1.   Relative Ranking of Professions in Two Studies

Profession	Benson and Benson Study	Dichter Study Group A	Dichter Study Group B
Physician	1	1	1
Dentist	—	2	2
Attorney	2	3	3
Pharmacist	—	—	4
Optometrist	—	4	5
School teacher	3	5	6
Clergyman	4	—	—
Druggist/pharmacist	5	6	—

Adapted from *Communicating the Value of Comprehensive Pharmaceutical Services to the Consumer.* Washington: American Pharmaceutical Association, 1973; and from *How to Win Friends and Influence Customers.* New York: Sterling Drug Co.

to coast. The number of respondents was not reported, but it is thought to include 200 or more.

RANKING OF PHARMACISTS

Both the Dichter motivational study and the Benson and Benson study attempted to rank pharmacists among other professions and occupations. Unfortunately, the two studies did not make congruent comparisons possible. The Dichter study used fifteen occupations, whereas the Benson and Benson study used eight occupations plus a "no opinion" category. The Dichter study included dentists and optometrists; the Benson and Benson study used clergymen. The latter researchers specified "high school teacher," but the former used the term "school teacher." The Dichter group divided the respondents into two groups. They used the word "druggist" with 218 respondents (Group A) and "pharmacist" with 229 respondents (Group B). In contrast, Benson and Benson used both words together as "druggist/pharmacist." Table 16–1 indicates the relative rank of the top seven professions in the Dichter and Benson and Benson studies. Bear in mind the many incongruencies in the techniques employed.

It is interesting that the combined term "druggist/pharmacist" ranked fifth among the top five occupations in the Benson and Benson study, while the term "druggist" ranked sixth among the top six occupations in group A and the term "pharmacist" ranked fourth among the same six occupations in group B of the Dichter study. People apparently perceive a difference between a "pharmacist" and a "druggist," and this perceived difference was verified in the Benson and Benson study. The respondents were asked whether, in their opinion, there was a difference between a druggist and a pharmacist. Forty-eight percent responded "yes," 42 percent said "no," and 10 percent had no opinion.[2] When the respondents were asked what the difference was,

Table 16–2. Pharmacists as Businessmen or Medical Men

Businessmen	1	2	3	4	5	6	Medical Men
% of Respondents	15	22	17	23	13	10	

Adapted from *Communicating the Value of Comprehensive Pharmaceutical Services to the Consumer.* Washington: American Pharmaceutical Association.

the answers focused on the pharmacist's roles of compounding and dispensing prescriptions and his education and licensure requirements; in contrast, the druggists had roles of ownership and dealing in many matters that were not health-related. The difference between the 48 percent and 42 percent would be statistically significant provided 600 or more persons were surveyed.

Paul interviewed 200 consumers in Pittsburgh concerning their patronage preferences.[9] He found that approximately 47 percent thought that there was a difference between a pharmacy and a drugstore. As the income of the respondents increased, the percentage of those who thought there was a difference between a pharmacy and a drugstore also increased.

ROLE AMBIGUITY

In Chapter 2 sociologic data were cited which indicated the divergent roles and role conflicts in pharmacy resulting from its institutional, professional, and business complexity. The Dichter group sought to determine the public's attitude toward a pharmacist as a professional versus a business person.[1] They used a modified version of the semantic differential technique, which positioned two opposing statements with a six-point scale between them. The two statements were as follows: "Pharmacists are more businessmen than they are medical men," and "Pharmacists are more medical men than businessmen." The results are shown in Table 16–2. In a more recent survey, 77 percent of the respondents thought of their pharmacist as a professional medical-person; 15 percent thought of him as "somebody in business,"and 9 percent thought of him "like a friend."[3] (Few gave multiple answers.)

The reasons given for the nonprofessional perception of pharmacists, shown via the probe technique, can be categorized as follows: (1) pharmacists were not professional in the sense that physicians, dentists, and attorneys are professional; (2) the place of practice is more a business than an office, usually have proximity to grocery and similar stores; (3) pharmacies sell many non-health products; (4) the attitude and behavior of pharmacists show a lack of concern, which seemed to be paramount to the respondents; and (5) the public doesn't expect the pharmacist to be *ultra* professional, but rather more concerned and helpful. Some of the respondents called this "professional interest," "common courtesy," and "devotion to duty."

In one study of 87 rural pharmacy patrons, 28 percent stated that the pharmacist was primarily professional, 23 percent indicated that he was a businessman, while 49 percent said that he was both.[10] This last assessment is probably a realistic appraisal.

One issue raised in Chapter 2 concerned career satisfaction and the internal role conflict of the pharmacist. The way the pharmacist feels about himself and his job determines, to a large degree, how he interacts and communicates with patrons and patients in the pharmacy. This interaction, in turn, affects their image of him and the pharmacy. Unfortunately, the level of career satisfaction has not improved, whereas the level of internal (psychologic) role conflict has remained about the same as 15 years ago. In an earlier study, 57.5 percent of the pharmacists indicated that they were satisfied with their career.[11] In a later study, 56 percent indicated that they were satisfied with pharmacy.[12] Again, 57.5 percent of the pharmacists in the earlier study indicated subjective role conflict; this finding is comparable to the 54 percent who have role conflict reported in the later study. There is a lesson in these observations for educators—to prepare students better for the real work-world—and to practitioners—to seek and to discover an adaptive role pattern that enables one to function optimally.

PERCEIVED ATTRIBUTES OF PHARMACISTS

For the pharmacist, professionalism is an elusive concept. It is a mixture of the friendly ''doc'' of past years and the knowledgeable, concerned modern pharmacist of today who gives advice about drugs, and watches for contraindicated drugs and drug interactions. The friendly, reliable, and helpful attributes of pharmacists were much in evidence in the Benson and Benson study,[13] as shown in Table 16–3.

In a more recent study, Zelnio and Gagnon found general support for the results of Benson and Benson.[14] The responses in this later study included a subsample of pharmacy patrons who gave ''a liking for the pharmacist'' as one of the three most important patronage motives. The following attributes, along with the percentage, were named by this subsample of 59 respondents: *Friendly,* 85 (percent); *helpful,* 83; efficient, 76; interested, 76; honest, 75; responsible, 71; clean, 71; concerned, 69; *sincere,* 63; informative, 64; knowledgeable, 64; *intelligent,* 63; careful, 59; personable, 53; and caring, 46. (Those attributes italicized were included in both studies.) Liguori found the following order of importance to be:[15] Friendly, courteous, sincere, liked in general, competent, professional, fast, and available.

These attributes may be categorized into four dimensions: (1) *friendly-personable,* with scores of 85 to 53 percent; (2) *professional concern,* with scores of 83 to 46 percent; (3) *professional integrity,* with scores of 82 to 59 percent; and (4) *professional competence,* with scores of 78 to 63 percent. The concept of a personal pharmacist who is friendly, concerned, responsible, and knowledgeable appears to be the answer to pharmacy's public image problem.

Table 16–3. Words Used to Describe Druggists/Pharmacists

Question to Consumers: Please go through all the cards and pick the ones that might be used to describe the average (druggist) (pharmacist).

Characteristic	%
Reliable	82.0
Friendly	82.0
Intelligent	78.0
Helpful	76.0
Hard working	63.0
Sincere	57.5
Public spirited	40.0
Clever	29.0
Generous	22.5
Charitable	19.5
Greedy	7.5
Crafty	5.5

(Multiple answers are included in the above table.)

Source: *How to Win Friends and Influence Customers.* New York: Sterling Drug Co. (in cooperation with the NARD), 1962.

Consumer Patronage

PATRONAGE MOTIVES

In the traditional context, patronage motives are primarily rational motives, although not entirely. Most textbooks on marketing or general retailing provide the following list of patronage motives: (1) *convenience*—rational, and traditionally the single most important motive in pharmacy patronage; (2) *reputation of the seller*—both rational and emotional motives; (3) *services rendered*—rational motive; (4) *breadth of assortment and quality of goods*—rational motive; (5) *price*—rational motive; and (6) *appearance and general appeal*—both emotional and rational motives.

Pharmacy is not an ordinary retail business, but is a professional institution as well. One might expect different factors to be influential in pharmacy patronage compared to grocery or department stores. The Benson and Benson research group sought to determine the reasons for consumers patronizing a particular pharmacy. The results of this research are tabulated in Table 16–4.

In comparing the results of the Benson and Benson study with the traditional and general patronage motives, there is remarkable agreement. Convenience stands out as the *single most important reason* for patronizing a particular pharmacy. If the various types of conveniences mentioned are additive, con-

Table 16–4. Reasons for Shopping at Pharmacy Patronized Most

Question to Consumers: What are your main reasons for shopping most at this drugstore?

Motive	Response item	%
Appearance and general appeal	Clean store, uncluttered	1.5
Breadth of **assortment** and quality of goods	Good, wide stock; have what is needed	12.5
	Has a soda fountain	.5
	Carries groceries	.5
Convenience	Close to home, neighborhood pharmacy	34.5
	Convenient, unspecified	19.0
	Close to doctor's office	5.0
	Close to other stores, shopping district	2.5
	Close to work	.5
Price	Reasonable prices, economical, sales	15.0
Friend	Know, friendly with owner, druggist, clerks	29.0
Reputation of the seller	Reliable, reputable, recommended to me	20.5
	Druggist is public-spirited	.5
Services rendered	Good service, prompt, helpful, courteous	15.5
	Have a delivery service	6.5
	Convenient hours	1.5
	Credit available	1.5
Other	No drugstore patronized most	4.5
	No reason	1.0

Multiple answers are included in this table.

Adapted from *How to Win Friends and Influence Customers.* New York: Sterling Drug Co. (in cooperation with the NARD), 1962, p. 9.

venience as a patronage motive totaled 61.5 percent, counting "convenient, unspecified," which had a 19 percent response. Most of the other reasons listed can be categorized under one of the other traditional motives. "Know, friendly with owner, druggist, clerks" drew a 29 percent response as a main reason for shopping most at a particular pharmacy. This reason had the *second highest* response rate, and when combined with the other reasons associated with reputation with a 21 percent response, the combined percentage was 50. Services had a combined response of 25 percent, and *ranked third,* followed by reputation, price and assortment of goods.

The Market Facts survey was conducted with telephone interviews of 998 heads of households who had purchased a prescription in a community pharmacy within the previous six months.[3] The sample was a scientific, random

Table 16–5.   Importance of Services and Features Influencing Pharmacy Patronage

Questions to Consumers: What features and services often available at drugstores would you consider very important in influencing your selection of a drugstore in which to trade?

Which one of these things is most important to you?

| | Consumers' Rating | | |
| | Most Important (%)* | Very Important (%)* | Important (%)† |
Features and Services			
Pricing	21	62	—
24-hour prescription service	21	47	15
Friendliness of druggist	12	61	41
Clean and neat inside	9	72	34
Delivery service	9	41	16
Quick service	8	55	55
Professional advice on health aids (OTC drugs)	8	38	(11)
Being open 7 days a week	6	41	—
Being open late at night	4	33	—
A wide variety of brands	3	32	—
A wide variety of types of merchandise	2	29	20
Availability of credit	2	18	18
Friendliness of clerks	1	46	31
Clean and neat outside	1	41	—
Ample parking space	1	25	25
Self-service	1	7	—
Professional advice on beauty aids	1	4	—
Trading stamps	—	4	—

Multiple answers are included in the table.

*Adapted from *How to Win Friends and Influence Customers.* New York: Sterling Drug Co. (in cooperation with the NARD), 1962, p.10.

†Reference 16.

sample of equal members of men and women. The fact that the respondents must have purchased a prescription made the sample a little different than the general population, but a more meaningful one for the purpose of the study. The maximum error was 4.4 percent with a 95 percent confidence level.

The Market Facts survey reported 51 percent of the prescription patrons indicated ''closeness to home or work'' was the one most important reason for patronizing their preferred pharmacy. This was followed by ''price of medicine''—19 percent, ''courteous and friendly service''—9 percent, and

Table 16–6. Factors Determining Choice of Pharmacy

Rank	Factor	Weighted Score	%*	%†
1	Professional service	2,302	100	18.5
2	Lower prices	2,192	95	17.6
3	Personal attention	1,970	86	15.8
4	A pharmacist who knows your MD	1,653	72	13.3
5	A ready source of drug information	1,632	71	13.1
6	A large variety of merchandise	1,437	62	11.6
7	Advertised drug prices	1,259	55	10.1
	TOTAL WEIGHTED SCORE	12,445	—	100.0

Adapted from *Communicating the Value of Comprehensive Pharmaceutical Services to the Consumer.* Washington: American Pharmaceutical Association, 19, p. 37, Table 13.

*Using 2,302 as the base.
†Using 12,445 as the base.

"reliable and dependable service"—6 percent. Comparing selected percentages from this survey with the Benson and Benson survey,[2] we found the following: convenience—51 vs. 61.5, price—19 vs. 15, service—15 vs. 15.5 (not including delivery, etc.)

The Benson and Benson survey also investigated a large number of services and features usually available in pharmacies. The respondents were asked which services or features they considered very important, and then which were most important in influencing their patronage of a particular pharmacy. These results along with comparable data from a study by Stewart et al.[16] were compiled in Table 16–5. The data in Table 16–5 are quite different from that in Table 16–4 because the focus and context of the questions are different. The focus of the question in Table 16–5 was on features and services other than the two dominant patronage motives—convenience and reputation of the pharmacist (although friendliness of pharmacist and clerks was included). Within this context, prices became the most important feature along with 24-hour prescription service. Friendliness of the pharmacist remained very important, and so did services, especially when combined, but these were segmented into various forms. In the context of Table 16–5, cleanliness became very important along with delivery and convenient (long) hours.

The above studies dealt with pharmacy patronage in general. A much different set of motives (reasons) would be expected to influence people in deciding where to purchase their prescriptions. This question was investigated in the Dichter study. The respondents were given a list of seven factors and requested to put the number corresponding to each factor in one of seven unequal segments of a circle or pie. The unequal segments were designed to give a relative weight to each factor. After all the computations were performed, the seven factors were ranked as shown in Table 16–6.

Perhaps more useful information could have been derived from the test shown in Table 16–6 if professional services had been divided into distinct and meaningful segments. Professional service is such a broad category. Also, the convenience factor should have been included as well. Convenience has been found to be a significant factor in nearly every research project on pharmacy patronage to date.

By way of comparison with the "high" score given professional service, a broad category, lower prices were only about one percentage point lower, and advertised drug prices, the lowest score of all, were only 8.4 percent lower than the professional service score. The personal attention score was 2.7 percent lower than professional services, whereas the ready source of information score was 5.4 percent below the professional service score. However, if the score for professional services (2,307) is used as the basis for comparison (100 percent), the differences are more pronounced. Advertised drug price has a score only 55 percent as great as that of professional services; a pharmacist who knows your physician has a 72 percent score, and lower price has a 95 percent score.

At least 24 studies of pharmacy patronage have been reported in the literature. Thirteen studies (in addition to those cited already in this chapter[1–4,7,9–11,14–16]) were reviewed.[17–29] Gagnon published a comprehensive review of 13 of them.[30] Many of the studies are not directly or completely comparable because of the differences in methodology. However, some broad generalizations may be made. In all but three studies, *convenient location,* or *convenience in general,* was the most important patronage motive.[15,22,28] Whereas *prices* or lower (better) prices were not rated as important as some other factors in the earlier studies, price has emerged as a significant factor in later studies, especially with patrons of chain pharmacies. On the basis of the median rank, price "nosed out" *"know* or *like* the *pharmacist,"* which, in turn "nosed out" *services.* Since direct comparison of these studies is precarious, it is safer to rank these patronage motives as equal in importance. The management/marketing strategy should be based on the strengths of the pharmacist and his pharmacy design.

Superior professional services probably would weigh more than any other patronage motive if the public could actually perceive, feel, and know that they were receiving that type of service. By superior professional service is meant a clinical encounter with each new prescription, with renewed prescriptions as circumstances warrant, and with each purchase of most nonprescription drugs. By clinical encounter is meant a consultation that has therapeutic significance and is so perceived by the patient. This particular type of service was not clearly defined or perceived by the respondents in most of the studies reported.

Confidence as a pharmacy patronage motive has been studied only recently. In one study, confidence in the pharmacist ranked second to convenience as a patronage motive,[29] whereas in another study, 70 percent of the consumers stated that they had confidence in the pharmacist's ability to detect errors in prescription, and 82 percent said that they accepted their pharmacists' rec-

Table 16–7.   Types of Pharmacies Consumers Preferred and Actually Patronized for Prescriptions

Type of Pharmacy	Percentage of Consumers	
	Actually Patronized	*Preferred*
Neighborhood, community	75.0	61.0
Prescription type	8.5	19.0
Chain type	13.5	8.5
Other types or no opinion	3.0	11.5

Adapted from: Paul, S.H.: Pharmacies: how do you know what the customer wants? *Marketing Insights,* pp. 12–14, Feb. 6, 1967.

ommendation on nonprescription drugs.[4] This same group of consumers rated prompt "filling of their prescriptions" as the most important factor in their relationship with the local pharmacy.[4] Fast prescription services ranked second, fourth, fifth, and sixth in four other studies. Confidence as a patronage motive is operative only if superior professional services are *provided, not just made available.*

In another semantic differential test, the Dichter study indicated that consumers are more concerned that prescription prices be posted than that they be advertised. Also, more people believe that they were being overcharged than believed that prescription prices were high. Price posting has been shown to be a weak patronage motive, and is probably of limited value,[25,29] but prescription prices are becoming an increasing concern of the public.[3]

Herman and Wills investigated community pharmacy patronage in a metropolitan city.[24] They found that people preferred an apothecary type of pharmacy to a traditional pharmacy, and a service-oriented pharmacy to a price-oriented pharmacy. However, these preferences were not indicated as being statistically significant. Older people appeared to prefer apothecaries over traditional pharmacies as indicated by the chi-square test. Paul sought to determine the type of pharmacy that consumers preferred and acutally patronized in purchasing their prescriptions.[9] The data from this research, although somewhat dated, are summarized in Table 16–7.

The difference between the preferences and actual purchases has a message that is consistent with the general theme of most of the data in the other studies. Pharmacists should emphasize their strong suit, namely, the provision of genuine professional service (for example, monitoring drug utilization and preventing therapeutic conflicts) in a warm, friendly manner, in pleasant surroundings, and at reasonable, defensible prices. This does not mean that every pharmacy has to divest itself of all nonhealth related products. On the contrary, it is attitude and behavior, and the actual delivery of true professional services that are important.

The Market Facts survey[3] indicated that 74 percent of the sample patronized only one pharmacy, 20 percent patronized two pharmacies, 4 percent patronized three, and 1 percent patronized four or more. Even among those who patronized two or more pharmacies, 81 percent traded at one pharmacy more frequently than the others.

Among all of the respondents, 24 percent had patronized the same pharmacy for five years, and 31 percent had patronized the same pharmacy for more than 10 years. The average (median) time the respondents had patronized the pharmacy where they preferred to trade was 6.1 years. Of those who had switched pharmacies, 37 percent did so because they had moved; 15 percent went to another pharmacy because it was less expensive; 13 percent went to another pharmacy that was more convenient or closer to home, and 8 percent traded at another pharmacy because the other pharmacy went out of business. This indicates that there is a very high level of patron loyalty of most pharmacies. Pharmacists should strive to deserve and enhance the level of patron loyalty.

To summarize, patronage motives in the order of perceived importance by the public are: (1) convenience, especially the pharmacy's location in respect to home, work, physician and other stores (in that order) as well as convenient parking and hours: (2) reputation and personal rapport, two different but complementary motives; (3) prices, especially prescription prices of popular drugs; (4) services, especially professional services, but convenient services are also important which include after hours prescription services, delivery, credit, and prompt and courteous personal attention (these latter three motives are ranked very closely); (5) confidence in the pharmacist, which may be really a part of motives 2 and 4, (6) assortment and quality of merchandise, and (7) appearance and cleanliness. Although appearance and cleanliness was ranked last, a sloppy, cluttered and dirty pharmacy can undermine all the other efforts by simply repulsing patrons.

DESIRED PROFESSIONAL SERVICES

The study by the Dichter Motivational Research Associates investigated respondents' awareness of, and desire for, a narrower range of primarily professional services. The people were asked which services they were most familiar with and which services they would most like to have. Each person was given a list of services to be evaluated. These results are reported in Table 16–8.

Comparison of Two Studies. The combined services of longer hours, deliveries, Sunday and emergency service in the Dichter study closely corresponded to the separate listing of being open late at night, delivery, being open seven days, and 24-hour prescription service in the Benson and Benson study. Fifty-eight percent of the Dichter respondents indicated that these were services they would most like to have, while a range of 33 to 47 percent of the Benson and Benson respondents indicated that these services were very important. Although these latter percentages are not additive, their combined effect probably would have matched the 58 percent in the Dichter study. Moreover, the respective percentages of people who indicated that these

Table 16–8. Consumer Awareness of and Desire for Pharmaceutical Services

Items Evaluated	A %	B %	Net Change B − A %
Maintains a complete inventory of drug products which physicians may prescribe for treatment.			
a. Properly stores same	62	47	− 15
Maintains a medication record for each prescription-filling customer.	57	57	None
Makes certain the prescription drug is "right" for the patient, questioning			
a. Drug conflict			
b. Patient allergies	30	70	+ 40
Guarantees drug's high quality and "freshness."	57	57	None
Packages, dates, and labels patient's prescription with directions.	87	39	− 48
Supplies patient with special information, i.e., to be taken on an empty stomach, X-times daily, and similar instructions.	51	62	+ 11
Dispenses information not directly related to prescriptions	24	48	+ 24
Provides credit and accounting services for tax purposes.	51	54	+ 3
Offers longer hours, deliveries, Sunday and emergency service.	48	58	+ 10

Note: Column A represents "services most familiar with" and Column B is "most like to have."

Source: *Communicating the Value of Comprehensive Pharmaceutical Services to the Consumer.* Washington: American Pharmaceutical Association, 1973.

services were most important totaled 40 percent, which probably are additive. It is interesting that only 48 percent of the Dichter respondents were aware of the availability of these services, while in fact they are available in most pharmacies, especially the neighborhood type of pharmacy. The conclusion that can be drawn from the foregoing data is that these services are traditional, but they are still considered important to the public.

It is obvious from the Dichter study that patrons want more professional services of the following nature than they perceive receiving from pharmacists:

Actual Medical or Drug Questions							
"I frequently consult a pharmacist on medical or drug questions."	1	2	3	4	5	6	"I never consult a pharmacist on medical or drug questions."
Percent of Respondents	12	17	17	12	18	23	

Potential Sources of Medical Information							
"Pharmacists are not physicians and, therefore, are not good sources of medical information."	1	2	3	4	5	6	"Because of their profession, pharmacists often are good sources of medical information."
Percent of Respondents	11	13	12	23	26	16	

Figure 16–1.   Pharmacists as actual and potential sources of health information.

(1) preventing drug conflict and allergies, (2) supplying information on how to take the medication, and (3) providing information about nonprescription drugs and health matters.

PROFESSIONAL CONSULTATION

The supplying of information about prescriptions and other health information was explored further by the Dichter motivational research group with the use of the modified semantic differential technique. Two sets of opposing statements dealing with the actual and potential use of pharmacists as a source of information were utilized. The results are shown in Figure 16–1. Obviously, more people think pharmacists are a good source of information than use them for this purpose.

A more recent study revealed that 52 percent of patients ask their physician when they have a question about their prescriptions, 16 percent ask their pharmacist, and 30 percent ask both.[3] In contrast, an investigation of rural pharmacy patrons disclosed that 46 percent consulted their pharmacist first, 51 percent consulted their physician first, and 3 percent consulted either one.[10] Forty-five percent of respondents of the national study stated that they had consulted the pharmacist when purchasing nonprescription drugs.[3] Also, 39 percent of the national sample asked their pharmacist about treating minor illness.[3] Additional data from the national study[3] appear in Table 16–9.

The data in Table 16–9 indicate that 53 percent of the people talked with their pharmacist the last time they had a prescription filled, and another 17 percent had talked with their pharmacist during the past six months. It should be noted that all of the people in this large nation-wide study had a prscription filled within the past six months, and more than one answer was given by some of the respondents.

Table 16–9. Selected Data from the Market Facts Survey

Overall N = 998		*No.*	*%*
When did you talk with your pharmacist?	N = 998		
Last time prescription was filled		531	53
Last six months		174	17
	N = 705		
While filling a new prescription		388	55
While getting a refill		304	43
Not specified, don't remember, etc.		14	2
What was discussed?	N = 705		
Instructions: how and when to take drug		159	23
About the medication		94	13
Side effects		77	11
Illness drug is for		16	2
Subtotal		346	49
Asked about refills		35	5
Asked what the prescription was (name)		19	3
Asked for generic/cheaper drugs		33	5
Asked how much it would cost		15	2
About price of drugs generally		9	1
Size/quantity of prescription		8	1
Strength of prescription		9	1
Availability of drug in prescription		7	1
General conversation about drugs		43	6
Illness, unspecified		6	1
Asked about OTC drugs		23	3
Other subjects, don't remember, etc.		316	45

Source: Adapted from referrence 3, p. 41

Not all of the conversations were clinical in nature, but 49 percent of the cases was clinical and drug related. When the last three specific items in Table 16–9 were included in the drug-related, clinical category, the percent was 59. In a direct observation study by Gambrell and Jackson,[31] only 23 percent of the questions asked of pharmacists was clinical in nature, 4 percent was of a personal nature, and 73 percent was administration in nature (N = 417 observations during 72 hours in one week in 18 pharmacies in a large southern city). There was no indication that pharmacists initiated any of the discussions in this latter study as was the case in the former study.

The respondents in the national study[3] were asked: Can you always talk to your pharmacist whenever you need to? A full 96 percent responded "yes," and only 4 percent, "no." In a survey of 221 shoppers (via questionnaire) in several shopping centers in a midwestern city, 67 percent indicated that they had experienced wanting information about a prescription but did not have the opportunity to disucss it with the pharmacist.[32] A similar response (61 percent) was given for nonprescription drugs. The primary reasons given for not consulting with the pharmacist were "too busy," "can't see him," and "not available."[3] Also, 28 percent stated they would like to be able to speak with their pharmacist (in private) where the conversation could not be overheard.[3]

There does not seem to be a ready explanation concerning the discrepancy among these studies; however, the nature and size of the sample indicate the national study[3] to be more valid.

Most assuredly, the message is clear that pharmacy patrons would like to have more information about their medication; many would prefer a measure of privacy in discussing their medication with their pharmacist; some feel that they cannot talk to their pharmacist because he/she is not available, and although the number of incidents may be small, it is still too many, and although pharmacists have a fairly good record on consultation with their patrons, there is still room for improvement by taking the initiative. *Management* should be cognizant of this potential, and plan to take advantage of this opportunity because it is *good professional and business practice*. Chain pharmacy managers and observers are now advocating that pharmacists counsel with their patrons concerning their prescriptions.[33]

Professional consultation should be provided, and it will be received if all the necessary ingredients are included. These ingredients include a knowledgeable pharmacist with a desire to provide consultation, empathy and communication skills, the necessary records and data, and the proper facilities for consultation. The reader is referred Figures 7–4 and 7–9 for designs of consulting facilities.

Purchasing Motives

CLASSIFICATION OF MOTIVES

Product purchasing motives may be classified along three dimensions or in three different ways. The first is time- and/or age-oriented. Therefore, the first classification of purchasing motives is *latent* or *dormant,* and *conscious* motives. Many motives are latent (lie dormant) in the mind until some effect, for example a display, arouses the desire to make the decision to purchase the item. The things that cause a latent motive to become a conscious one vary with circumstances and especially with age. See Chapter 10 for a fuller discussion of motivation. As other types of motivations are discussed, it should be apparent that these have greater impact on each of us at various ages and circumstances.

The second way to classify purchasing motives is related to the primacy of the motive. Thus, a purchase may be classified as either *primary* or *selective*. These two types of motives have their counterpart in the context of the *generic* versus *branded* product controversy. A good example of this classification is the purchase of a headache remedy. The first or primary motive is to purchase a remedy to relieve the headache. Because of the influence of an advertisement or advice, the purchaser may become selective and demand a particular brand of aspirin. The technique of product differentiation, both real and contrived via advertising, is the basis of actuating a selective purchase motive.

The third classification, and perhaps the most pertinent of all, is based on the rationality of the purchaser's behavior. Thus, purchasing motives are classified as *rational* or *emotional*. Most of us think we behave rationally almost all of the time, including the way we spend our money. Not so! Research has shown that the majority of purchases are really actuated by appeal to our emotional motivations. A careful study of advertisements, using the technique of content analysis, would reveal the degree to which emotional appeal is used in the majority of the ads. The complexity of the entire purchasing process must be recognized, and it must be noted that a combination of motivational appeals, both rational and emotional, is used in most advertisements.

RATIONAL MOTIVATIONS

Rational motivations may be further classified and described in the following manner:

1. *Dependability* or *confidence* is one of the strongest rational motives.

2. *Economy* refers to the "best buy" or "greatest value," not necessarily the lowest price. People often confuse economy with the lowest price.

3. *Low price* (or simply *price*) is an appeal to the rational process. Although people are sometimes misled, it is still a rational appeal, and only the lack of information is the basis of a "bad buy."

4. *Money gained* is related to the economy motive above, but it differs in that the appeal is to future gains or benefits to be derived from the purchase. An example would be a well-fitted suit for a salesman.

5. *Convenience* is rational in nature and it relates to the ease of use, repair, and related characteristics. This is one of the strongest motives for patronage of a pharmacy, as previously discussed.

EMOTIONAL MOTIVATIONS

Emotional motivations are numerous and complex. They are designed to appeal to both our innate and our acquired appetites and desires. Not all appetites and desires are bad, and values are not to be inferred from this classification. However, our value system will play a large role in the effectiveness of emotional appeals; in fact, it may completely negate the effect of certain advertisements or displays on some people. Emotional motives may be classified as follows:

1. *Pride* traditionally has been one of the most common and strongest

emotional motives among Americans. It may focus on the individual, his family, an organization, or any entity with which a person identifies.

2. *Emulation* is the basis of fashion changes. The expression, "keeping up with the Joneses," is a good illustration of this motive, which may well replace pride as the number one motive in this country.

3. *Innovation* probably is the second fastest growing motivational appeal in the advertising industry. The concept of avant-garde, borrowed from the French, plays an important role in modern American life. Many advertisements appeal to this type of life style, which, of course, is symptomatic of the affluence of our society.

4. *Comfort* and *recreation* are two somewhat related motives. One may argue that they contain an element of rationality, and they probably do. They are not identical, but both theoretically are directed toward a sense of well-being. However, neither, and especially recreation, may produce the desired results. Many purchases are based on these two appeals.

5. *Conformity* or *sameness* is still a common motive among Americans. This motive is related to emulation, but it goes one step beyond. It is based on the desire to be "lost in the crowd" as opposed to emulating the new or the lastest style.

6. *Sex* is the most used motivational appeal today. The term is not even listed in the older marketing textbooks. The use of this basic and often base appeal is a matter of concern among a portion of our society, whereas other parts of our society see sex and its use in motivating as a "healthy liberation" of humanity. The manner in which sex appeal is used in advertisements is to draw attention to a product, and to this end it no doubt is successful. The interactive mode of sex appeal is the implied association among the product, the personification of the appeal and the person to whom the appeal is made. Whether such appeals have long-term or even actuating force is a subject that awaits interesting and profound psychologic research. Its continued use indicates it is successful.

7. *Love* is the last of our emotional motives in this classification. Love is a complex emotion and is represented by two opposite extremes—*self-love* or *ego,* and *altruism.* Self-love cuts across and underlies all of the above ego-oriented motives. Altruism is somewhat old-fashioned, but it is a force that happily still exists in our society. For example, if not from habit, then altruism is the motive underlying the sale of many boxes of Valentine candy.

With a basic understanding of product purchasing motives, the pharmacist is better qualified to construct an advertisement or display. He certainly will be able to consult with the advertising manager of his local newspaper. This latter statement is particularly important, since most pharmacists do not have either the time or sufficient knowledge to develop their entire advertising program.

INTERRELATIONSHIP OF MOTIVES

The public's image of pharmacy, pharmacy patronage, and product purchasing motives are all interrelated. The understanding of each, in turn, has

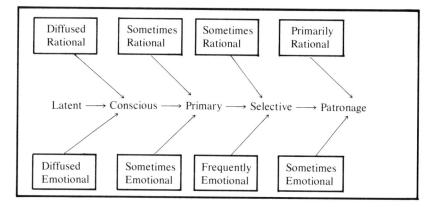

Figure 16–2.   The interrelationships among the various purchasing motives.

an effect on the efficient application of the other and implications for the development of promotional strategies. The interrelationships are depicted in Figure 16–2.

GENERAL MODEL OF CONSUMER MOTIVATION AND BEHAVIOR

Motivation actuates people to behave as they do, and thus *behavior,* as it is generally understood by psychologists, is the final result of motivation. Neither of these phenomena just happens without some underlying set of circumstances and conditions. Behavioral scientists have studied these phenomena and their underlying circumstances and conditions and have elucidated them to a degree; yet there are many facets that we do not fully understand. Sufficient evidence enables us to construct a general model of the various factors involved, which are depicted in Figure 16–3.

The model is composed of three basic elements—the psychologic processes, the social/cultural environment, and the basic core of motivation and behavior. The last element is more psychologic than social, but it has a social component. There is a state of dynamic equilibrium among the various factors that is constantly changing, though often imperceptibly. *Attitudes* represent a frame of mind, that is, a combination of innate propensity and learned predisposition to think and to behave in a particular manner when faced with a given set of circumstances. The *value system,* on the other hand, represents a social/cultural constraint, which exerts pressure to think and to behave in a certain way under given conditions. These two factors, individually and collectively, form a buffer system that provides stability to the state of equilibrium.

The intended meaning of most, if not all, of the factors in Figure 16–3 is the commonly understood definition. Among the psychologic factors, perception is achieved through one or more of the senses; impulse refers to the physiologic as much as to the psychologic process; reasoning comprises the analyzing, classifying, ordering, and interpreting processes; cognition/learn-

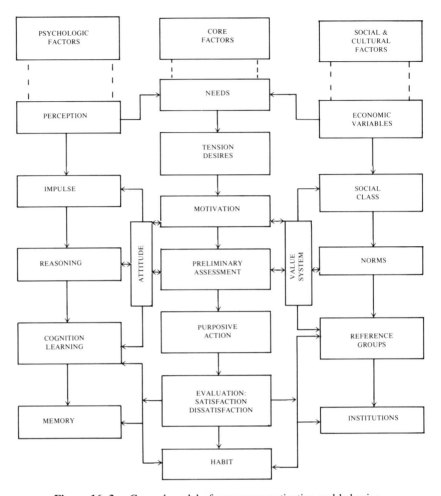

Figure 16–3.   General model of consumer motivation and behavior.

ing includes the integrating and synthesizing processes; memory is the store of knowledge. For the meaning of needs and motivation, the reader is referred to Chapter 10. In Figure 16–3 "tension" is used to denote the psychologic tension manifested for the purpose of actuating a person to meet the needs. The remaining factors are used in their ordinary sense.

A study of and reflection on this general model should provide a fair understanding of the motivational-behavioral process by which consumers are moved to purchase, or to refrain from purchasing, products and services. Such an understanding is a requisite for any professional or promotional program designed to meet the needs of consumers. It should be apparent that efforts to influence the purchase-decision process, that is, the core factors, must be directed primarily through the psychologic (factors) process. It takes long-term efforts to influence the purchase-decision process through social factors. Of course, significant changes in personal economic status may drastically change the *perceived* needs. It should be noted that the change in needs is through the psychologic process; the need must be perceived. Even professional efforts to meet the needs of patients, e.g., consultation with patients, will be mediated through the psychologic process, and a satisfactory evaluation is necessary for a successful intervention.

The subject matter of this chapter is one of the most complex of all the facets of pharmacy management and practice. More definitive research is needed. Past research has produced a great amount of data and some much needed insight into the general subject; however, much more research is needed. There are many facets of public image and consumers' motives about which we know little.

REFERENCES

1. *Communicating the Value of Comprehensive Pharmaceutical Services to the Consumer.* Washington: American Pharmaceutical Association, 1973.
2. *How to Win Friends and Influence Customers.* New York: Sterling Drug Co. (in cooperation with the NARD), 1962.
3. *Market Facts: National Prescription Buyers Survey.* Kalamazoo: The Upjohn Co., May, 1983.
4. *Pharmacists and the Consumer: A Fresh Look from Both Sides of the Counter.* The Schering Report, Schering Corp., Kenilworth, N.J., 1979.
5. Sigerist, H.E.: The medical student and the social problems confronting medicine today. *Bull. Inst. Med., 4*:411–22, 1936; also Sigerist, H.E.: *A History of Medicine.* Vol. 1, New York: Oxford Press, 1955, pp. 3–37.
6. Jang, R., Knapp, D.A., and Knapp, D.E.: Reactions of the public to the pharmacist as drug advisor. *American Pharmaceutical Association.* Unpublished paper, 1970.
7. Yellin, A.K., and Norwood, G.J.: The public's attitude toward pharmacy. *J. Am. Pharm. Assoc.,* NS *14*:61–65, 1974.
8. The Gallup Poll is widely published in newspapers and magazines; present source: Rubin, I. Stat-O-Grams column, *Pharmacy Times, 47*(11):1, Nov., 1981.
9. Paul, S.H.: Pharmacies: how do you know what the customer wants? *Marketing Insights,* pp. 12–14, Feb. 6, 1967.
10. Atkins, P., and Smith, H.A.: Profile of patrons' attitudes and preferences in three rural pharmacies. *Kentucky Pharmacist, 41*:17, 24–26, 1978.
11. Quinney, E.R.: Adjustments to occupational role strain: the case of retail pharmacy. *Southwestern Soc. Sci. Quart., 44*:367–376, 1964.
12. Smith, H.A., Branecker, J., and Pence, B.S.: Role orientation, conflict and satisfaction among pharmacies and students, *J. Soc. Adm., 3*:18–19, 1985.
13. *How to Win Friends and Influence Customers, op. cit.,* p. 5.
14. Zelnio, R.M. and Gagnon, J.P.: What patients like about pharmacists. *Apothecary, 89*:11–13, 55, 1977.
15. Liguoir, S.: The image of community pharmacies: a study of patron image. Doctoral dissertation, Purdue University, 1972. University Microfilm No. 72–30–928.
16. Stewart, J.E., Kabat, H.F., and Purohit, A.: Consumer-pharmacist congruence: understanding consumer wants and needs. *J. Am. Pharm. Assoc.,* NS *17*:358–361, 1977.
17. Ohvall, R.A.: Prescription patronage motivation. Seminar paper, University of Wisconsin, 1959.
18. Jowdy, A.W., and Smith, E.M.: Factors influencing the choice of a drugstore. *Carolina J. Pharm., 43*:6, 7, 1962.
19. Myers, J.M.: The patterns of prescription patronage. Master's thesis, University of Wisconsin, Madison, 1968.
20. Kabat, H.F.: Choice of source of pharmaceutical services. *J. Am. Pharm. Assoc.,* NS *9*:73–78, 1969.

21. Willis, R.H., Jr.: Patient loyalty in the purchase of prescription medications. Paper presented to the Academy of General Practice of Pharmacy, American Pharmaceutical Association, Annual Meeting, Boston, Mass., July 23, 1973.
22. Jackson, R.A., et al.: A study of pharmacy patronage motives and price awareness in a small town. *Bull. Bureau Pharm. Services. 10*:1–4, 1974.
23. Gagnon, J.P.: Consumer receptivity to pharmaceutical services. Final report to National Association of Chain Drug Stores, Arlington, Va., 1974.
24. Herman, C.M. and Willis, R.A., Jr.: Community pharmacy patronage, *J. Am. Pharm. Assoc.,* NS *14*:66–70, 91, 1974.
25. Keckler, D., Gagnon, J.R., and Nelson, A.A.: Does price posting influence pharmacy patronage? *Apothecary. 87*:10–12, 30–34, 1975.
26. Amarinthnukrowth, P.: The community-pharmacy: a quantitative study of its image and consumer selection process. Doctoral dissertation, University of Minnesota, Minn., 1975.
27. Parker, G.R.: Consumers' views of pharmacy. *Iowa Pharmacist, 30*:14, July, 1975.
28. Zelnio, R.M., and Gagnon, J.P.: Pharmacy image and marketing strategy. *Pharm. Management, 151*:127–133, 144, 1979.
29. Baldwin, H.J., Riley, D.H., and Wojcik, A.F.: Prescription purchasers' patronage motives. *Pharm. Management, 151*:185–190, 1979.
30. Gagnon, J.P.: Factors affecting pharmacy patronage—literature review. *J. Am. Pharm. Assoc.,* NS *17*:556–559, 566, 1977.
31. Gambrell, J.E. and Jackson, R.A.: The community pharmacist as a source of information for the patient. *The Apothecary, 90*(5):10–12, 56–69, 1978.
32. Hall, E.L., Holt, G.A., and Baker, D.E.: Patron choices regarding drug counseling. *Calif. Pharm., 30*(6):20, 21, 25, 28, 1983.
33. Bolger, R.J. and West, J.P.: *Chain Drug Store Management and Operations,* Ithaca: Cornell University (production by Symons, Brown and Neimeroff, New York, NY), 1984, pp. 156–168.

REVIEW

1. Discuss the purposes of wave I and wave II of phase I of the Dichter motivational research and explain the technique(s) used in phase I and phase II of the research.

2. What was the key concept that emerged from the Dichter motivational research?

3. Explain how this concept developed over the years and the basic instinct underlying the feelings of consumers.

4. Explain the interdependence of the performance of the modern professional service the consumer desires and the role of the friendly pharmacist of past decades.

5. What are the public's most prevalent perceptions of the modern pharmacist? How does the pharmacist rank among members of other vocations in terms of honesty and ethical standards?

6. Given the various professional categories used in the Dichter and Benson and Benson studies, rank pharmacists and/or druggists in reference to the other occupations.

7. What are the five major categories or reasons why pharmacists are not considered by consumers to be professional, as shown in the Dichter study? Are these valid?

8. Discuss role ambiguity from the perspectives of rural patrons, patrons generally, and the pharmacist.

9. How does career satisfaction affect role ambiguity and, in turn, the public's image of pharmacy?

10. What were the terms used to describe the average druggist/pharmacist by over 50 percent of the respondents in the Benson and Benson study?

11. What are the four basic dimensions of the perceived attributes of pharmacists? Categorize the various perceived attributes into four basic dimensions.

12. What are the six traditional patronage motives?

13. Identify the 17 reasons for patronizing a pharmacy given in Table 16–4 with the 6 traditional patronage motives. Rank these according to frequency.

14. Rank the patronage motives in the Market Facts Study and compare these to the results of other studies.

15. What were the top seven services or features that the respondents in the Benson and Benson study considered to be most important in selecting a pharmacy?

16. Rank the patronage factors in the Dichter study and compare these with other studies of patronage factors or motives.

17. Discuss prices as a factor in patronage motivation and any change in its importance.

18. Discuss the role confidence in the pharmacist plays in pharmacy patronage and how the pharmacist improves this factor.

19. Is it the high prices of prescriptions or the feeling of being overcharged for prescriptions that concerns consumers the most? Or both? Discuss the implication.

20. Give an overview of patronage motives and be able to "defend" each of the following as the most important: Convenience, price, reputation of the pharmacist, convenience services, professional services, and confidence.

21. Evaluate the level or status of pharmacy patronage according to the Market Facts study and explain why these results are or may be consistent with previous research.

22. What factors did Yellin and Norwood find to be the most significant in improving patrons' attitudes toward pharmacy?

23. In the Dichter study, the respondents were asked which of nine services they were most familiar with and which they would most like to have. Which services did the respondents have greater expectations than awareness?

24. Discuss professional consultation in terms of the frequency with which it is currently done, the receptivity of the public, and the necessary requisites; state how you would improve the present situation.

25. Distinguish between (a) latent (dormant) and conscious; (b) primary and selective; and (c) rational and emotional purchasing motives and show by a schematic diagram the relationships among these motives.

26. Given a list of emotional and rational purchasing motives, identify them as either rational or emotional.

27. Discuss the motivation process, including the general model and all its elements and components and their interrelationships.

28. Based on the data in this chapter, and especially but not exclusively Table 16–9, develop a professional promotional strategy.

29. Based on the data in this chapter, develop a promotional plan including objectives, data base, analysis, strategy, plan format or protocol, and evaluation for a traditional pharmacy practice.

30. Discuss (or debate between two students or teams) the notion that good business is good professionalism and vice versa.

17 | Promotion/ Merchandising

The age of consumerism is here and likely to stay.[1] Advocates of consumerism, as exemplified by Ralph Nader, have obtained a high degree of sophistication and acceptance. The new consumerism has taken many forms including picketing, boycott, publicity of various causes, legal actions, and lobbying for legislation. Two well-known expressions are indicative of the public's concern for health or the lack of it, namely, "health as a fundamental right" and "the right to know." It should be apparent that the public will have input into the decisions affecting matters related to health. This principle should be in the minds of pharmacists, both individually and collectively, as a philosophic guide when they are developing promotional programs of all types.

With this increase in consumerism and the public's awareness of health needs and costs, it is more important now than ever before that pharmacists begin to communicate with their patrons and develop positive promotional programs.[2] Pharmacists need to implement innovative services, and make these, as well as traditional services, visible to the public through all the various media of promotion. If pharmacists choose not to advertise prices, they should be prepared to defend them.

Objectives

The specific objectives for a particular pharmacy depend to a large degree on the type of pharmacy or practice and location. However, there are general promotional objectives for any pharmacy in any location: (1) to develop a public image and public acceptance of the pharmacy; (2) to attract new patrons to the pharmacy; (3) to maintain patronage of present patrons and thus maintain a competitive position; (4) to gain acceptance of a new service or line of goods; and (5) to induce both new and old patrons to purchase more merchandise and services.

359

Classification of Promotions

All of the various types and modes of promotion are either *institutional* or *merchandising* in nature. The former tend to be *professional* and the latter *commercial,* but not necessarily.

INSTITUTIONAL APPROACH

Institutional promotions focus on the firm or organization and its services and characteristics. An institutional advertisement is used to tell the public of a new service such as a patient medication record system, or it may make the public aware of a unique characteristic such as "Serving the community for over 100 years." Direct patient contact by the pharmacist is the most effective means of institutional promotion, although the promotional program may well use other methods simultaneously.

MERCHANDISING APPROACH

In contrast, merchandising promotions focus on merchandise offered for sale, depicting special features as dependability or convenience of use, or a special price. Merchandising advertisements may emphasize weekend specials, special events, such as anniversary or holiday sales, a new line of goods, or a combination of products. The term *sales promotion* is used synonymously with merchandising promotion because of its familiarity and similarity in most contexts.

MODES OF PROMOTION

There are several modes of promotion, each with its purpose, advantages, and disadvantages.

Public Relations or Publicity. Public relations and publicity are used synonymously in most instances. One technical difference is the case in which a public relations program is launched with the expenditure of funds, whereas publicity, by definition, is free. This criterion also distinguishes publicity from advertisements.

A public relations or publicity program is community oriented. It may be a local program such as sponsorship of a local civic event or program, which may be either athletic, academic, or cultural in nature. Other types of programs support national drives or campaigns, usually health-related. National Poison Prevention Week, National Diabetic Week, and National Pharmacy Week are just a few of the many examples a pharmacy can use as a basis for a good public relations program.

Personal Selling. Personal selling may range from ordinary sales activities of clerks to professional consultation with patrons by the pharmacist. The public is hungry for this type of personal attention, as documented in Chapter

16. The success of professional consultation depends on: (1) genuine concern or empathy, (2) friendliness and accessibility of the pharmacist, and (3) a patient medication record system, especially when the consultation involves prescriptions or other drugs that may interfere with their effectiveness.

Sales Promotion. The term ''sales promotion'' is used to provide a convenient label or umbrella for a large number of specific promotional activities. Sales promotion may be defined as the coordinated use of advertising, displays, direct mail, and miscellaneous promotional activities such as contests, coupons, and trading stamps. These activities usually are directed toward the sale of merchandise and should be coordinated with personal selling efforts.

Developing a Promotional Program

The first decision in developing a promotional program is to determine the type of promotional program that is most compatible with the type of pharmacy, its location, its layout and its objectives. Basically, the pharmacist-manager must decide whether to use the institutional or merchandising approach, or a combination of the two. The promotional program must be compatible with the philosophy of the pharmacist, the pricing policy and strategy of the pharmacy. To do otherwise may dilute the promotional efforts, confuse the public image, and nullify the results of the promotional program. However, traditional pharmacies have used a combination of the two approaches, placing the greater emphasis on the type of promotion that best characterizes the practice, and the dual approach historically has been successful.

PROMOTIONAL STRATEGY

Based on the aforementioned considerations, the pharmacist-manager should devise a general promotional strategy. The strategy normally is determined by the following three factors: the *services offered,* the *physical facilities* and the *image* these project, and the *market* and *market position* of the pharmacy. At this point, the manager should analyze his/her entire practice and assess the many characteristics and features of the practice with the view of meshing these into a well-integrated promotional strategy and plan. The *first* consideration is the match between the type and size of the pharmacy and its market. For example, the pharmacy may be located in a fairly large and active shopping center with a potentially large and varied clientele (age, income, singles, married, etc.) but with a small traditional pharmacy space of 2,000 sq. ft. This is not a good match. In the ordinary course of events, the match would have been achieved as discussed in Chapters 5 to 8.

If for any reason the match is a poor one (you may have purchased the pharmacy at a good price but with high rent), this should be corrected first of all. You may need to expand the facilities or relocate. Trying to make a success under such conditions is very difficult. THIS IS FUNDAMENTAL. A market analysis using a sample of patrons from the prescription files, accounts receivable or both should be performed annually to determine market as outlined in Chapter 6. You should be drawing 50 to 60 percent of your clientele from the area of a mile radius and 40 to 50 percent from beyond that area. Note the distribution of patrons throughout the market area.

The *second* consideration is the services provided by the pharmacy. Do they include all the traditional services of credit, delivery, record of prescriptions purchased for tax and insurance purposes, and prompt and courteous clerk service? These should *not* be featured unless they are fully delivered.

Professional services should also be featured if they are expertly provided. Pharmacists, especially independent pharmacists, must realize that neither their financial welfare nor the profession is served by "hiding their light under a bushel." As a corollary, there is no justification for advertising a professional service, or for the use of a professional fee for that service, if all the pharmacist does is deliver the right drug, in the right dosage, to the right patient, with the correct directions on the label, basically a marketing function. Professional services should include screening for drug compatibility, proper drug use, and meaningful consultation with the patient, all of which should be performed with the aid of a medication record system.

Special professional services should definitely be promoted. These may include the fitting of trusses and other orthopedic or surgical appliances, screening for certain diseases such as diabetes, hypertension, or cancer, counseling patients on diet and exercise, for example. One service, the counseling of patients on the proper use of nonprescription drugs, is one for which the pharmacist is uniquely trained, yet it is poorly executed for the most part. Pharmacists generally have neglected to develop and to promote their professional skills. Both pharmacy and society would be better served if pharmacists were aggressive in developing their marketing and professional skills. The promotional strategy and the general approach, institutional or merchandising, are determined primarily by the services provided by the pharmacy.

A *third* consideration is the physical facilities of the pharmacy and the image they project. A pharmaceutical center or a prescription shop should use the institutional approach and feature professional services. A super pharmacy (drugstore) should use the merchandising approach. As stated previously, a traditional pharmacy may use a combined approach. If a combination is used, the pharmacy's sales activities should be segmented into three major areas, as a basis for developing a promotional strategy. Generally, the emphasis of the promotional plan should be proportional to sales activities in the three areas.

The *first segment,* the professional areas, includes the prescription department, prescription accessories, orthopedic and surgical supplies and appliances, home health care aids, and "ethical" nonprescription drugs.

The *second segment,* the general merchandise departments, includes proprietary drugs, cosmetics, toiletries, and traditional drug sundries. Special skill departments also may be included in this segment or in the professional segment, depending on the nature of the department and the promotions used.

The *third segment*, the promotional and traffic-building departments, includes special promotional merchandise, the tobacco department, magazines, candy, and the fountain.

In order to know how well your layout design and promotional strategy are working for you, a qualitative traffic flow analysis should be conducted annually. (See Chapter 7 for the methodology for conducting a traffic flow analysis.) This will enable you to detect bottlenecks in your layout that impede traffic flow and the relative productivity of the three segments and various departments. It will provide an indication of where to enhance displays and other merchandising techniques. In addition, sales analysis via cash register readings should be conducted to determine traffic levels and patterns of sales productivity. This should be done hourly over a week period on a quarterly basis. Records of analyses should be kept to establish trends. If the register has departmental keys, this analysis will be very useful for various purposes, including promotional strategy and staffing patterns.

Based on these data, the pharmacist selects one of the major segments as the primary basis of his seasonal promotional strategy, depending on the type of pharmacy. Some pharmacists-managers utilize all three segments when developing a promotional strategy, especially in a large traditional or super drugstore. The promotional strategy incorporates the pricing policy and competitive strategy, discussed in Chapter 15. The amount of market segmentation and quasi-price reduction, and the amount and type of direct price reduction also must be included in the promotional strategy.

The *fourth* consideration is the market position the pharmacy presently enjoys or the market position that you, as the pharmacist-manager, would like to achieve. Market position means the relative share of the market. This share must be considered in light of the promotional emphasis, institutional (professional) or merchandising (commercial). If the emphasis is professional, then the market share of those products and services featured is the relevant consideration. Moreover, the immediate trade area is the relevant market, not the entire city. Another related consideration is the goal of either maintaining a market position in an expanding market or increasing the share of a market that is steady, expanding, or decreasing. The latter goal requires a much more aggressive strategy than the former, especially for a merchandising strategy, and demands that the pharmacy manager penetrate the market, that is, reach more persons than before.

PROMOTIONAL BUDGET

Developing the promotional budget is one of the most important but difficult steps in the promotional plan. The problem is to budget enough money to get the market penetration desired without overspending, which is wasteful. There is not a magic formula to use in developing a budget. Using an average

Table 17–1. Promotional Planning Calendar

Date/Period	Theme and Events	Featured Products/Service
SUMMER	"Fun in the Sun"	Professional services, tanning/sun burn products, and sun glasses
June	"Wedding Bells"	Wedding accessories, gifts
6/14	Flag Day	Assorted flags; books on flags
	Father's Day	Gifts, men's toiletries
July	"Independence," "Liberty"	Picnic and vacation goods, skin care, and first aid
7/4	Independence Day All Star Game	Books on history of revolutionary war and heroes
August	"Dog Days"	Foot care and pet supplies
	"Back to School"	School supplies
	"Check-up Time"	Dental care and toothbrushes
FALL	"Harvest Time" Cornucopia	Professional services, allergy and cold products and vitamins
September	Football "School Spirit" Labor Day "Let's Rest"	Sports medicine and first aid products

American Heart Food Festival Week (mid month)
Unofficial Muscular Dystrophy Week (Labor Day Telethon)

October	"October's Bright Blue Weather"	
	World Series	Shaving products
1,2 Tishri	Rosh Hashannah	Books on Jewish history and heritage
10 Tishri	Yom Kippur	
10/12	Columbus Day	Books on Columbus and exploration
10/24	U.N. Day	
10/31	Halloween	Poisonproof candy

Alzheimer National Awareness, Immunization, and Drug Abuse Prevention Campaign Month

November	"Thankfulness," "Sharing"	Professional services, baby care, vitamins, ℞ accessories, cough and cold and skin care products
	Election Day	
11/11	Veteran's Day	
	Thanksgiving Day	Boxed nuts

National Diabetes and National Epilepsy Month   Diabetes screening program

Great American Smoke-out Day (Third Thursday); Launch Christmas Seals Campaign—American Lung Association—continues through December—"It's a matter of life and breath"

Date/Period	Theme and Events	Featured Products/Service
WINTER	"Guard Your Health"	Prescription/professional services; cough and cold, cosmetic, skin protection and vitamin products
December	"Cheerfulness and Hope-fulness for Mankind"	
25 Kislev	Hanukkah (Channukah)	Candy, cards, gifts, seasonal decorations and ornaments
12/25	Christmas	
January	"Start the New Year Right," "Keepin fit"	Party goods, antacids Exercise equipment and books, home health care
Birth Defects Prevention Month and March of Dimes		Article on birth defects
February	Honesty/Integrity	Article based on Gallup Poll
2/12	Lincoln's Birthday	Log cabin craftwork items
2/14	Valentine's Day	Candy, cards, and gifts
	Presidents' Day	Books and biographies on presidents; chocolate cherries
2/22	Washington's Birthday	
National Children's Dental Month		Dental products and dental check-up ads
March	"Ill Wind Bloweth No Good?"	Skin care, lip ice, and cold remedies
3/15	Ides of March	Roman calendar replicas
3/17	St. Patrick's Day	Green shamrocks
National Poison Prevention, National Red Cross, and National Kidney Month		Article on poison prevention
SPRING	"A New Beginning"	Professional services, books and products related to gardening, flowers, herbs, lawns and allergies
	Passover	Kosher candy/food package
	Easter	Baskets, candy, cards and candles.
April	"April Showers, May Flowers"	Allergy and baby care products. Books on income tax, cancer, and diet aids
National Cancer Awareness Month		Article on cancer
May	"Freedom," "Memories"	Books on wars, heroes and patriotism
	Mother's Day	Candy, flowers and gifts
	Armed Forces Day	
5/30	Memorial Day	Flowers and wreaths
	Graduation	Gifts
National High Blood Pressure, National Arthritis, National Better Hearing and Speech, and National Mental Health Month, National Asthma/allergy Awareness Week (2nd week)		Blood pressure screening program Articles and displays promoting the prevention or cure of these diseases and disabilities

percent of sales, as reported in publications such as *The Lilly Digest,* is not the answer, although it is better than a "guesstimate." *The Lilly Digest* for 1984 reported a range of 1.0 to 1.4 percent of sales, while the *NACDS-Lilly Digest* reported a range of 1.2 to 2.3 percent of sales.

The first step is to estimate the full market potential for your location and type of pharmacy. If the full market potential has not been reached, an upward adjustment in the budget is indicated. If, on the other hand, the full market potential has been obtained, a "set" promotional budget should be used to maintain the competitive position.

Next, the budget should be segmented into seasons and months based on a calendar of events. Generally, the monthly budget should correspond to the monthly percentage of annual sales. The pharmacist-manager should consult with a local advertising agency or with the advertising manager of the local newspaper. Extra money should be budgeted for certain months because of special events such as "back to school days" for a merchandising promotional plan, or National Diabetic Week for an institutional-professional promotional plan. Then the budget should be divided according to the major segments of the pharmacy or departments that will be featured each month. Finally, the budget should be divided between money spent on displays and the various advertising media. Once the budget has been established, adherence to it is recommended, unless something unusual develops that requires an additional advertising expenditure.

CALENDAR OF EVENTS

The calendar of events is the master guideline for the week-to-week promotions. The National Wholesale Druggists Association (NWDA) publishes a Planning Calendar which can be used or easily adapted for most pharmacies. The Planning Calendar indicates all the special weeks and months, such as National Pharmacy Week, National Cancer Month, and many more. It also indicates national and religious holidays and the birthdays of important people. In addition, the calendar lists four departments or lines of products that are suitable for promotion each month. With the addition of local events and the anniversary of the pharmacy, the NWDA Planning Calendar provides the basis for developing an excellent promotional calendar of events.

The NWDA Planning Calendar, or the one in Table 17–1, should be selected to provide the detailed guidelines of the promotional strategy. This in turn will depend on the type of pharmacy and promotion, institutional or merchandising. Professional and health related events and campaigns naturally should provide the basis of a promotional program for a pharmaceutical center or apothecary shop. A traditional pharmacy could use both health-related and other special events, with the emphasis dictated by the percentage of sales derived from the prescription and other health-related departments. A large super pharmacy would make more use of Valentine's Day, Mother's Day,

Father's Day, "Back to School" events, weekend specials, and related types of promotion.

Executing the Program

STEPS IN IMPLEMENTATION

After developing the promotional program, including the strategy, budget, and calendar of events, specific steps have to be taken to put the program into effect. The promotional budget should indicate the amount that has been budgeted for displays, the various advertising media, direct mail, and miscellaneous promotional methods. If not, this is the *first step* in executing the promotional program. The selection of the primary medium or media is important. This medium should be, first of all, affordable, on a weekly basis, within the promotional budget. It is better to use one medium that reaches most of the target market on a consistent basis than to "hop, skip" with several or many media.

The *second step* is to select the proper mix of products and/or services to be promoted. If promotional or seasonal merchandise is selected, the best source of supply must be sought. The amount to be purchased should be based on experience. This points to the importance of *step three,* complete records of promotions, including the amount purchased, the cost of the promotion, and the success in terms of the sale of promotional and staple merchandise.

The *fourth step,* and the most critical, is to inform all sales personnel of the details of the promotion. Without the knowledge and energetic support of the sales personnel, any promotion will fail to achieve the desired results. Failure to keep all personnel informed happens in too many instances.

Finally, a schedule, including the date of each step, should be developed and followed. Execution of the promotional program may be summarized as follows: (1) selecting and stocking the appropriate merchandise or service; (2) selecting the various modes of promotion; (3) informing the sales personnel; (4) making and following a schedule; and (5) keeping records of the results.

ADVERTISING

Advertising is any paid publication of information, which reaches beyond the confines of the pharmacy, and appeals persuasively to the public to patronize a pharmacy and/or purchase its merchandise or service. Any of the various media may be used. The pharmacist may select from newspapers, direct mail, handbills or circulars, billboards on highways or moving vehicles, radio, and television. The pharmacist must select the medium or media which will serve his purpose best. This depends largely on the type of promotion and pharmacy practice, but it also depends on the scope of the circulation and the hearing or viewing area as compared with the pharmacy's trading area. The key is to match the circulation, hearing, or viewing audience with the target market. Whereas a regular or cooperative chain may use a large advertisement in a large city newspaper or on television profitably, the small independent pharmacy cannot.

Selecting the Media. Certain criteria can be used to evaluate the efficiency of the various media. These are (1) cost-per-thousand (CPM), a measure of general cost efficiency; (2) modified cost-per-thousand (MCPM), a measure of the cost efficiency for the target market, and (3) "punch," a measure of the drawing power of the medium. The medium can be evaluated in terms of the last criterion only with experience; therefore, it will be discussed under promotion evaluation. Initially, the decision has to be made on the basis of the two measures of cost of the potential media.

The first step is to compare the general cost efficiency, using the following formula:

$$CPM = \frac{\text{Cost of the Ad}}{\text{TA} \div 1,000}$$
$$TA = \text{the total circulation or audience}$$

On determining the CPM values for several media, compare the modified cost efficiency, using this formula:

$$MCPM = \frac{\text{Cost of the AD}}{\text{TMA} \div 1,000}$$
$$TMA = \text{the total target market audience or circulation}$$

The latter measure of cost efficiency is more direct and specific for the pharmacy's particular needs. After the pharmacist-manager has had some experience with several media and has evaluated their respective drawing power, he can select the best media mix, using the above three criteria.

Smaller pharmacies may profitably use radio spot announcements, sponsor a short, community-oriented radio program such as birth announcements or hospital news, use "shoppers' news" and place small institutional ads in the larger papers. Rural pharmacies can profitbly use the weekly county newspaper.

Direct mail is one of the best media for professional, institutional ads directed to either lay patrons or prescribers. Direct mail costs more than prepared handbills or circulars, but it can be better controlled to reach the specific target people.

The use of announcement cards, which may be reproduced in the newspaper or used as a spot announcement on television, is an ideal method for introducing a new service such as a patient record system, diabetes screening program, or the monitoring of hypertension for selected patients with approval of the patient's physician.

Media Cost. Newspapers generally charge by the column inch. Some charge by the agate line, and there are 14 agate lines per inch. Rates vary with the geographic area, circulation of the newspaper, weekdays versus Sundays, and the amount of annual advertisements contracted. Readers should check with local newspapers for prevailing local rates. Circulation and rate cards are available from these sources.

As a general guide, rates for a medium-sized newspaper in a medium-sized mid-American city (circulation: 112,000 Sunday, 106,000 weekdays) in 1985 are as follows: Open rate (no contract) $21.60/column inch for daily and $24.56/column inch for Sunday. In addition to the Sunday subscribers, another 50,000 households receive the advertisement in a special Sunday advertising supplement at a combined rate of $28.28/column inch. A contract for only 100 column inches per year reduces the rate to $19.84 for a daily edition, $22.80 for Sundays, and $26.52 with the special advertising supplement. A larger contract (500 column inches) reduces the rates to $19.48, $22.44 and $26.16, respectively. The rate for a weekly newspaper averages about $2.60/column inch with a range of $1.75 to $4.00 in 1985 in Kentucky. A newspaper advertisement should be two columns wide at a minimum to receive the attention of the reader.

Typical rates for advertising on radio and television are depicted in Table 17–2. These are shown as a model or guide for selecting times for spot commercials; the figures may not be accurate for your market area. As with anything we pruchase, the price varies with the value of the product—in this case, the size of the viewing or listening audience.

Other media costs vary so widely that it is difficult to provide any guidelines. Generally, these media cost less than those just discussed. A small, independent pharmacist can use these miscellaneous media to great advantage, both because he can tailor them to his particular needs and because the cost usually is less.

Types of Advertisements. Merchandising advertisements are one of three types: *omnibus*—made up of many unrelated items; *related items* or product line advertisement; and *single product* advertisement. As previously stated, an advertisement may be institutional, which informs the public of one or more services or unique characteristics of a firm.

Larger merchandising independents and the regular or cooperative chain drugstore most often use the omnibus ad. Frequently, these contain an institutional component, usually relating to services of the prescription department. Often a product line or a single product ad is a cooperative advertisement paid for wholly or in part by the manufacturer.

Psychology of Advertising. The psychology of advertising can best be illustrated by the use of the acronym AIDA, the title of a well-known opera.

A—Attract attention, usually with headline and sometimes an illustration.

Table 17–2.   Typical Radio and TV Ad Rates[a]

	R A D I O							
	5,000 W Day;		*1,000 Night AM*		*10,000 W AM;*		*3,000 W FM*	
Time	*Open 30″*	*Rate 60″*	*Contract 30″*	*Rate 60″*	*Open 30″*	*Rate 60″*	*Contract 30″*	*Rate 60″*
6–10	$55	$59	$42	$46	$13	$18	$11	$16
10–3	24	27	19	21	11	13	9	11
3–7	33	37	27	31	12	16	10	14
7–	18	20	8	10	9	10	7	8

WKYT TELEVISION[b]						
Time:	6:00	7:00	9:00	12:00	12:30	4:00
	7:00	9:00	12:00	12:30	4:00	5:00
Rate[c]$:	20	40	60	75	50	75
Time:	5:00	5:30	7:00	8:00	11:00	11:30
	5:30	7:00	8:00	11:00	11:30	X:XX
Rate[c]$:	115	240	250	540	250	50

[a]These are typical rates in 1985, which are presented for the patterned variation and not as specific rates for a particular market.

[b]A CBS affiliate in a metropolitan area (200,000 people) with a median viewing audience of 90,000 households.

[c]These rates are for a 30-second commercial; for 10-second spot the rate is 50% and for a 60-second spot the rates are 200%. The $540 rate is average across prime time.

I—Induce interest, usually with an illustration, price, or overall layout design.

D—Develop desire to buy, appealing to the various purchasing motives.

A—Actuate to buy, usually with special message, e.g., "Available only through _____."

Preparation of the Advertisement. The first step is to decide on the type of advertisement and the general message or theme that is to be conveyed. The theme may be institutional in nature, a special event, an anniversary sale, a weekend special, or a value or price reduction message. This may involve one or more services, a product, a product line, or group of unrelated products. Once this decision is made, it is necessary to select the appropriate products for the ad. This step is critical.

Common sense indicates many of the products to select for seasonal and special events promotions. However, there are some *criteria for selecting promotional products* in general. (1) The product should have general *sala-bility,* that is, it should have *wide appeal* and usage among the general public. This criterion is especially important for weekend specials. The product may be staple, such as hand lotion, or it may be a fad, as were hula hoops and skateboards a few years ago. (2) The product should have high *quality.*

Nothing destroys goodwill faster than to advertise a product that turns out to be poor in quality when used. (3) The *price* of the product must be right. If it is a well-known product, the sale price should be significantly below the regular price. (4) A fourth criterion that may be used is *promotional "tie-ins."* An example of this would be an ad and a display of Gillette razor blades during the World Series. It is desirable that the product have three of these four criteria to be a good candidate for promotion.

Next, the copy is written and it may be elaborate, constituing the major portion of the ad, or it may be as simple as notice of a reduced price. In most cases, the copy must be concise and direct. The headline for the written ad should be simple, but it should attract the attention of the reader and should announce the theme of the ad.

The logo, which is the one permanent or constant component of every ad, is the trademark that identifies the pharmacy or firm. It is usually placed at the top or bottom of the ad and must be well coordinated with the headline. Illustrations, if they are to be used, must be drawn or selected from available sources. Illustration can brighten an otherwise dull ad.

Finally, the layout of the various components of the advertisement must be arranged: the headline, the logo, the size and shape of the ad, the arrangement of the illustration. Product, price, and message must be arranged to meet the four criteria of advertising psychology. The visual ad should be clean, not cluttered. Not only should the ad catch the reader's attention, it should hold it long enough to cause the reader to peruse through the entire ad and to remember it. Obviously, this requires talent when one considers the great amount of competition for the reader's attention. Most pharmacists should consult with an expert in advertising when developing any other than a simple ad. For further discussion of advertising for a pharmacy, consult a reference on advertising and your local newspaper, radio and TV stations.

DISPLAYS

Displays are known as point-of-sale advertising. There are various types of displays, each serving different secondary purposes with the one common purpose of increasing impulse sales.

Types of Display. The more common types of display are: (1) window displays, (2) "shadow-box" displays, (3) showcase displays, (4) counter displays, (5) "hot-spot" or high-traffic displays, and (6) mass displays.

Window displays are used for professional displays and seasonal merchandise. It is recommended that window displays be kept sufficiently low to provide full view of the interior of the pharmacy. The "shadow-box" displays are small window displays, usually 3 feet by 4 feet or less located on the side of the store. They are frequently used to display a line of cosmetics or some other special line or service.

Showcase displays are the oldest type of display and are used for cosmetics, costume jewelry, cameras, and other expensive items.

Counter displays have been used for years and may be used for seasonal products, a new product or product line, and fast-moving staple goods. These are often the three- or four-tier displays adjacent to the cash register, often referred to as a "selling console."

"Hot-spot" displays are usually carton or floor displays placed in high-traffic areas. They are often specially built by manufacturers to display their seasonal or new products. This type of display is used for special promotional merchandise—nonstaple merchandise purchased in large quantities at a special reduced price. There are several types of "hot-spot" displays, many of which are provided by the manufacturer. These include the floor stand, the dump, the end-cap, and the carton displays. The floor stand display is made of cardboard and is normally placed in a high traffic aisle. It is appropriate for seasonal merchandise and for special sales. The dump is a variation of the floor stand. It consists of a cardboard box or a wire basket in which the merchandise is literally dumped. It is appropriate for seasonal and irregularly shaped merchandise, and for goods sold at a low, special price. The end-cap is a display placed at the end of a gondola. This is effective for both staple and promotional merchandise, especially on the front end of the gondola and near the cash register and the prescription department. The carton display is effective when placed near the cash register, wrapping counter, or check-out counter. It is useful for small convenience goods often purchased on impulse.

Mass displays are used on gondolas, on the top of the wall shelving, and sometimes on the "selling console." A large amount of merchandise is normally displayed with multiple facings of each item and each size of an item. The theory is that the massiveness of the display will attract attention of patrons and create the image that it is a popular and highly desired product. This image is often enhanced by a price reduction or a special sale. The floor-stack display, one of the most effective, is a special type of mass display made by stacking full cases of a product with the top and front panel of the top case cut away to expose the merchandise.

All displays should have a header card (corresponding to the headline in an ad), which announces the special features and the name of the product, the price, and any other special feature.

Psychology of Displays. The basic psychology of displays is the same as that for advertising and is also illustrated by the acronym, AIDA. There are additional psychologic factors of which the pharmacist should be aware in construcitng displays. The display should have one dominant theme. Good use should be made of color and lighting effects, and the display should reflect order but not necessarily symmetry. Most displays, especially mass and "hot-spot" displays, should implement the *buying-break* concept, which simply means that two or three packages are missing. This practice has a definite, positive psychologic effect on the purchaser. The number of *facings* (the number of packages with the front panel facing the purchaser) of a product in a display, or on the shelf, should be proportionate to the relative sales volume of the item, up to about four facings, as a general rule. Each size is considered to be an individual item or product.

Another psychologic principle is *to position* a product *according to the size,* with the smallest size to the left and the larger sizes to the right. Since most people are right handed, they will tend to pick the larger size on the right. A related principle is to position the most popular brand at eye level on the shelf. Within a department or product section, there is a hypothetic *"hot-spot cross configuration."* The vertical stem of the cross is in the center of the section, and the horizontal arm of the cross is the shelf at eye level. The cross is used as a guide to display related products according to their relative popularity and sales volume.

Sales are stimulated by displaying products adjacent to related products. This is called *related-product* merchandising. A similar technique is the *cross-merchandising* of products. The placing of a display of an antacid product near a stack of party goods is an example of cross-merchandising. These are not related products, but overindulging may cause heartburn and hence the association between the products. For a more complete discussion of merchandising over-the-counter drug products, the reader should read several issues of pharmacy trade periodicals.

Constructing the Display. The *first step,* trite and simple as it may be, is to remove the old display and thoroughly clean the display area.

The *second step* is to select the theme, which usually includes the merchandise to be displayed or the service to be illustrated or demonstrated.

The *third step* is the assembly of the physical materials for the display, which may include: background material (especially in window displays), fixtures (regular or special such as boxes), accessory items (cloth, paper, show cards, price tickets, professional equipment, or animated devices), and the merchandise.

The *fourth step* is to sketch the display on paper when appropriate. Sometimes the display can be visualized without the benefit of a sketch.

The *fifth step* is to arrange the display as sketched or planned. Often this may require that parts of the display be rearranged several times to obtain the desired effect.

Selecting the Merchandise. There are several factors influencing the choice of merchandise, the most obvious being the nature and type of display. There are other factors to be considered such as the value, bulk, perishability, and attractiveness of the merchandise. Other factors such as the season, the calendar of events, and "tieing in" the display with national promotion should also be included in the consideration.

DIRECT MAIL

Direct mail normally is used for personalized and professional messages. It is one of the most effective methods of reaching a particular group of people, and is the recommended method of reaching prescribers in the area.

Professional newsletters or bulletins are included in this category. Direct mail is an excellent means of introducing a new line of goods or services. Some examples include a new line of cosmetics, a new and complete line of orthopedic and surgical appliances and supplies, a medication record system, or a screening or diagnostic laboratory service. It is perhaps the best single promotional method for a pharmaceutical center or a prescription shop. The American College of Apothecaries (ACA) provides its members with excellent materials for a professional newsletter for prescribers and a health newsletter for patrons. The ACA and NARD have published a book on advertising and promotion.[4] A good up-to-date mailing list is an essential part of all direct mail promotions.

MISCELLANEOUS PROMOTIONS

There are dozens of promotional methods that fall into the miscellaneous category. This broad category includes samples, gifts for babies, posters and banners, push merchandise (PMs), drawings for prizes, coupons, trading stamps, brochures or package inserts, and contests, just to name the more common forms. Some are useful; others are not recommended.

Most of these promotional methods have their place in the various types of pharmacies; however, trading stamps are neither profitable nor economic in the long run except for the trading stamps producer and the manufacturers of the premium products. Trading stamps are an expensive means of promotion, and they lose their competitive advantage as soon as the competitors adopt other stamps. The producers of the stamps and the premiums reap a windfall from the unredeemed stamps alone. The goods offered as premiums usually can be purchased at a lower price in regular stores.

In my opinion, PMs are not a good method of promotion because of the tendency to divide loyalties and to promote an overly aggressive attitude among the sales personnel.

It is suggested that banners and window signs be used judiciously, if at all, so that they do not lose their effectiveness when the full impact is needed. Less frequent use prevents a continuous cluttered appearance which obscures the total effect of well-organized displays and a good layout design of the pharmacy.

The miscellaneous professional promotional programs are excellent. These include patient medication record system, a record of the expenditures for drugs for income tax deduction, health information brochures on various diseases, record of immunization, special printed instructions for medications with complicated instructions, standardized measuring spoons, and a list of prescription accessories that may be needed with certain prescriptions. This list is only the more common means of professional promotion.

Coupons in newspaper ads can be valuable in measuring market penetration and the effectiveness of a promotion.

PERSONAL SELLING

Personal selling is the personal assistance given a patron to achieve his desired satisfactions and to meet his real needs. Of course, this ranges from the simple act of taking his money to the complicated process of helping the patron select the proper product and providing the appropriate advice.

Fundamentals of Personal Selling. The fundamental principles of professional personal selling or consultation are: (1) know your patrons and patients; (2) know your drugs and other products; (3) understand and use patronage and purchasing motives; (4) develop empathy; and (5) provide prompt, courteous, and helpful service.

A person's name is to him one of the sweetest sounds on the earth. Forgetting the names of the people who patronize our pharmacies is one of the most common failings among a large majority of pharmacists. There are a few rules, *if used,* that will greatly assist in overcoming this problem. The first rule is to have a personal interest in the patron as an individual. The second rule is to be sure to understand his name, even if it requires his repeating it several times. Repetition of the name is itself the third rule. The fourth rule is to write or type the name. Seeing the name in print is a powerful reinforcement in the remembering of names. Last, associate the name with something about the person, his appearance, his occupation, or something such as an event that is *unique,* not something that is common.

Pharmacists should know the products they sell and should know drugs thoroughly. The important thing is to think of the indications, side effects, dosage, and other information in terms of the individual. For example, a drug is contraindicated because a particular patient, Mrs. Clark, has diabetes; this should be remembered or available for recall from the patient medication record. A superior professional consultation requires an appropriate facility that provides a degree of privacy, which is not presently available in many pharmacies. The pharmacist should strive always to be judicious, as well as objective and truthful, in consulting with patients and patrons.

Patronage and purchasing motives have been discussed in the previous chapter. The important point is to personalize this knowledge and understanding when dealing with clients. It should be realized that it is the results—the ease of pain, comfort, attractiveness—not the product, that the patron is really buying.

Developing empathy is not easy for most of us. We are too self-centered. Empathy comes from really putting oneself in the place of the other person. Some will argue that one loses objectivity when this happens. It is my contention that sufficient objectivity *can* be retained while one is developing empathy for another.

With genuine interest in the objectives of the pharmacy—achieved via MBO (management by objectives)—and empathy, pharmacists and clerks alike are ready to provide prompt, courteous, and helpful service. The process is almost automatic and supervision is reduced to a minimum.

Meeting Objections. There are at least three methods of answering objections. First is the "yes, but" method which consists of agreeing with a customer as far as possible without argument. The clerk then proceeds to present the goods from another perspective and to obtain the patron's agreement on as many points as possible, while developing and maintaining an affirmative attitude toward the patron and the product.

Second, the person may ask a patron to explain her objections. This must not be done in a critical or haughty fashion, but must indicate a sincere desire to learn from the objections of the customer. The salesperson must treat all patrons' prejudices and fears with sympathy and alleviate them if possible.

Finally, the sales person may strive to turn the objections into a selling point. For instance, if a customer indicates that he hasn't time, the clerk may suggest that a few minutes' time now may save the customer more time by eliminating a second trip.

Meeting Price Objections. The clerk may emphasize the value of the article and show the difference between it and less expensive but similar merchandise. He may demonstrate the superior quality and workmanship necessitating higher cost and selling price. A thrifty customer may be convinced of the long-run economy resulting from the purchase of an article of higher quality.

If the clerk is convinced that the patron actually believes he cannot afford the higher-priced merchandise, the clerk may turn to a lower-priced similar article. But, while discussing that article, he ought to keep the higher-priced and higher-quality product in sight in case the customer changes his mind.

In case of a new, high-priced prescription drug, the obvious suggestion is to point to the savings to the patient now possible with the new drug, i.e., he is spared a protracted period of hospitalization with its accompanying expenses and loss of income.

The patron may claim that he can buy the articles more cheaply elsewhere. A pharmacist and his clerks should be acquainted with competitors' prices and know whether there is a real difference in price or quality. He may need to adjust his pricing policy if he cannot defend it in terms of quality or superior services.

In general, the best rules to follow are: (1) be positive and give encouragement; (2) avoid contradictions, superiority, discouragement, overgeneralization, and too much personal opinion; and (3) if the patron does not buy the product, try to cultivate an atmosphere that will induce the patron to return for the goods later.

LIMITING FACTORS

The success of promotional programs is limited by such factors as: (1) the overall market potential and market saturation, which may have been affected by various promotions; (2) the law of diminishing return, which is a formal expression of the aforementioned factor; (3) the chance that special promotions may "borrow" from future sales at regular prices; (4) the possibility of increased pilferage resulting from the crowded conditions; and (5) the possibility of having unsold merchandise that may have to be sold at less than sale price, or not at all.

Evaluation of Promotion

Most pharmacists no doubt would like to know whether their promotional campaigns are successful. Some are less concerned about measuring the results of the money they spend on advertising and promotion, but they spend the money out of a sense of being competitive. They somehow feel they need to spend 1 to 1½ percent of their sales on advertising and promotion because most pharmacy proprietors and managers feel that is what is required to be competitive. This is indicative of the intuitive, nonscientific approach to pharmacy management and practices. For pharmacists who are concerned with the results achieved from the advertising budget, the measuring of results is not an easy task. The institutional type of advertising produces results much more slowly, but its effects last longer than the merchandising type of promotion and vice versa. There are techniques available that will provide some measure of the results achieved through advertising and promotion.

GENERAL METHODS

The general method of measuring the results of promotion involves measuring the increase in sales over a base line previously established. The sales of the same period a year before generally are insufficient to serve as base line data. Some event, such as a special sale, a flu epidemic, or extremely bad weather, could have influenced the sales for that period of the previous year. This possibility should be investigated and adjustments made as necessary. The pharmacist must establish the sales growth trend resulting from general economic and/or inflationary growth and from the pharmacy's own sales growth data resulting from its own relative market strength. The inflationary rate for products normally sold in pharmacies increased by 10 to 15 percent per year between 1980 and 1984. Prescription drug prices increased by 13 percent annually, OTC drug prices by 11 percent and all items in CPI by 7 percent between 1980 and 1983. Independent pharmacy sales increased by 10.5 percent annually during the 1974–1983 period, and chain pharmacies sales increased by 7.6 percent annually during the same period. The sales data were derived from the *Lilly Digest*. The inflationary rate must be exceeded if the pharmacy is to have any real growth.

Once the overall annual sales growth trend for the pharmacy has been established, seasonal adjustments should be computed for each month and week, especially for those weeks or months with large sales variations, such as December. This is accomplished in the following manner. Let us assume that the last five years have been used to establish the annual sales growth trend. Using the figures for the last five years, we compute a monthly, or weekly, sales index as follows: (1) compute the average sales for each month, or week, for the last five years; (2) compute the average annual sales for the past five years; (3) divide the average annual sales by 12 to compute a hypothetical average monthly sales figure for the past five years; and (4) divide the average five-year monthly sales for each month by the overall monthly average to determine the average monthly variation from the overall average for each month. Let 100 represent the overall monthly average, and the average sales for each month will be represented by an index number in relation to 100.

An example will illustrate the technique. Let us assume the overall monthly sales average $20,000 over the last five years. Further, let us assume that the average sales for December for the last five years were $22,400. Dividing $22,400 by $20,000 gives a quotient of 1.12; thus, December has a monthly seasonal index of 112 after multiplying 1.12 by 100, a 12 percent variation from the overall monthly average. If the average sales for June for the past five years were $18,000, then the index for June would be 90 ($18,000 ÷ $20,000 = .90 and .90 × 100 = 90).

Accurate records of advertising and promotion budgets and expenditures are necessary to determine whether extra expenditures for a particular month, week, or special event had an effect on the sales for a particular period. Allowance should be made in computing seasonal (monthly or weekly) indices or adjustments. If the annual five-year growth trend and the seasonal, monthly, or weekly indices are developed during a period of typical or normal advertising and promotion expenditures, then the base line data should be adequate to measure a significant sales increase resulting from a special promotional campaign supported by increased expenditures. This method may be used for a major department or the entire pharmacy.

SPECIAL METHODS

There are some special methods or techniques for measuring the success of a special promotional campaign. By placing in an ad a coupon that is to be detached and presented to receive a discount or a prize, the pharmacist can determine how effective the ad has been. The ratio of the number of "redeemed" coupons to the total market potential would be indicative of the degree of success of the promotion. Different types of promotion or advertisements could be compared as a measure of the effectiveness of promotion or the design of the advertisement.

Perhaps a better technique is to require the name and address to be completed on a coupon in a newspaper advertisement, circular, or direct mailing for a drawing for a prize. By charting the addresses on the redeemed coupons, the pharmacy manager can measure the market penetration as well as the geographic location of the market. He can also determine whether he has made contact with new patrons.

Summary

Extending the advertising and promotional program through the point of sale is essential. No advertising program is complete without it. An ad cannot make the sale, only the salesperson can. Unfortunately, many pharmacists fail in their advertising campaigns precisely at this critical point. Their salespeople frequently do not know what is going on, are limited in their ability to do the job, or are not properly motivated to do the job. Therefore, a final admonishment should be made to pharmacist-managers regarding a successful promotional program. It should include the following: develop the budget, establish the objectives, prepare the theme, select the media, and most important, do not forget that salespeople make the sale!

The role of advertising and promotion in our economy has become controversial. Many say that advertising is an unjustifiable social cost which does nothing more than switch people from one brand of merchandise to another. Others who support advertising claim that it does provide a service to our society, and it does justify all the expenditures made. Furthermore, they argue that advertising also keeps the economy strong by encouraging expenditures, which in turn increase or keep employment high. The controversy over advertising continues, and there certainly is merit in both arguments. It may be true that advertising cigarettes does nothing more than encourage people to elect between several equally bad alternatives. On the other hand, advertising does increase consumption and demand in our free economy. Advertising *is* a form of *communication* and pharmacists should be good communicators.

Rather than pursue the argument whether advertising and promtion are worthwhile expenditures of funds, the general philosophy of this chapter rests on the following assumptions: (1) the pharmacist-manager's competitors will advertise, (2) if the pharmacist intends to make a go of his enterprise, he, too, must advertise, and (3) advertising is an additional cost of doing business. As for the moral or ethical considerations of advertising, the general tenor of this chapter is to consider advertising and promotion as a means of communicating information that will have a positive effect on the health and well-being of the public. Other references should be consulted for additional information on promotion.[6-10]

REFERENCES

1. Consumerism vs. professionalism: a panel discussion. *J. Am. Pharm. Assoc., NS 12,* 356–366, 1972.
2. *Communicating the Value of Comprehensive Pharmaceutical Services.* Report of the Dichter Institute for Motivational Research, Inc., Washington: American Pharmaceutical Association, 1973.
3. Gulick, G.E.: Advertising. In *Effective Pharmacy Management.* Kansas City, Mo.: Marion Laboratories, Inc., 1979, pp. 279–307.
4. Farr, G., Huffman, D.C., and Ryan, M.R. (Eds.): *Professional Promotion for Pharmacy Managers.* 2nd ed. Memphis: American College of Apothecaries, Aug., 1976.
5. *How to Win Friends and Influence Customers.* New York: Sterling Drug Co. (Co-sponsors— NARD, Chicago), 1962.

6. *How to Promote Your Retail Pharmacy.* Chicago: NARD, 1969.
7. Sawyer, W.E.: Sell as Customers Like It. 7th printing, New York: Dell Publishing Co., 1971.
8. McMahon, J.L., Baldwin, J., and Sawyer, W.E. (Eds).: *Sales Management.* Vol. 1, New Burnswick, N.J.: Johnson & Johnson and Co., 1971.
9. Huffman, D.C., Jr., and Smith, H.A.: *Building A Successful Pharmacy Practice: A Case Study.* Memphis: American College of Apothecaries, 1972.

REVIEW

1. What are the five general objectives of pharmacy promotion?

2. Discuss the differences between institutional and merchandising promotions.

3. Which types of pharmacies can best utilize the institutional and the merchandising type of promotions?

4. Describe the several modes of promotion.

5. Discuss the promotional strategy.

6. Discuss how a pharmacist can develop a promotional budget and a calendar of events.

7. Discuss the five steps in implementing a promotional plan.

8. Define advertising.

9. What are the three basic types of merchandising advertisement?

10. Discuss the major types of media available for advertising, their cost, and their use for different types of pharmacies.

11. Discuss the steps in preparing an advertisement, including guidelines for selecting products.

12. Outline the basic psychologic principles of display and advertisements keyed to the acronym AIDA.

13. Discuss the various types of displays and how they are best used.

14. What are some of the major factors influencing the type of merchandise used in displays?

15. Outline the steps in constructing a display.

16. List and discuss several examples of types of miscellaneous promotions, both professional and nonprofessional.

17. Describe professional personal selling.

18. What are the five fundamentals of professional personal selling?

19. Discuss the methods of answering patrons' objections generally and to price specifically.

20. What are the factors limiting the success of a promotional program?

21. Discuss the methods of evaluating promotion.

22. Discuss the ethical aspects of advertising by pharmacists.

23. Who are the critical people at the end point of the chain of events in the promotional program?

CONTROLLING

Controlling is the fifth section and the fourth major function of management. In the introduction to the previous section, we made a distinction between directing, on the one hand, and planning and organizing, on the other hand, based primarily on the continuity of effort given to the function and the process itself. A similar comparison places controlling between directing and organizing. The controlling function must be continuous in its influence to be effective; also frequent and regular attention must be given to it for it to be effective. Whereas directing activities will be performed many times each day, controlling activities normally will be performed only several times daily. The process of controlling is continuous, but the effort given to it is intermittent and frequent. Three chapters, financial analysis, control mechanisms, and risk management and insurance are included in this final section. Financial analysis is a necessary component of control as well as providing the data for progress assessment and overall management. Although market or entrepreneurial risk can be factored into the planning function and controlled, to a degree, with planning and control systems, exogenous risk can be managed only by certain preventive measures *and* insurance.

18 | Financial Analysis and Management

Once a pharmacist has established a pharmacy practice, he is faced with the task of managing the various components in a manner that fosters growth and maximizes profit in the long run. All aspects of management are important to a successful practice. Some phases of management focus on the initial establishment of a practice, whereas other phases are either a continuous process, for example personnel administration, or a continuing periodic process, such as financial and profit analysis. A thorough financial and profit analysis is a necessary precursor to the discovery of problem areas and of the nature and source of problems.

Analysis Objectives

Profit and financial analysis is directed toward one or more of several objectives. Obviously, one of these is the *profit* objective. Another objective is the *liquidity* objective. Liquidity, as the term is used in financial management, indicates the ability of a firm to meet its current debts without jeopardizing its existence or profit potential. Another important and related objective is *solvency*. Solvency is defined as the capability of meeting current debts and recallable long-term debts from available current assets and avoiding bankruptcy in the meantime. Another objective is a good *financial* and *credit position*. This objective balances all the owner's net assets, his equity or net worth, against all the debts, both long- and short-term. It is desirable that the owner's equity equals or exceeds the total liabilities if at all possible. *Efficient operation* is the fifth objective.

The objectives are self-explanatory for the most part. The interrelationships that exist among these objectives are less obvious. Profit is necessary under most conditions to achieve the other objectives, and conversely, achievement of the other objectives enhances the prospects of profit. Greater liquidity

383

usually increases the solvency, which, in turn, enhances the financial position in time.

There are several financial ratios that indicate achievement of the various objectives, or the failure to achieve them. Some ratios are more indicative and significant than others; however, a conclusion relative to a problem should be supported by several ratios pointing to the problem area. Some ratios point toward more than one objective and to more than one problem area. In addition, the analyst must look beyond the ratios themselves to the actual data and the economic and social environment of the pharmacy for a final determination.

Definitions and Standards

Some ratios are derived from the profit and loss statement, while others are derived from the balance sheet, but the most significant ratios are derived from a combination of the two financial statements. The various terms and classifications of the two financial statements are defined in this section.

LIQUIDITY AND SOLVENCY RATIOS

Current Ratio. To determine this ratio one divides the current assets by the current liabilities. It is an old and time-honored ratio which is indicative of *solvency.* The minimum desirable ratio is 2:1. The 1984 *Lilly Digest* average was 3:1. This ratio means that, if the current assets exceed the current liabilities by a margin of 2 to 1, sufficient cash, together with credit if necessary, should be available to meet current debts due within a year.

Acid Test Ratio. One can arrive at this ratio, which is often referred to as the *liquidity ratio,* by dividing the current assets less the inventory value (at cost) by the current liabilities. The minimum desirable ratio is 1:1. The 1984 *Lilly Digest* average was 1:1. The ratio is a more rigorous test of the pharmacy's ability to meet its current obligations. When inventory has to be sold under adverse conditions, it frequently is sold at a sacrifice in value. Thus, inventory is not included in this ratio. Although it may be that accounts receivable may not receive dollar for dollar if sold to a financial institution, it is the usual practice to balance accounts receivable against accounts payable. Therefore, cash plus accounts receivable should equal accounts payable at the very least. This assumes accounts receivable will be collected at about the same rate as current debts become due.

Net Working Capital (NWC). This term is the excess of current assets over current liabilities. The amount of working capital varies with the size of the pharmacy and more particularly with the sales volume. As a rule, older pharmacies have a greater amount of net working capital than do newer ones. Also, net working capital usually is somewhat less than net worth, but the two values are close in a well-established pharmacy. The most definitive statement one can make about net working capital is that it should fall within the range of 50 to 60 percent of total assets, with an average of approximately 55 percent for established pharmacies.

Inventory To Net Working Capital. This ratio, which is often abbreviated as Invt./NWC, is simply the ratio of inventory to the net working capital. It usually is expressed as a percentage. The ratio normally falls within the range of 75 to 125 percent, with a desirable target of about 90 to 100 percent. *The 1984 Lilly Digest* average was 102 percent. The ratio is indicative of two aspects of management—liquidity and inventory imbalance. If an inordinate amount of net working capital is invested in inventory, the pharmacist may experience difficulty in meeting current debts. Under normal conditions, the ratio obviously is indicative of efficient use of capital. On the one hand, too little inventory results in out-of-stock situations and loss of sales, whereas too much inventory decreases the rate of return on the investment. A high Invt./NWC ratio correlates positively with a large difference between current and acid test ratios, both of which are indicative of a liquidity problem.

Current Liabilities (CL) to NWC. This ratio, expressed as a percentage, is another measure of solvency. A ratio of 50 percent or less is desirable, with a critical value at 100 percent. New pharmacies usually have a higher percentage than older pharmacies because of high start-up cost and current debts. A pharmacy with a current ratio of 3:1 normally has a CL/NWC ratio of about 50 percent; a current ratio of 2:1 is approximately equivalent to a 100 percent CL/NWC. The 1984 *Lilly Digest* average was approximately 50 percent.

FINANCIAL POSITION RATIOS

Ratio of Current Liabilities to Net Worth. This ratio indicates the pharmacy's capability to meet its current obligations by utilizing all of its net worth or equity capital if necessary. This ratio normally is expressed as a percentage. Obviously a high percent, above 80 percent, is undesirable and indicative of *undercapitalization*. Undercapitalization is another term for a poor financial or credit position, which frequently is accompanied by liquidity and solvency problems. A ratio less than 50 percent is desirable. The 1984 *Lilly Digest* average was 47 percent.

Ratio of Funded Debt To Net Working Capital. This percentage is calculated by dividing the sum of the long-term liabilities (those debts not due within a year) by the net working capital. The ratio is normally expressed as a percentage. This ratio is indicative of two aspects of financial management. A low percentage indicates a good financial position and ability to borrow money if necessary. A high ratio indicates a poor financial position and that the interest charge on the debt will continue to diminish working capital and net profit. This ratio may range from zero to over 100 percent. A value above 50 percent is undesirable. The 1984 *Lilly Digest* average was approximately 29 percent. If a pharmacy's net worth and net working capital are such that the pharmacy is in a sound financial position, a limited amount of funded debt (10 to 20 percent of NWC) with a reasonable interest rate is desirable. It is assumed the pharmacist will be able to use the borrowed capital to generate net profit in excess of the interest charge. This technique is referred to as the use of capital leverage (see Chapter 8).

Ratio of Total Liabilities to Net Worth. Again, this ratio indicates the overall financial and credit position of the pharmacy. It is indicative of whether a pharmacy can meet its financial obligations in due course of its operation. It also indicates the distribution of the capital between owners and creditors. The ratio is usually expressed as a percentage. If total debts exceed net worth, a ratio above 100 percent, the pharmacy is quite vulnerable to sharp changes in its operation, such as a sudden or prolonged drop in sales or a rise in expenses. Fifty percent or less represents a desirable target value. *The 1984 Lilly Digest* average was approximately 75 percent.

Ratio of Fixed Assets To Net Worth. The ratio is indicative of the degree to which scarce capital has been invested in fixed assets, which precludes alternate use of the capital. This ratio is expressed as a percentage. A percentage of 60 or more indicates that too much money is tied up in fixtures and other fixed assets and not available as working capital. Such a condition is often accompanied by a large long-term note with the concomitant high interest charge, which reduces profit and further encumbers management. A figure as high as 50 percent may represent too much investment in fixed assets. *The 1984 Lilly Digest* values ranged from 17 to 43 percent with an average of approximately 24 percent.

New pharmacies have a higher percentage for each of the four ratios discussed, as compared with older pharmacies. This is because debts, both short- and long-term, are usually higher in new pharmacies, whereas both net worth and net working capital are usually lower.

PROFITABILITY RATIOS

Percent of Net Profit to Net Sales. This ratio (NP/NS) is the one most frequently used to indicate the profitability of a pharmacy. Financial analysts generally have preferred to use other ratios to measure profitability, especially net profit to net worth or net profit to total assets. However, in the recent era of inflation, the NP/NS ratio is probably the most useful profitability ratio, since the inflated profit is measured against an equally inflated sales figure. In time, net worth and assets are only moderately inflated. Profit before income tax, rather than after income tax, is used for a better comparison among pharmacies with varying income tax rates. Net profit does not include the proprietor's salary. Corporations frequently report net profit when corporate income tax has been deducted, and this should be taken into consideration when comparing corporations with other types of legal organizations. *The 1984 Lilly Digest* average for independent pharmacies has decreased from 3.7 to 2.9 percent over the past decade. The average percent net profit to sales as reported in *The 1984 Lilly Digest* was 2.9 percent for independent pharmacies and 5 percent for chain pharmacies. A target percentage should be 5 percent or greater.

Percent of Net Profit to Net Worth (NP/NW). This percentage is most indicative of the overall profitability and operational efficiency of any single ratio under normal, noninflationary times. This ratio relates *net* profit to the *net* investment in the pharmacy and thus measures how well funds, as supplied by the owner(s), are being utilized. *The 1984 Lilly Digest* average was approximately 21 percent. A 20 percent or better figure is considered a realistic target. In a new pharmacy with a relatively small net worth, this ratio may distort the profit picture. In corporations with a considerable amount of outstanding preferred stock, debentures, and long-term notes, the use of net worth or stockholders' equity as the denominator may distort the picture also. For these reasons the next ratio should be used to supplement the NP/NW ratio.

Percent of Net Profit to Total Assets. This ratio has come into greater use in recent years for the reasons cited above. The rationale for using this ratio is that it measures the efficient use of *all* the assets under the control of management. The formula for calculating this ratio is known as the duPont formula.

$$\frac{NP}{Net\ Sales} \times \frac{Net\ Sales}{Total\ Assets} = \frac{NP}{Total\ Assets}$$

The first ratio in the formula has been discussed already and the second will be discussed later and shown to represent the velocity of utilizing assets. When the two ratios are combined, both *profitability* and *efficiency* are being measured. A minimum desirable value is 10 percent. *The 1984 Lilly Digest* value averaged approximately 12 percent.

Percent of Net Profit to Total Investment. By total investment (TI) is meant the net worth, which is the net investment, in addition to the funded (long-term) debt, which is the borrowed investment. The difference between total assets and total investment was $33,000 for the 1984 *Lilly Digest* sample of pharmacies. The target return on total investment is 15 percent, compared with 20 percent on net investment (NW) and 10 percent on total assets (TA). The 1984 *Lilly Digest* average NP/TI was 17 percent.

Net Profit Per Dollar of Inventory. This ratio is calculated by dividing net profit by the ending inventory. The ratio is expressed in the following manner: $.20/$1.00. While some might suggest using the average inventory as more comparable to the time span the net profit was earned, the more important consideration is the most current valuation of the inventory. The ratio measures both profitability and the efficient use of inventory. Proper management and control of inventory is one of the most challenging aspects of management. This ratio is indicative of how well this is being accomplished. The range of this ratio for independent pharmacies as reported in *The 1984 Lilly Digest,* when data were arranged by sales volume, was $0.01 to $0.24 per $1.00. The average was $0.20/$1.00. The minimum desirable value is $0.20/$1.00. The average for chain pharmacies as reported in the 1984 *NACDS-Lilly Digest* was $0.36/$1.00.

EFFICIENCY RATIOS

Inventory Turnover Rate (TOR). The TOR is calculated by dividing the cost of goods sold (CGS) by the average inventory (Avg. Invt.) at cost. The average inventory is computed from the beginning and ending inventory for the accounting period. The ratio may be calculated from sales and average inventory at retail value. This widely used ratio is indicative of efficient purchasing and inventory control. A minimum desirable ratio is 3, that is, the average inventory value is purchased and sold three times a year. The theoretic maximum TOR is 24. Under the current policy of issuing monthly statements during the last few days of the month with payment not due until the tenth of the following month, a pharmacist with good inventory control theoretically could operate on the average monthly cost of goods sold. Only one-half of this amount would be the average inventory investment, providing 24 TOR/year. However, a more realistic target falls within a range of 8 to 12. With computerized inventory control, EOQ and frequent cyclic billing, the maximum efficient TOR *may* reach 24 turns per year in the future. *The 1984 Lilly Digest* average for independent pharmacies was 4.6. Chain pharmacies as reported in the 1984 *NACDS-Lilly Digest* registered 5.1 on the average.

Ratio of Net Sales To Inventory. This ratio is only a modification of the inventory turnover rate, in which sales are substituted for cost of goods sold. The ratio obviously will be greater by the amount of gross margin. Again, this ratio is indicative of inventory management with a minimum desirable figure of 5. The target value is in the range of 12 to 18. *The 1984 Lilly Digest* average was approximately 6.7.

Net Working Capital Turnover. One can calculate this turnover rate by dividing sales by the net working capital (NS/NWC). It is indicative of the efficient use of working capital. Like other turnover ratios, there is a desirable range, not just a single critical value, which is 4 to 8 turnovers per year. The *Lilly Digest* average was 6.7. If the value is low, below 4, it is indicative of either low sales and inefficient use of working capital or too much working capital for the sales generated. This may be the result of too much inventory and/or accounts receivable in relation to the sales volume. This condition is known as *undertrading.* If the value is high, over 8, the opposite condition is the case—too little working capital for the amount of sales, which frequently is caused by excessive trade credit. This is known as *overtrading* due to *undercapitalization.* New pharmacies can expect to have a rather high net working capital turnover during the first few years. The 1984 *Lilly Digest* value ranged from 7.2 for young pharmacies to 6.5 for older pharmacies in the $400,000 to $600,000 sales range.

Capital Turnover Rate. This ratio is calculated by dividing net sales by net worth (CNS/NW). This ratio is similar to the one discussed above except that desirable range is 3 to 8. *The 1984 Lilly Digest* average was 6.3. This ratio normally is somewhat less than working capital turnover because net worth usually is greater than net working capital. Again, new pharmacies normally have a higher turnover rate during the first few years. A high value, above 8, definitely is an indication of *undercapitalization,* a case in which the firm is being financed by excessive credit, both short- and long-term. It is also indicative of *overtrading.* A low value indicates just the opposite, a sluggish, inefficient operation.

Average Accounts Receivable Collection Period. This value is a useful figure in identifying good or poor credit management. The figure indicates how long, on the average, it takes for the outstanding accounts receivable to be collected during the course of the usual accounting period. The average collection period is computed in the following manner: (1) credit sales for the year are divided by the outstanding accounts receivable at the end of the year to arrive at the average accounts receivable turnover rate, and (2) the 365 days of the year are then divided by the accounts receivable turnover rate to ascertain the average collection period in days. An example will illustrate the procedures: Annual charge sales were $120,000 and the outstanding accounts receivable were $10,000. (1) $120,000 ÷ $10,000 = 12 turnover rate. (2) 365 days ÷ 12 = 30.4 or 30 days to the nearest whole day. Since credit is usually granted on a monthly basis, a 30-day average collection period is considered a reasonable period. A period up to 40 days is acceptable, whereas an average collection period of more than 40 days indicates attention should be given to credit management.

Average Time To Pay Accounts Payable. This value measures how well the pharmacist is meeting his current obligations. It is indicative of solvency, and it also may indicate whether the pharmacist is receiving his cash discounts. The value is calculated as follows: (1) All purchases of merchandise are divided by the outstanding accounts payable at the end of the accounting period. This determines the accounts payable turnover rate. (2) Then 365 days are divided by the accounts payable turnover rate and this gives the average collection period for accounts payable expressed in days. Again, a value of 30 days is very good and indicates that cash discounts normally are being received. A longer time period, for example more than 40 days, is not good, and a 60 day period indicates that the pharmacy is operating on "borrowed" trade capital and may not be solvent.

Methods of Analysis

There are several methods of financial analysis. After analysis, interpretation of the significance of the financial ratios and related values follow. The first step is to compute the financial ratios and arrange them in a *matrix* or *paradigm* in which those ratios that point toward management objectives or problem areas can be identified. Next, an internal analysis of data should be made to confirm the identity of specific problem areas, such as inventory or accounts receivable, and to determine if the profit, efficiency, liquidity, and solvency objectives are being met. The analysis of internal data should include a *trend analysis* for the past three years if the pharmacy is that old. Unfavorable trends of a ratio or a set of related ratios are a good indication that steps should be taken to reverse the trends. As stated previously, the raw data in the profit and loss statement and the balance sheet should be examined carefully to identify weak spots and unfavorable trends in that data.

Another method of analysis is to *compare the ratios with external standards*. Some of the best known standards are described and reported in the *Lilly Digest*. It should be noted that averages do not represent the best a pharmacy can or should do, but they represent a base against which to compare a pharmacy's performance as about "average." The analyst should look beyond the pharmacy to the economic condition of the community and the nation for possible causes. Are the economic indicators on the upswing or downswing? What about trends in population, per capita income, business, industrial and agricultural growth? The trend in number of prescribers in the community is another significant indicator. A pharmacist must judge his sales, profits, and pertinent ratios in light of the economic trends.

RATIOS AND PARADIGM

Table 18–1 illustrates a useful arrangement of ratios to identify specific problem areas and to determine whether management objectives are being achieved. The matrix in Table 18–1 shows the relationship between the various ratios and management objectives. It also indicates those ratios that are interrelated and point toward one or more problem areas. An "X" with "(?)" indicates a probable, but not definitive, relationship.

A study of the relationships in Table 18–1 shows that most ratios point toward more than one management objective or problem area, and that any problem area will be reflected by two or more ratios. As one would expect, any ratio containing net profit as a factor indicates profitability and often efficiency. Those ratios categorized as turnover rates indicate management efficiency and frequently liquidity, solvency, and/or overall financial position. Ratios with inventory as a component reflect the state of inventory management. The average collection periods are indicative of credit problems, but they may also support the identification of other problems. The fixed assets to net worth ratio indicates overinvestment in fixed assets.

COMPARISON WITH STANDARDS

The following example of a three-year-old traditional community pharmacy is used to illustrate the application of external standards. It is one of four

Table 18–1. Paradigm for Ratio Analysis

RATIO	Profitability	Efficiency	Liquidity	Solvency	Financial Position
		Management Objectives			
NP/NS	X				
NP/NW	X	X			
NP/TA	X	X			
NP/TI	X	X			
NP/Invt.	X	X			
Invt TOR		X			
NS/Invt.		X			
NS/NWC		X	X(?)	X(?)	
NS/NW		X		X(?)	X(?)
Invt/NWC		X	X		
Acid Test			X		
Current				X	
CL/NW			X(?)	X	X
CL/NWC				X	
TL/NW				X	X
L-TL/NWC					X
FA/NW		X			X
Avg. A/R CP		X			X(?)
Avg. A/P CP	X(?)	X	X(?)	X	X(?)

pharmacies in a small town of 7,000 people with a total trading area of 15,000. There are four physicians practicing general medicine, who are average prescribers. The proprietor is a pharmacist 27 years of age who practiced in another pharmacy in this town for three years before starting his own practice. The pharmacy occupies 2,400 square feet of selling area with 400 square feet and $28,000 worth of inventory in the prescription department. The pharmacy dispensed 12,600 prescriptions last year at an average charge of $11.50. Last year's credit sales amounted to $126,000. The first year the pharmacy nearly broke even, and last year the pharmacy realized a net profit of $2,000.

Figures 18–1 and 18–2 are the Income and Expense Statement and the Balance Sheet, respectively, for the third year of operation. Table 18–2 is a comparison of the ratios calculated from this pharmacy with comparable *Lilly Digest* averages and with standards.

Utilizing the ratios and data generated and tabulated in Table 18–2, the analyst should proceed with further analysis and interpretation. Comparison of the computed ratios with standards, averages, and critical values will identify certain financial and managerial problems.

Profitability. The net profit commands the focus of our attention. In financial jargon, "It's what's on the bottom line that counts." It is obvious that the present pharmacy was not very profitable. This is indicated by the dollar amount of net profit, percent net profit to sales, percent net profit to total

BROWNSVILLE PHARMACY
BROWNSVILLE, KENTUCKY
DECEMBER 31, 19XX

			%
Net Sales		$290,000	100.0
Cost of Goods & Services:			
Beginning Inventory	$ 60,000		
Purchases	204,000		
Total		$264,000	
Ending Inventory		70,000	
Cost of Goods Sold		194,000	66.9
Gross Margin		$ 96,000	33.1
Prop. Salary	$ 24,000		8.3
Employee Wages	40,000		13.8
Rent	12,000		4.1
Heat, Light & Power	3,000		1.0
Interest	4,800		1.7
All Other Expenses	4,000		1.4
Total Expenses		87,800	30.3
Net Profit		$ 8,200	2.8
Add Prop. Salary		24,000	8.3
Total Prop. Income*		$ 32,200	11.1
Income Tax*		6,200	2.1
Net Discretionary Income*		$ 26,000	9.0

* These figures are not used in computing any of the ratios

Figure 18–1.   Income and expense statement.

(gross) investment in assets, and net profit per dollar invested in inventory. This conclusion is not supported by percent net profit to net worth because net worth is reduced drastically by the large amount of liabilities, both current and long-term. Of course, one must look further to determine the cause, or contributing factors, of the low profits. One may begin with current items and work backward, as it were, but perhaps a better picture can be gained by beginning with the older or long-term items.

Initial Capitalization and Investments. The ratio of fixed assets to net worth at 89.5 percent is much higher than is desirable, even for a pharmacy only three years old. This indicates the strong possibility of overinvestment

BROWNSVILLE PHARMACY
BROWNSVILLE, KENTUCKY
DECEMBER 31, 19XX

Assets

Current Assets:

Cash	$ 6,000	
Accounts Receivable	19,000	
Inventory	70,000	
Total Current Assets		$ 95,000

Fixed Assets:

Fixtures & Equipment	$33,600	
(Net after reserve for depreciation)		
Total Fixed Assets		33,600

Other Assets:

Prepaid Expenses	$ 3,000	
Total Other Assets		3,000

Total Assets	$131,600

Liabilities

Current and Accrued Liabilities:

Accounts Payable	$24,000	
Notes Payable (within one year)	8,000	
Accrued Expenses	14,000	
Total Current and Accrued Liabilities		$ 46,000

Long-Term Liabilities:

Notes Payable	$48,000	
Total Long-Term Liabilities		48,000

Total Liabilities	$ 94,000
Net Worth	37,600
Total Liabilities and Net Worth	$131,600

Figure 18–2. Balance sheet.

in fixed assets, a common error. It further indicates a small net worth, which is the case in this instance. It also suggests a high amount of liabilities, especially long-term liabilities. By correlating the ratio of funded debt to net worth with the ratio of fixed assets to net worth and considering the dollar values involved, the conclusion becomes apparent—overinvestment in fixed assets financed by a large funded debt. This leads to a chain reaction.

Payments on the funded debt reduce the available cash for current operations and thereby causes an accumulation of accounts payable and accrued expenses.

Table 18–2. Comparison of Financial Ratios with Comparable Lilly Digest Averages and Standards

	Computed Values	The 1984 Lilly Digest Average*	Standard	Position of This Case
Current ratio	2.1:1	2.9:1	2:1	Just above the minimum
Acid test ratio	0.54:1	0.8:1	1:1	Below the minimum
Current debt to NW	122%	62%	50%	Above critical value of 80%
Inventory to NWC	143%	111%	90–100%	Above critical value of 125%
Inventory turnover rate	2.98	4.2	3–12	Below the minimum of 3
Total debt to NW	250%	132%	100%	Above critical value of 100%
Funded debt to NWC	98%	59%	50%	Above critical value of 50%
Fixed assets to NW	89.5%	42%	20–50%	Above critical value of 75%
Net working capital turnover	5.9	6.9	4–8	Within standard range
Capital (NW) turnover	7.7	8.2	3–8	Within standard range
Net profit/$1.00 inventory	$0.12	$0.22	$0.20	Below minimum standard
Net profit to NW	21.8	30%	20%	Above the minimum standard
Net profit to total assets	6.2	13%	10%	Below critical value of 10%
Average A/P remittance period	43 days	21 days	30 days	Above critical value of 40 days
Average A/R remittance period	55 days	NA†	30 days	Above critical value of 40 days

*Most comparable group.
†Not available.

In addition, interest charges on these debts further reduce cash, and worse, profits are decreased. This point is supported by the ratios of current liabilities to net worth, total debt to net worth, funded debt to net working capital, and to a lesser degree by the current ratio.

Inventory Management. The problem is compounded by an overinvestment in inventory, a $10,000 increase over the previous year. However, sales were doubled. This fact is indicated by the ratio of inventory to net working capital, inventory turnover rate, and a comparison of the current ratio of 2.1:1 with the acid test ratio of only 0.54:1. The acid test ratio does not utilize inventory in the numerator, thus pinpointing the high proportion of capital invested in inventory. Again, the net profit per dollar of inventory is further indication of the problem.

Solvency and Liquidity. The combined economic factors discussed above can be expected to produce an adverse effect on the solvency and liquidity position of the pharmacy. This fact is indicated by the following ratios: current ratio, which is just above the acceptable minimum value; acid test ratio, which is about one-half the minimum value; current debt to net worth; inventory to net working capital; and the average remittance period for accounts payable of 43 days. This latter ratio is indicative of the pharmacist's inability to meet accounts payable on time and earn the cash discount. There is strong indication that the pharmacy is losing up to $4,000 a year in cash discounts, which is nearly one-half the amount of annual net profit.

Four ratios—current ratio, net working capital turnover, capital (NW) turnover, and percent net profit to net worth—seem to indicate a healthy financial condition for the pharmacy. It was noted that the current ratio was just above the minimum. The other three ratios appear normal only because of the fact that low sales and profits are counterbalanced by low net worth and net working capital.

Conclusion. This case illustrates the chain reaction that takes place when a pharmacy is undercapitalized and begins operation at a disadvantage. When this is complicated by poor management, the pharmacy stands to suffer economic loss, even possible bankruptcy. Such is the case with this pharmacy. Large fixed investment financed by a large amount of long-term indebtedness, reduced cash reserves for current operation, and overinvestment in inventory (apparently attempting to "buy" himself out of the hole) result in a precarious financial position and reduced profits from interest charges, loss of cash discounts, and salaries and wages which are too high.

The remedy lies in: (1) obtaining some ready cash, if the pharmacist can obtain a bank loan, (2) reducing the inventory as rapidly as possible without jeopardizing sales, and (3) reducing expenses, especially salaries and wages. The extra cash can be used to reduce accounts payable and accrued expenses which will permit the pharmacy to realize cash discounts and increased profits.

TREND ANALYSIS

It is possible, indeed it frequently happens, that a firm may be making a profit and be in a precarious financial position with its creditors. Conversely, a firm may operate at a loss for a relatively short period of time and still maintain a sound financial position with its creditors; however, it should be obvious that a deficit operation cannot continue indefinitely. Trend analysis will identify those problems that develop gradually over time.

Of the several methods of financial analysis, year-to-year trend analysis is perhaps the best single technique. This technique, however, is strengthened significantly by the use of comparative data from *The Lilly Digest*.

ILLUSTRATION OF TREND ANALYSIS: A CASE STUDY

Data for three consecutive years were selected from a traditional community pharmacy and are shown in Figures 18–3 and 18–4 to illustrate year-to-year analysis. The values were rounded for ease of computation. The pharmacy, in its sixth year of operation, is located in a community of 5,000 inhabitants. There is one other pharmacy in the community, and there are approximately 10,000 people in the trading area. The size of the pharmacy is 70 feet by 40 feet with the prescription department occupying 400 square feet.

Sales, both prescriptions and other, show a favorable trend about 7 percent per year increase. The percentages of prescription sales and gross margin also show a favorable trend. Gross margin nearly always increases with increased prescription sales. Net profit has *not* increased proportionally, however. Expenses have increased proportionally more than gross margin, providing a slight dollar increase in net profit but a percentage decrease. Employee wages, delivery, advertising, bad debts, and miscellaneous expenses are significant because these expenses are variable or semivariable costs, and can be controlled and brought into a better relationship with sales. Although advertising and delivery are variable or semivariable expenses, these expenditures are needed to sustain sales growth.

This pharmacy is still in the critical *growth profit interval* (G-P-I) of operations—time in which expenses should become stabilized while sales are still increasing. The period before a profit is realized is the *growth loss interval* (G-L-I). The problem in this case is to hold employee wages to about 10 percent, reducing bad debts to about 0.1 percent and miscellaneous expenses to approximately 1.5 percent, while increasing sales another 5 to 10 percent. Of course, all of the other expenses must be kept at about the present level.

The income statement will not provide all the information necessary to reveal the ''soft spot'' in a practice. Comparative data from the balance sheet and other data provide additional signs of mismanagement. Let us examine the comparative balance sheet data for this pharmacy.

While net working capital increased steadily ($54,250, $66,920, and $70,740), there were some undesirable trends among the current items. Cash steadily decreased, while accounts receivable, inventory, accounts payable, and accrued expenses increased. Although net working capital increased, it became increasingly less accessible and manageable. Let us examine the interrelations among these items and certain items of the income statements.

	3rd Year	%	4th Year	%	5th Year	%
Sales:						
Prescription	$152,000	39.0	$168,000	40.0	$184,500	41.0
Other	238,000	61.0	252,000	60.0	265,500	59.0
TOTAL	$390,000	100.0	$420,000	100.0	$450,000	100.0
CGS	253,500	65.0	269,000	64.0	283,500	63.0
GM	$136,600	35.0	$151,000	36.0	$166,500	37.0
Expenses:						
Proprietor's Salary	30,000	7.7	36,000	8.6	40,000	8.9
Employee Wages	48,000	12.3	52,200	12.4	59,000	13.1
Rent	7,800	2.0	7,800	1.9	7,800	1.7
Heat, Light & Power	3,900	1.0	4,200	1.0	4,500	1.0
Legal & Acct. Fees	1,170	0.3	1,260	0.3	1,350	0.3
Taxes (except income)	5,850	1.5	5,880	1.4	5,850	1.3
Insurance (except bldg)	2,340	0.6	2,520	0.6	2,700	0.6
Interest Paid	2,220	0.6	1,680	0.4	1,400	0.3
Repairs	1,170	0.3	1,700	0.4	2,250	0.5
Delivery	1,560	0.4	2,100	0.5	2,250	0.6
Advertising	5,070	1.3	5,900	1.4	6,750	1.5
Depreciation	5,400	1.4	5,400	1.3	5,400	1.2
Bad Debts charged off	390	0.1	840	0.2	1,350	0.3
Telephone	1,170	0.3	1,250	0.3	1,340	0.3
Miscellaneous	5,190	1.3	6,930	1.7	8,760	1.9
TOTAL	$121,230	31.1	$135,660	32.3	$151,200	33.6
NET PROFIT	$ 15,270	3.9	$ 15,340	3.7	$15,300	3.4
TOTAL INCOME	45,270	11.6	51,340	12.2	55,300	12.3
Income Taxes	13,570	3.5	15,120	3.6	16,650	3.7
Net Profit, after taxes	$ 10,670	2.7	$ 10,820	2.6	$ 10,690	2.4
TOTAL INCOME, after taxes	31,700	8.1	36,220	8.6	38,650	8.6

Figure 18–3. Comparative income statement data.

ASSETS	3rd Year	4th Year	5th Year
Current Assets:			
Cash	$ 15,860	$ 13,660	$ 10,980
Accounts Receivable	12,690	17,090	18,970
Inventory	57,100	74,345	79,830
SUBTOTAL	$ 85,650	$105,095	$109,780
Fixed Assets:			
Fixtures & Equipment	23,000	20,000	17,000
(net after depreciation)			
TOTAL ASSETS	$117,650	$125,095	$126,780
LIABILITIES			
Current Liabilities:			
Accounts Payable	$ 17,150	$ 22,100	$ 22,935
Accrued Expenses	4,250	6,075	6,105
Notes Payable (within year)	10,000	10,000	10,000
SUBTOTAL	$ 31,400	$ 38,175	$ 39,040
Long-Term Liabilities:			
Notes Payable	20,000	10,000	– – – –
TOTAL LIABILITIES	$ 51,400	$ 48,175	$ 39,040
NET WORTH	66,250	76,920	87,740
TOTAL LIABILITIES & NET WORTH	$117,650	$125,095	$126,780
RELATED DATA			
Credit Sales	$162,000	$191,100	$197,100

Figure 18–4.   Comparative balance sheet data.

Increased credit sales without proper management produced an increase in accounts receivable and bad debts. Inventory build-up caused a reduction in the turnover rate and an increase in accounts payable. Increased expenses produced a backlog of accrued expenses. All these factors reduced the cash available for paying bills, earning cash discounts and reducing the notes payable.

As previously stated, trends are useful to determine the direction a practice is taking and reveal a deteriorating situation. An analysis of the data for one year will not. Financial ratios are especially useful for trend analysis and this is illustrated in the present case.

The acid test ratio for the third, fourth, and fifth years was 0.91, 0.81 and 0.79, respectively. An acid test ratio below 1:1 is considered to be below the minimum safe level. Similarly, the following ratios evidenced an unfavorable trend:

Inventory to Net Working Capital:	105%	111%	113%
Net Profit to Net Worth:	23.0%	19.9%	17.4%
Net Profit to Total Assets:	13.0%	12.3%	12.1%
Net Profit Per Dollar of Inventory:	0.27	$0.21	$0.19
The Average Time to Remit Accounts Payable	25 days	28 days	29 days
Inventory Turnover Rate	4.5	4.1	3.7

Three other ratios were outside the acceptable range for one or more of the years, and they also manifested an unfavorable trend: inventory to net working capital, net profit to net worth, and accounts receivable remittance period. In addition, four other measures demonstrated unfavorable trends. The average collection period for accounts receivable should be maintained at about 30 days. This ratio increased from 29 days to 33 days to 35 days during the three-year period. Finally, net profit to net sales ratio was not very satisfactory and decreased each year.

When the income and expense data from this pharmacy are compared with data from *The Lilly Digest,* this pharmacy on balance compares favorably with the exception of employee wages and bad debts. After analyzing this case, it may be concluded that the proprietor, encouraged by the apparent success of the pharmacy during the first three years, employed more help than was necessary and failed to watch closely his credit extension. These are two items that can readily get out of control. Under present economic conditions, a traditional community pharmacy should keep the payroll, including the proprietor's salary, at 20 percent of sales or less; the payroll for this pharmacy was 22 percent of sales the previous year.

Summary of Case Study. This pharmacy illustrates improper management of credit, inventory, employee wages, and bad debts. A selective, controlled reduction of inventory could easily support the sales volume. This would free sufficient cash to liquidate notes payable and accrued expenses and reduce accounts payable. Better management of credit and expenses generally will not produce as spectacular results, but it will increase profits and place the pharmacy in a much better financial position. If the pharmacist could maintain the expenses at 30 percent of sales, the resulting net profit would be nearly doubled. This amount of net profit would produce a net return on sales of 7 percent and a net return on the net investment (net worth) of 36 percent. This would represent a profitable operation and a stable financial position.

BREAK-EVEN FINANCIAL ANALYSIS

Break-even analysis focuses on cost factors as reported in the profit and loss statement. The objective is to determine the point at which the pharmacy breaks even. The break-even point may be determined in terms of sales volume or time in months. Sales volume is most often used. Break-even analysis assists the pharmacist in making decisions that affect costs and/or sales in his pharmacy.

Break-even analysis is based on the anticipation of a probable future performance and assumes certain mathematical relations and a cost classification based on past experience. The analysis determines the outcome of a decision that changes one or more variables. With this analysis, certain questions can be answered and decisions made more intelligently. Some examples of such questions follow. What will be the profit or loss with a change in sales volume? What additional sales volume will be required to cover certain additional fixed costs of modernizing? How will the addition of another staff pharmacist affect the profit, or what are the necessary sales to cover the additional expense? What will be the effect on profit of reducing the percent gross margin? What will be the effect on profit of a change in a fixed rent to percent-of-sales rent?

Procedure for Break-Even Analysis. The following steps provide the procedure and framework for break-even analysis.

STEP 1—Classify all operating expense items into two groups: (a) *fixed* and (b) *variable*. Some expenses are semivariable, that is, they contain fixed elements, but vary with sales to some extent. For example, as the number of prescriptions dispensed and delivered increases, the expenditures for gasoline, oil, and repairs increase, but the depreciation, taxes, and insurance costs remain the same.

STEP 2—Determine the amount of *variable expense* as a *percent of sales*. For the purpose of this analysis, the following expense items are classified as *variable expenses,* even though they may be fixed to an extent for a given pharmacy: advertising, bad debts, employees' wages, and miscellaneous expenses. Employee wages and miscellaneous expenses are semivariable, but they are classified as variable expenses for the purpose of delineating all expenses into two categories.

STEP 3—Determine the amount of *fixed expenses* in *dollars*. Fixed expenses include proprietor's salary, rent, heat, light and power, accounting and legal fees, taxes, interest paid, repairs, insurance, delivery, depreciation, and telephone. Delivery expenses, and perhaps others, are actually semifixed, but they are classified as fixed expenses for convenience.

STEP 4—Determine the *marginal income ratio*. This is done by subtracting the percent of variable expenses from the percent of gross margin. This is the percentage of sales left to cover the fixed expenses and net profit, if any.

STEP 5—Compute the sales volume at the *break-even point*. This is done by dividing the amount of fixed expenses by the marginal income ratio. At this point no profit or loss is realized.

Table 18–3. Data for Break-Even Analysis

	Dollars	% of Sales
Sales	$ 180,000	
Gross margin	64,800	36.0
Fixed expenses	28,800	– – – –
Variable expenses	25,200	14.0
(Total expenses)	(54,000)	(30.0)
Marginal income ratio	– – – –	22.0
(Net profit)	(10,800)	(6.0)

This procedure is illustrated by the following example:

Fixed expenses	$27,000
Variable expenses	14.4% of sales
Gross margin	36.2% of sales
Marginal income ratio	21.8% of sales (36.2% − 14.4%)
Break-even point	$\dfrac{\$27,000}{.218} = \$123,853$

This technique may be applied to any fixed investment or expense. Modifications are necessary when the technique is applied to a variable expense. Break-even analysis is based on historical percentages and data, which may change during the experimental year. These changes are usually minor for a well-established pharmacy because of the inherent stability of the pharmaceutical profession.

It should be noted that cost of goods sold is a *variable* cost, but it figures only indirectly into the computation of the break-even point. This is true because it is the *gross margin* that is available to meet the fixed and variable expenses and to provide a net profit, if any.

Application of Break-Even Analysis. Miller's Pharmacy is located in a town of 10,000 people and a total trading area with a 20,000 population. There are four other progressive, modern pharmacies in this town. This pharmacy is old and has not been remodeled in several years. The sales volume is $180,000. The pharmacist would like to know approximately how much additional sales will be required to pay for remodeling, which will cost $4,000. Table 18–3 gives the pertinent data derived from his last profit and loss statement.

Figure 18–5 shows the break-even point when these parameters are plotted.

Since the marginal income ratio is 0.22 expressed as a decimal, the additional sales needed to pay for the remodeling are $18,182 ($4,000 ÷ 0.22). This amount of sales will pay for the additional cost incurred for remodeling and permit the same net profit as for the year before, assuming all other factors remain constant.

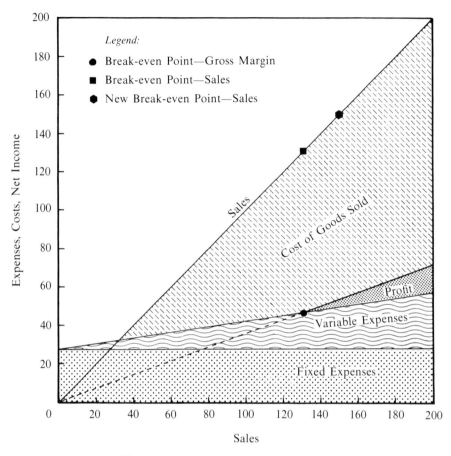

Figure 18–5.   Graphic break-even analysis.

Summary

Financial management requires thorough analyses, and financial analyses should be guided by analysis objectives. Some 19 financial ratios or values should be computed and compared to standard and/or average values to further the analysis process. By relating these various financial ratios to one or more of the analysis objectives, specific financial and managerial problem areas may be identified.

After these initial calculations, analysis may proceed with one or more methods. The first method logically is to arrange the various ratios in a paradigm. In this manner, those ratios which manifest a specific objective or problem area can be readily identified. When two or more ratios point to the same problem or weakness, they usually confirm the problem. This is an internal analysis. Next, the analyst will compare the ratios to external standards and averages for further confirmation. When data for two or more years are available, a trend analysis will not only confirm a problem area, but it will also point to impending problems.

Break-even analysis is used to predict the outcome of certain decisions. More specifically, break-even analysis will indicate the amount of new sales necessary to pay for a fixed investment.

Careful interpretation of the various methods of financial analysis often indicates the necessary steps to solve the problem.

REVIEW

1. What are the five objectives of financial analysis and which ratios relate to or are indicative of each?

2. Define net working capital and four ratios that are indicative of liquidity and solvency. Give the acceptable limits or standards and the desired target value, if applicable, of the four ratios.

3. Define the four ratios that are indicative of the financial position of a firm. Give the acceptable limits and the desired target values, if applicable, for the four ratios.

4. What is undercapitalization?

5. What is meant by capital leverage?

6. Define the five profitability ratios. What are the minimum desired values of each? Which two of the four ratios measure both profitability and efficiency?

7. Define the six efficiency ratios. Give the usual acceptable range or value for each.

8. What are the maximum potential and the realistic target values for inventory turnover?

9. Explain why a very high turnover rate is undesirable as well as a low value.

10. Explain the significance of net working capital turnover and how it differs from capital (NW) turnover.

11. Explain undertrading and overtrading and relate these to undercapitalization and overcapitalization.

12. Explain the significance of the average accounts receivable collection period and the average time to pay accounts payable.

13. Given the appropriate data, calculate all of the ratios discussed.

14. Describe each of the methods of financial analysis: Internal using Paradigm; Comparison with External Standards; Trend Analysis; and Break-even Analysis. Using real data from a pharmacy, hypothetical data, or average data from *The Lilly Digest*, apply each of the above analyses.

19 | Control Mechanisms

Control mechanisms include many techniques that fall into one of two general categories, budgetary and nonbudgetary controls. The former deals primarily with financial controls, the latter with a variety of functions and activities that lend themselves to extra-budgetary controls. This does not suggest that these latter activities are devoid of financial implication. On the contrary, they definitely do have financial implication, but the functions cannot be controlled by budgets alone.

Any control mechanism is composed of two primary elements: (1) procedures or guidelines for controlling activities, and (2) a feedback mechanism to communicate the results in order to assess the effectiveness of the control mechanism. These two elements have been previously depicted in Chapters 9 and 10. Control mechanisms are necessary at several levels of the firm, as is control of the firm itself in relation to society. Management by objectives (MBO) provides the broad framework for overall control without the oppressive influence of most of the older approaches to management and control.

Through MBO, realistic goals and objectives are established that are consistent with the goals of society and the economic environment in which the pharmacy operates. Measurable criteria are established to determine which objectives are being achieved and to what degree. This provides the broad and basic framework for all the control mechanisms. The organizational structure, legal form, and policies are then formulated within the basic framework provided by MBO. Objectives, policies, and the various coordinating and control mechanisms form an integrated management system.

Budgets are related to, and form a necessary part of, the *financial control* of any organization. However, overall control encompasses a wider scope, reaching beyond the activities reflected by financial data alone. *Overall control* includes every aspect of an organization—objectives, policies, personnel, professional activities, inventory, credit, fixed assets, and security. Some of the mechanisms necessary to control the various aspects of management have been discussed in previous chapters, including objectives, policies, personnel, and inventory. The computer can provide the means for superior control of all facets of a pharmacy practice.

404

Role of the Computer

Modern-day business could not operate at the present high level of productivity without the computer. The major contributions of the computer are (1) its rapid computation and retrieval of data, (2) its extreme accuracy, and (3) its capacity for storage of a vast quantity of data. This third function is often provided, in part, by ancillary equipment. The computer cannot, however, perform any function that has not been programmed and/or designed into the computer by persons. Of all the functions in pharmacy management, the control function benefits the most by computerization.

In addition to regular accounting and business functions, the computer is useful in the professional function, especially for screening patients' medication records for drug interactions, contraindications of drugs, and drug utilization. Moreover, the repetitious and detailed record processing of third-party-pay prescriptions is greatly expedited by the computer. There is ample justification for a computer in most community pharmacies. Although 100 prescriptions per day have been used as a rule of thumb for the economic justification of the computer, as few as 60 to 75 prescriptions per day *might* be sufficient to justify a carefully customized comptuer service. Of course, the percentage of third-party prescriptions is a major factor to consider.

There are, in general, three types of computers—the small microcomputer, in-house minicomputer, and the large, high-volume mainframe computers. The small microcomputers are designed to do the work that a small firm, such as a pharmacy, can use. These computers have become available in recent years as a result of electronic technology. The large computers are designed to do the work a large firm or a university would need. A combination system is available—a small, self-contained computer to assist the pharmacist in many functions, especially professional ones, and a terminal connected to a large computer by telephone lines for large-volume processing, such as accounts receivable.

COMPUTER COMPONENTS AND TERMINOLOGY

A computer system may be divided into two major components: the actual physical equipment, called the *hardware,* and the programs or instructions to the computer equipment, called the *software.* The computer hardware is a rapid counting or adding machine. The hardware is designed to perform some basic procedures, whereas the software tells the hardware what to do. Some of the software forms a part of the basic computer system, and other software can be developed for many different data manipulations.

Hardware Components. The hardware component, in turn, is composed of four basic units or components. The first, and certainly the heart or core of the computer, is the *central processing unit,* abbreviated as CPU. The CPU is made up of an *operations* component, a *temporary storage* unit (or *main memory* unit) for the storage of data to be used at one point or another in the processing of the data, and *operating systems* software, which controls the processing of the data. (In a system as complex as the computer, one can expect some ambiguity, such as a CPU that contains a software component.) The temporary data storage unit is analogous to the memory bank in a calculator.

The other hardware units collectively are called the peripheral devices, which are further classified as input devices, output devices, and storage devices.

Input devices are either a card reader, a punched paper tape reader, an optical scan device, a magnetic tape reader, a disc reader, or a direct digital (cathode ray tube, or CRT) input terminal device. Before the card reader can read the data into the CPU, the data must first be "punched" on the computer (IBM) card with a card-punching device, which looks like, and is used much as, a typewriter. In a similar manner, the data must be "punched" on a paper tape before being read or transmitted into the CPU. The optical scan device optically reads the data, which may be regular alpha or numeric characters, or codes. (More on magnetic tape later). The digital input device permits the input of data in a readily usable form.

Output devices provide the user with the information the computer has processed. The information may be either in printed form or displayed on the CRT device. Pharmacies using a CRT device will probably need a printer to produce "hard" copy of the data. If the pharmacy has a high volume of printing, such as accounts receivable statements, a high-speed line printer may be required. Otherwise, a low-speed character printer may be sufficient.

Storage devices are means of storing data in a ready, or nearly ready, to use form. These devices are also data media for input purposes. Thus punched cards and tapes are both data media and storage devices, but not in a readily usable form. Other storage devices or media include magnetic tapes and magnetic discs. These are said to be "on-line" because the data are in a form that is readily "called up" and used by the computer. The disc is similar in construction to a phonograph record, and the data are available by random access. There are two types of discs, floppy and hard discs. The latter are more expensive, but they store more data. Data on the magnetic tape are not as readily accessible, because the data are in sequential order and must first be located on the reel.

Data Component. The key to data accessibility depends as much on the form of the actual data as on the form of the devices or media. The CPU manipulates data in the form of electronic impulses as 0 (absence of impulse) and 1 (impulse). The computer uses the binary system of arithmetic. Using its internal systems software, the computer translates the decimal data (i.e., base 10 numerals) into the binary system and then processes the data. Early computers translated only decimal numerals; later ones translated alpha and numeric forms. Computers can now translate bar codes and process data that are coded within a set of bars. If one looks at nearly any consumer goods, he will find the bar code. This code is read by a photoelectric light, using the same principles as optical scan reading. The bar code with the photoelectric wand or "pencil" is the most efficient method for handling a large amount of complex data. There may be one hazard in using some wands and translation system, viz., in sweeping across two sets of bars too quickly, the data are confounded.

Another facet of data processing is the "batch" or "on-line" approach. The batch approach uses data on a medium such as punched cards or punched tape (paper or magnetic), and the entire data set is read into the computer in one huge "gulp," is assimilated, and is then processed. With the on-line approach, the computer assimilates the data and updates files as the data are entered and read. This latter approach requires a CRT type of input/output device. The real advantage of this approach, and device, is the ability to retrieve data from the computer on-line, i.e., immediately. This speed is a must for computer-assisted professional functions, such as screening for drug interactions.

Software Component. The software is the "brains" of the computer system. There are two types of software, systems software and applications software. We have already alluded to the internal systems software that controls the internal operations of the system. All other data manipulations—ranging from printed statements, to reports in every imaginable format, to every known mathematic or statistical function or process—are controlled by applications software. Much of this software has been developed and is available in a "packaged" form. Sometimes, packaged software needs to be modified for a particular purpose, and occasionally the software has to be developed for some particular purpose. Computer programmers are trained to develop (write) or to modify applications software. Generally, the hardware manufacturer develops all the systems software needed (this was not so in earlier days), whereas applications software often is developed by a computer service organization. These organizations can customize the software for a client. However, the greater the modification and/or the development of software, the more the software component costs.

The most important facet of the software, for a particular pharmacy, is probably the *references files*. Again, there are two types of files, permanent, actually semipermanent, and tailored files. The former includes the drug file (with name, dose, contraindications, interactions), the sig file, MAC file, drug (wholesale) price file, and basic accounting files. The tailored files include prescribers, patients and their medication profiles, accounts receivable, pricing formula, and many others. In addition, the pharmacy's name, address, and other specific information must be programmed into the system's software.

Additional terminology is included in a glossary of terms at the end of this chapter.

FUNCTIONS OF A COMPUTER

Several computer functions have been alluded to already. Here, we want to classify and to describe these functions briefly within the context of management control. For our purposes, the functions are classified into managerial and professional categories.

Managerial Control Functions. The accounting system forms the ''back-bone'' of the financial control system. If the pharmacist-manager computerizes his pharmacy, the entire accounting system should be computerized. In addition, several special controls should be programmed.

Sales analysis is a particularly important control device, and should include the following: sales by department, by product group, by manufacturer's lines, by individual salesperson, and comparisons made with previous month and the same period a year before. *Inventory control* (perpetual, with monthly summaries) is especially important, and has been discussed in detail in a previous chapter. *Credit control* with age analysis, to be discussed in detail later, is also important. *Personnel records,* including complete payroll and FICA records, should be included. A *productivity index,* using individual sales, may be constructed.

A summary of each third-party-paid prescription program, including the number of prescriptions processed and the dollar volume processed and outstanding, should certainly be included.

Monthly *financial reports,* along with selected *financial ratios,* complete the computerized controls. The following are recommended monthly financial ratios: NP/NS, NP/$/inventory, acid test, current ratio, inventory/NWC, inventory TOR, NWC/NS, A/R avg. collection period, and A/P avg. remittance period.

Professional Control Functions. A complete discussion of these functions is beyond the scope of this book. However, the professional functions should include, at a minimum, the following: label preparation, assignment of prescription number, computation of price (cost of ingredient plus fee), special notations on the prescriptions, receipt, refill status, third-party billings, and all clinical support functions, e.g., drug interactions.

SELECTING A COMPUTER SYSTEM

The *first step* after studying this (or other text) text material is to see several computer systems demonstrated. This provides one with a better ''feel'' of or insight into what computers will do. The *second step* is to review this (or other) material to be sure that one understands the basic functions and performance of the computer. The *third,* and most *crucial,* step is to make careful analysis of one's pharmacy practice to determine which functions and activities should be computerized. This analysis of functions should lead to two lists: (1) the minimum functions that need to be computerized to make one's practice efficient, and (2) the maximum or deluxe list of functions that one would like to computerize.

The *fourth step* is to consult with several computer service firms to obtain preliminary estimates of the cost for each of the two lists of computer functions. Based on these estimates, one should decide whether one can afford to computerize. Will it be cost-effective to computerize? If so, then one should proceed with *step five,* which is a detailed study of the computer services available in terms of one's needs, and the quoted cost for the minimum and maximum list of functions.

The *final step* is the decision of which system to purchase. Before deciding, one should visit pharmacies that are using the various systems under consideration. Talk with the pharmacist-manager or proprietor and "test" the various procedures and results (reports, for example). This careful, step-by-step procedure should provide the means for making a good decision. See Figure 19–1 as a guide for selecting a computer. For a more detailed discussion of the selection of a computer for a pharmacy practice, the reader is referred to *Computers for Pharmacy.*[1]

Nonbudgetary Controls

The personnel area of management has been discussed in Chapter 12. It is only necessary here to reiterate how MBO—when extended to all managerial, professional, and supervisory or key employees—and policies and procedures provide excellent control mechanisms. Implicit in MBO are good two-way communications, a philosophy of participatory management, and measurable criteria to determine when objectives are, or are not, being met. Such criteria should consist of performance measurements such as sales increase, expense decrease, and mutually agreed rating scales for less tangible achievements of employees such as improvement and development. It should be noted at this point that nonbudgetary control is complementary to budgetary control. Since inventory control was discussed in Chapter 14, only a reminder that inventory control is a part of the overall control procedures in this chapter.

PROFESSIONAL FUNCTIONS

Control of professional functions is an important area of nonbudgetary control. One specific example is the control of drugs and pharmaceuticals subject to the drug laws. The control of these items exceeds ordinary inventory control methods and includes the necessity of accurate records of receipt and dispensing of all substances subject to these laws.

The monitoring and control of the utilization of all prescription and non-prescription maintenance drugs falls within the scope of the control of professional functions. The proper management of all facets of drug utilization—over- or underutilization, allergic reactions, drug-drug interactions, and drug-food interactions—requires the use of a medication record system. The professional and public health reasons for maintaining a medication record system have been well documented.[2–6]

A medication record system provides appropriate control over drug utili-

INSTRUCTIONS: Make a column for each computer and enter the data (yes, no, or quantity) for comparison. See Glossary for meaning of terms.

CPU   Capacity in Ks
External disc drives, number and capacity in megabytes each.
Number of work stations accommodated.
Number of prescriptions processed per day.
Number of new prescriptions before purging is necessary.
Number of refills before purging is necessary.
Number of patient profiles before purging is necessary.
Number of accounts receivable before purging is necessary.
Number of drugs in file before purging is necessary.
CRT Screen Size.
Character Printer?_____ No. of character/second.
Line Printer?_____ No. of lines/minutes
Prints labels_____ Receipts_____
Third Party: floppy diskette_____ tape_____ Printed copy_____.
Accounts Receivable_____ age analysis_____.
Inventory Control: EOQ____ Reorder Point & Quantity____ Usage Report____.
Summary of prescriptions dispensed.
Writes purchase orders; tracks orders_____.
Payroll: _____FICA_____ Tax Reports _____.
Writes Checks.
Accounts Payable.
General Ledger.
P & L Statement.
Balance Sheet.
Operational Reports.
Price Updating _____how_____ frequency _____.
Prescription Pricing_____ how_____ No. of formulas/tables _____.
Nursing Home Package and functions.
Durable medical equipment records.
Counseling tips_____ how/form_____.
Drug interactions.
Adverse Reactions.
Cost for comparable set of components.
Cost of each of the other components.
Lease per month.
Lease applies to purchase price.
Service contract for hardware: cost, service time, down time.
Service for software: cost____ frequency of updates____ what is included____.
History of down time and service.

Figure 19–1.   Check list for comparing computers.

zation as enumerated above and should meet certain criteria. First, an individual record should be maintained for each patient. Only then can the pharmacist efficiently monitor the drug utilization of the patient. Individual patient records are also more efficient for insurance purposes. Second, the record should include nonprescription drugs used as maintenance medication. Third, the record should include personal and health data as exemplified in Figure 19–2.

The medication record cards should be filed alphabetically by family with

NAME		BIRTHDATE
ADDRESS		
CHRONIC DISEASES		
ALLERGIES: Drugs-	Foods-	
IMMUNIZATION DPT		
Polio	Typhoid	

Date	℞ No.	Drug	Str.	Form	Amt.	Prescriber	Price	Renewal Dates

Figure 19–2. Medication record system card.

the head of the family first, followed by the remainder of the family filed in the order of spouse and then children from the oldest to the youngest. If manual, the card for the head of the family should be of a different and distinct color.

There are economic considerations of medication record systems. Smith reported a cost-to-effectiveness ratio of 1 to 2.54 for a medication record system.[7] In other words, each dollar spent to implement, maintain, and promote the medication record system yielded $2.54 in net profit during the first year following its implementation. The same study found that the cost of the system was approximately 3.5 cents per prescription dispensed.

In a study of the use of medication profiles in one of the Appalachian Regional Hospital outpatient pharmacies, it was estimated that it cost 5 cents per prescription to maintain the system.[8] The significance of the study,[9] however, was the effectiveness of the medication record system in controlling the use of drugs, especially overuse. Overuse was by far the greatest problem, followed by underuse. The former problem was more prevalent among patients whose drugs were financed by a third party, whereas the latter was more prevalent among private patients. Misuse of drugs of all types was more prevalent among those aged 65 years and over. Overuse occurred more often among users of psychotherapeutic and antihypertensive drugs when compared with eight other categories. These differences were significant as indicated by the chi-square test.

CREDIT CONTROL

The decision by the independent pharmacist to offer credit to selected patrons is almost automatic. The practice is widespread, and refusing credit, at least to good risk customers, would place a pharmacist at a distinct disadvantage. Credit is widely practiced among most retail establishments and it is expected by the general public. Because of the nature of pharmacy in providing health maintenance and even lifesaving drugs and services, it has a long history of offering credit to those who request it. Although it is true that some of the larger chain drugstores and discount houses with prescription departments do not yet offer charge service, in recent years some of these establishments have provided credit through one of the several charge cards.

In an economic sense, the decision to establish a credit program involves a cost-benefit analysis. In other words, the earnings in net profit derived from the extra sales resulting from the charge service must be compared with the potential earnings from the working capital funds tied up in accounts receivable at the going interest rate. In computing the net profit from the charge sales, the additional expense of bookkeeping, administration, collection, and bad debts resulting from extending credit should be included. Such computation is an easy task for pharmacists with computers.

In a 1964 study of 26 pharmacies in a Midwest city with a population of 100,000, the average accounting cost was 2.7 percent of the average credit sales of $80,530.[10] In another study, Doerr and Evanson reported an average accounting cost of 3.9 percent on $32,428 credit sales.[11] These findings compare favorably with the estimated cost of 3 to 5 percent on credit sales reported by Kelly and Lawyer.[12] In the 1964 study, bad debts averaged 0.2 percent of total sales and 0.84 percent of charge sales. *The Lilly Digest* reported a range of 0.1 to 0.2 percent of sales for many years.

It might appear on superficial analysis that credit sales were not profitable, since the average net profit reported in *The Lilly Digest* for 1964 was only 5.1 percent of sales.[13] However, without the charge sales, which averaged almost one-third of total sales in one study, many of the pharmacies would have lost money. This is true because the marginal income produced by credit sales exceeded the marginal cost of these sales. The excess of marginal income over marginal cost was more than could have been derived from the interest on the money invested in accounts receivable.

The *first step* in setting controls for a credit sales program is the decision to extend credit at all. An actual cost-benefit analysis or an intuitive estimate is implicit in this decision. Once the decision has been made, control procedures should be established. Controls should be predicated on the following questions: What type(s) or form(s) of charge accounts will be utilized? What limitation, if any, will be placed on the amount of credit? What collection procedures will be used? Finally, what criteria will be used for charging off bad debts?

Types of Charge Accounts. What types of charge accounts should a pharmacist use? There are four types: (1) the ordinary open account, (2) the installment account, (3) the budget account, and (4) the revolving account. The *open account* is the most common in pharmacy practices. It simply involves charging merchandise and services when purchased, with payment due when the bill is sent to the customer, usually at the end of the month. In the past, pharmacists seldom charged interest or a service fee on delinquent accounts. In recent years, however, a service and/or interest charge of 1 to 1½ percent per month has been assessed on the unpaid balance after the regular 30-day credit period has elapsed.

The *installment credit* plan is seldom used in pharmacy, although it is sometimes used by some pharmacists for expensive items such as a hospital bed. A down payment of 10 to 30 percent is collected, and the remainder is paid in equal payments, usually monthly, over a period of six months to a year. Again, an interest or service charge may or may not be used for installment credit.

The *budget account* is simply a short-term modification of the usual installment plan. Usually, a larger down payment is required, and the balance is paid in equal installments within a period of two to four months. This plan is used for substantial purchases, such as a wheelchair. A service charge may be used at the discretion of the pharmacist.

The *revolving account* has become popular in recent years, especially with department stores. Pharmacists have not used this approach to a great extent, but some chain drugstores are using this method. The revolving account permits the consumer to purchase up to a designated limit, for example $300, and the consumer pays a specified amount each month, for example $50 to $100. A service charge as high as 1½ percent per month is paid on the unpaid balance.

Credit cards are popular today, and many pharmacists believe that they should participate in these plans. Any or all of the above credit plans are available from one or more of the various credit card services. In every case, a service and interest charge, usually 1½ percent per month on the unpaid balance, is charged the consumer. With many of these plans the pharmacist (or other vendor) is charged a service fee for delinquent accounts. This charge is imposed to cover interest and collection cost, and may range from 3 to 5 percent.

An informal plan is the so-called *lay-away plan*. The consumer pays a nominal amount to have the pharmacist hold an item to be purchased by a designated time. If the customer does not purchase the item by the designated date, he forfeits the initial payment. This is often used at Christmas time to hold an item intended as a gift.

The pharmacist must decide first of all whether to offer credit to his patrons and then which credit plan or combination of credit plans to use. It should be obvious that the greater the number of credit plans used the more difficult it will be to control credit.

Investigating the Credit Applicant. Investigation of the credit applicant is the *second and* most *critical* step in credit control procedures. Several sources of information may be used to gather pertinent information, including a credit application form, the local credit bureau, banks, and other creditors. The credit application form should request the following types of data:

1. *Personal data*—name, address, how long the applicant has lived in the city or county, age, and names of the members of his or her family.

2. *Employment*—the employer, position, immediate supervisor, previous employer, and names of other employed members of the family.

3. *Bank*—the name of the bank or banks the applicant patronizes.

4. *Other firms* at which the applicant has charge accounts.

After the applicant has completed the credit application form, he should be told when he will be notified of his credit status. After examining the information on the application, the pharmacist should check with the credit bureau to determine whether the applicant has been reported delinquent by any of his other creditors. Every pharmacist who contemplates considerable charge sales should belong to the local credit bureau; otherwise, the information requested from the bureau will be rather expensive. Members of the local credit bureau usually are sent weekly bulletins, which list poor credit risks and other related information. It is a good policy to check with two or more other creditors to determine more precisely the payment record of the applicant. The banks are reluctant to provide much financial information about a client because they consider this to be confidential information. However, they do provide some general information that can be useful in deciding the credit risk of an applicant.

Form letters should be carefully composed for acceptance or rejection of a credit applicant. Both letters should be as pleasant in tone as possible. The acceptance should indicate your appreciation to the person for selecting you as his family pharmacist and enumerate all the special services and merchandise lines you feature. The credit policies and terms should be explained in such a manner that the patron will understand and accept them.

It should be noted at this point that as a professional person, licensed to provide critical health services, the pharmacist should not let his credit policies preclude the dispensing of a prescription on credit *in an emergency.*

Monitoring Charge Accounts. This procedure is an important phase of credit control. There are two basic techniques of monitoring charge accounts: *account age analysis* and the *average collection period of accounts.* The latter technique was described in Chapter 18. Ideally, the average collection period should not exceed 30 days, but a 40-day average period is not too critical. An average collection period of 50 days or more is too high and indicates that concerted steps should be taken.

The average collection period is a control check on the credit management as a whole, but it does not indicate which accounts are delinquent. Account age analysis will indicate the status of each account in terms of rate of payment related to rate of credit. Account age analysis provides information on the overall balance at the end of the month, the amount purchased and paid during the past month, and the amount that has been due 60 days, 90 days, and over 90 days. Some account age analyses classify the amount due 120 days and over.

As a general rule, debts more than 90 days old are difficult to collect. As a significant portion of a current balance is revealed by the age analysis to have been due for 90 days or more, steps should be taken to collect the account. Depending on the history and circumstances of the particular client and the general reputation of the people in the trade area, debts of 60 days' duration may be considered as doubtful in terms of collection.

A related question concerns the time when a pharmacist has to write off an account as a bad debt. As a general rule, a time period of one year is reasonable. If an account, or a significant portion of it, has been due for a year, and all attempts to collect have failed, it would be wise to write off the acocunt as a bad debt and take the income tax advantage.

Collection Procedures. Although investigating and selecting charge customers is the most critical phase of the credit control procedure, efficient colleciton procedures are the *most difficult* phase. A system should be devised to prevent credit extension from getting out of hand and to treat all patrons fairly. Again, the cost-benefit analysis approach should be used in determining how far one is willing to go to collect a debt. For example, it is unprofitable to spend $25 to collect a $10 account.

A good collection procedure should include the following steps. *First,* an invoice or ''charge ticket'' for each charge purchase should be given the customer at the time of the purchase, and two copies of the invoice retained in the pharmacy. Regular statements should be mailed to all charge customers. The statement should include a duplicate copy of each invoice or ''charge ticket'' for all purchases listed on the invoice. Statements normally are mailed monthly; however, in rural areas statements may be mailed quarterly, semi-annually, or sometimes annually. Statements are sent less frequently in the rural areas because rural patrons receive most of their income once or twice a year, when they sell their major cash crop, and because charge sales generally constitute a smaller percentage of total sales.

As a *second step,* some pharmacists stamp a notice of ''past due'' on the second mailing of the statements. Other terms used are ''Please remit (or pay) promptly,'' or ''Kindly send us your check for this statement.'' This type of reminder generally is used only if a significant payment has not been made during the previous month.

The *third step* in the collection procedure is to send a personal letter requesting payment of the past due bills. This type of letter should be firm, but not offensive. According to Steinmetz et al.,[14] this type of letter should have two objectives: ''(A) Bring the debtor to a conviction that the bill must be paid, and (B) secure the debtor's action by the shortest possible route and still retain his goodwill." The same authors further state that "the collection letter should start out as a reminder, then become firmer, and as a last resort indicate drastic action."[14] However, several other authorities recommend three different letters, emphasizing the same three separate points stated in the order above. The last letter, however, should end on a conciliatory note after indicating whatever drastic action is comtemplated. Sometimes the telephone is used in place of the initial letter to provide a more personal touch. A set of prototype letters is provided here:

FIRST LETTER

Dear Mrs. Jones:

It has come to my attention that your account (in the amount of $_____) is past due. We are pleased to have had the opportunity to serve you and extend credit as an additional service. As you know it costs our pharmacy a great deal to provide our many services and this is especially true of our credit service.

Will you not pay your bill promptly in order that we may continue to serve you and our other clientele as efficiently and professionally as we have in the past? Your thoughtful consideration of this matter will be appreciated.

Sincerely yours,

SECOND LETTER

Dear Mrs. Jones:

This is the second reminder of your past due bill in the amount of $_____ including the interest charge. I cannot overemphasize the seriousness of this matter. Failure to pay your bill has added to our operating cost and could jeopardize your credit status in our community. I urge you to remit the above amount within the next ten days.

Sincerely yours,

THIRD LETTER

Dear Mrs. Jones:

I regret to say that our previous appeals have failed, and you have not responded in any manner to our request that you pay your bill. If you do not pay your account within ten days, I will turn your account over to a collection agency. Needless to say, I am reluctant to do this, but you have left me no alternative.

We have cherished your patronage in the past and will continue to do so if you will pay your account in full, or arrange to pay a substantial amount now and the remainder within an agreed period of time.

I trust you will act promptly on this proposition and re-establish our long-standing and mutually beneficial relation.

Sincerely yours,

The *final* and *most drastic step* is to utilize a free-lance collector, a regular collection agency, or an attorney to collect the bill. The pharmacist has more control over the proceedings if he uses an attorney, but it usually costs him more. A regular collection agency normally is the most efficient because these organization are specialists in this particular activity.

As a final note to the collection procedure, it is the consensus of most experienced people that the customers are more likely to continue to give a firm their patronage after they have been coaxed, pressured, or forced to pay their bill. There are two reasons given for this theory. First, people stop patronizing a place after they have accumulated a sizable bill because they are embarrassed to face the proprietor. After the bill has been paid, this barrier is removed and they often return to the pharmacy for their pharmaceutical needs. Second, the pharmacist often gains additional respect for his forthright business-like practices. As a professional person and humanitarian, a pharmacist should give proper consideration to hardship cases. Historically, this has been one of the hallmarks of the pharmaceutical profession.

STORE SECURITY

Burglaries and Robberies. Security has become one of the major problems in pharmacy with the increase in both burglaries and robberies, which have been motivated primarily by the need for dependence-producing drugs. With the passage of the Controlled Substance Act in 1965, and the more stringent law, the Comprehensive Drug Abuse Prevention and Control Act in 1970, "street drugs" have become more expensive to obtain. Consequently, there has been an increase in robberies and burglaries of pharmacies to obtain these drugs, reaching "epidemic" proportions in the last five years.

First, the burglaries and robberies began in the large metropolitan cities, but they soon spread to the rural towns throughout the United States. The problem has become so serious that a bill has been passed by Congress to make burglaries and robberies of pharmacies a Federal offense. Some pharmacies have been burglarized more than six times.

Pilferage. Pilferage is another serious problem for pharmacists. It costs them more than burglaries and robberies combined; however, it does not have the attendant danger of homicide or serious injury and the social problem of drug abuse and dependence.

Pilferage is committed by both employees and "outsiders." The former source of pilferage can be controlled by good personnel administration practices, especially with good selection techniques and appropriate compensation. Some pharmacists use the polygraph in selecting employees or in suspected cases of pilferage.

Security Measures. As previously mentioned, good employee selection procedures and personnel relations can control, if not completely eliminate, the problem of pilferage by employees. Controlling pilerage by the public is much more difficult. The use of large mirrors in the front of the pharmacy has reduced pilferage only to a nominal degree.

A system of closed-circuit television cameras and monitors has proved to be effective in reducing pilferage. In the mid-1970s, one small drugstore chain of 35 units installed a closed-circuit television system with excellent results.[15] The system was installed on a lease and purchase agreement. The cost averaged between three and four dollars per day per pharmacy over a period of 36 months, depending on the number of cameras and monitors required. This cost included the rental and service for four cameras and one to three monitors. One monitor was placed in or near the prescription department, and one was placed in the center of the pharmacy. This latter monitor was used for its psychologic effect because customers could see people over the entire pharmacy as the scene switched from one camera view to another. At the end of 36 months, the system could be purchased for a nominal fee of about $100. No doubt these costs have increased two- or three-fold since that date.

The cost for an individual pharmacy would be considerably more. However, a cooperative group or a group of pharmacies in a city or a cluster of neighboring towns could negotiate a favorable contract based on the economics of servicing the equipment. In either case, the pharmacist will have to pay for service calls after he purchases the system.

Most pharmacists have burglary and robbery insurance, but these policies are usually cancelled after two or three burglaries or robberies. There are several variations in burglary alarm systems. Originally, an alarm (bell) sounded when the circuit around the door and safe was broken. This was refined to a remote alarm at the nearest police station but silent in the pharmacy. This was designed to apprehend the burglars before they finished the burglary. An infrared-sensitive device and a noise-sensitive device have been incorporated into the newer systems. Like participants in the cold war, the burglars have learned to avoid every alarm innovation.

Probably the simplest and most effective technique available to prevent burglaries is the dispersal of controlled drugs throughout the prescription department and their frequent relocation, together with a remote alarm. Before the burglars can find enough drugs to make the burglary worthwhile, the police can apprehend the culprits. After all, arrest and conviction are much more effective than sophisticated gadgets, which most burglars learn to foil.

The 1973 September issue of *Pharmacy Times* listed 20 techniques to improve security. The major items have been discussed above, but the various other techniques, such as checking that the pharmacy is free of customers before it is locked each night, are common sense, and worthwhile practices.

Budgetary Controls

Any budgetary control procedure requires a working knowledge of basic accounting concepts and procedures. Accurate records are necessary to the successful operation of any organization, either profit or nonprofit. In fact, the evidence indicates a close relationship between inadequate accounting records and business failures.[16] A well-designed accounting system is necessary for a budgetary or financial control system. It also serves other purposes. An accounting system has four objectives. The first objective is to provide the financial information necessary for bank or trade credit. The second objective is to provide the basis for income tax returns. The third objective is to protect the firm's assets from careless errors and frauds and to provide a systematic method of depreciation of fixed assets. The fourth objective is to serve as a basis for financial and business planning. It is the last two objectives that are the primary focus of the remainder of this chapter.

The overall control budget is divided into two primary sections, the income or revenue section and the expenditures section. The latter is further divided into fixed and variable costs.

Usually nonprofit organizations develop an expenditure budget based on goals or planned services and hope the revenue will be sufficient to meet the budget. This is not the case in institutional pharmacies, generally speaking, because the pharmacy, along with the clinical laboratory and the x-ray department, are the departments that most consistently show an operational surplus.

REVENUE COMPONENT OF THE BUDGET

This portion of the budget is both the most critical and most difficult to project. Yet it is a vital and necessary part of budgetary planning for both profit and nonprofit organizations, if either a balanced budget or profit is to be achieved. Projection of revenue usually is based on data from past experience. Too frequently the projection for the next fiscal year is based on the change between the year ending and the previous year. This is sound under stable conditions. The simplicity of this approach ignores two important variables, one internal and one external.

Internal Variable. This variable is the growth curve of the pharmacy. One normally would anticipate a rapid growth rate for a newly established pharmacy. An in-depth location analysis will provide a basis for the early growth rate projections, which should be adjusted annually according to the actual sales data. Of course, if a large error is made in estimating the potential volume and growth rate, not only will the adjustment be large, but relocation should be considered, especially if the error was made on the optimistic side. Normally, the early growth rate of a pharmacy begins to plateau in about four to five years, followed by a normal growth pattern corresponding to the general economic conditions of the market.

External Variable. This is the overall economic growth (or inflation) curve, or decline, of the market in which the pharmacy is located. The market conditions include a multitude of factors, such as the general economic condition of the country as measured by the gross national product (GNP), local economic variations, and both seasonal and random or nonpredictable fluctuations. Local economic variations may include strikes, new industries, droughts, and the like. Seasonal variations have little or no effect in predictions covering a period of more than one year. Random, nonpredictable variations include such factors as epidemics, unusual weather, an increase or decrease in prescribers, and the introduction of a new drug for the treatment of a disease

Table 19–1.   Sales Forecast for 19XX Based on Five-Year Data

Year	Y*	x	x²	xy
1980	$ 416,000	− 2	4	− $832,000
1981	439,000	− 1	1	− 439,000
1982	498,000	0	0	- - - -
1983	529,000	+ 1	1	529,000
1984	563,000	+ 2	4	1,126,000
- - - -	$2,445,000	0	10	$ 384,000

*Sales for the respective years.

for which no adequate treatment previously existed. Obviously, these non-predictable factors cannot be used in the projection of the revenue or sales portion of the budget.

The pharmacist can use the GNP growth trend to make appropriate adjustment in his pharmacy's growth trend, based on a broad consensus among the professional economists concerning the national trend. The pharmacist should take note of the local economic trends and development and make appropriate adjustments in his income projections.

Income Projection. Income projections should be based on at least five years' data when available. One can use as a guide a well-established pharmacy under normal economic growth conditions, or *The Lilly Digest* average sales during a similar period. A straight-line equation is used to establish the trend. Table 19–1 shows the average sales volumes, as reported in *The Lilly Digest.*[17]

The data may be used to illustrate income projection. The technique is the simple least-squares method for a five-year trend using the middle year as the origin or pivotal point of the trend line.[18] The equation is:

$$Y' = a + bx$$

where: Y = the actual sales
Y' = the estimated sales volume for the respective years
x = the deviation in terms of the number of years from the mid-year
a = the average annual sales for the period
b = the rate of change in the sales volume or the slope of the trend line.

The computations are as follows:

$$a = \frac{\Sigma Y}{N} = \frac{2{,}445{,}000}{5} = 489{,}000$$

$$b = \frac{\Sigma xY}{\Sigma x^2} = \frac{\$384{,}000}{10} = \$38{,}400$$

Substituting in the equation, $Y' = a + bx$, the estimated sales volume for 1985 is calculated as follows:

$$Y'(1985) = \$489{,}000 + 3(\$38{,}400) = \$604{,}200$$

EXPENDITURE COMPONENT OF THE BUDGET

The expenditure component of the budget is composed of two parts, variable expenses and fixed expenses.

Variable Expenses. Since variable expenses, by definition, vary proportionally with sales, it would appear that they could be projected by multiplying the percentage for each by the projected sales. This procedure is acceptable, however, only after each expense item has been analyzed carefully and compared with some standard, such as a comparable group of pharmacies as reported in *Heart of the Lilly Digest*. The percentages of the several variable expenses change with the level in sales volume, as shown by a study of *The Lilly Digest*. Based on data from this source, a range of percentages for the several variable expenses applicable to most pharmacies has been constructed.

Employees' wages	7.0–13.0%
Advertising	1.0– 2.0%
Bad debts	0.1– 0.3%
Miscellaneous expenses	2.0– 4.0%
Total	12.1–18.3%
General average	15.0% (rounded nearest 1%)

Fixed Expenses. Fixed expenses are constant for a given fiscal period, normally a year, but they may increase with time as the pharmacy grows significantly in sales volume, or by enlarging the facilities or services provided. Unless a significant change has taken place, the pharmacist may plan for the same fixed expenses as budgeted and/or expended the previous year. Sometimes, however, on close examination, he may see the need to alter certain items.

Some fixed expense items are not absolutely fixed, but vary to a degree with sales. Delivery costs, for example, vary to a degree with an increase in sales, but the larger portion of the costs—depreciation, insurance, property taxes, and repairs—is fixed for the most part, at least for a given year. Although inventory can be expected to increase with sales, and thus the insurance premium and property tax on inventory; insurance premium and property tax on fixed assets, however, would decrease because of depreciation. This decrease in insurance and property tax through depreciation usually equals or exceeds the increase due to increased inventory.

Most pharmacists pay a fixed rent per month. Some pay rent as a percentage of sales. In this case, rent is certainly a variable expense. This situation occurs more frequently in medical clinic buildings and in large shopping centers. Normally, the lessor requires a minimum monthly rent, which covers sales up to a designated amount; then the lessee pays a percentage rent, which again may decrease at various intervals up to a specified sales volume. The latter feature, a decreasing percentage rent with increasing sales volume, should be included in all percentage rent leases, and the pharmacist should negotiate for an upper dollar limit on the rent.

Nearly all other expenses are fixed, at least in a given fiscal period. The proprietor's salary should be realistic—the amount one would have to pay a manager to perform comparable work.

After making the aforementioned analyses and projections, an overall budget may be constructed as in Table 19–2.

A more detailed budget should be constructed for each month, as illustrated in Table 19–3. This table provides the mechanism for the control of expenses, of other expenditures, and of the flow of cash.

CASH FLOW CONTROL

The proper management of the cash flow of a pharmacy is important at any time and is vital in periods of inflation and high capital cost. Figure 19–3 illustrates the key role that cash flow plays in the normal operation of a pharmacy.

There are many reasons for a pharmacy manager to be concerned with maintaining an appropriate cash flow. Cash flow, for example, can provide sufficient funds to (1) pay accounts payable and other bills on time in order to earn cash discounts; (2) pay normal day-to-day expenses; (3) maintain a good credit rating; and (4) take advantage of special-purchase opportunities.

In order to maintain adequate cash flow, several potential problem areas should be monitored closely and continuously. These sensitive areas are (1) inventory control, (2) accounts receivable, (3) fixed and variable expenses, and (4) debt service or loan interest expenses.

Fluctuations in cash flow occur when there is an unusual decrease in cash receipts or an increase in expenditures brought about by the stockpiling of seasonal merchandise, an unusual extension of credit, an extraordinary disbursement for expenses or equipment, or the periodic remittance of taxes.

Certain purchasing practices may lead to a low cash level or even to a cash deficit. Such practices include: buying too much unprofitable merchandise, failing to use postdating opportunities, timing purchases improperly, and failing to take cash discounts.

One of the biggest contributors to an unfavorable cash flow position is the time it takes to collect accounts receivable on third-party programs. Aside from political activity and continual negotiations with the third party, the pharmacist-manager can do little to speed the process. His best recourse is to complete the required forms promptly and meticulously to avoid unnecessary payment delays and claim rejections. A computer system is valuable in this respect.

The pharmacy manager should anticipate cash flow fluctuations and should maintain a cash reserve to meet expenditures as they arise. In addition, the pharmacy manager should establish a mechanism that will help to track cash flow and to predict accurately cash requirements on a month-to-month basis. Table 19–2 represents such an overall budgetary control mechanism.

In Table 19–2, the budgeted amount for cash outlays is projected from data from the previous few years, taking into consideration trends such as inflation, market conditions, and anticipated sales increases. These amounts are targets, and the objective of the control mechanism is to keep expenditures within

Table 19–2.   Overall Control Budget

Month	Total Sales	Cash Sales*	Received On Acc't.	Budgeted Cash†	Mdse. Purchases	Expenses & Other Expenditures‡	Cumulative Deficit or Surplus
January	$28,500	$14,850	$12,800	$29,000	$18,525	$11,033	$442§
Total	$326,270	$169,150	$156,450	$325,000	$212,075	$113,499	$1,026

*Includes actual cash sales, rebates, commissions, and other similar cash income.
†Budgeted cash is projected based on a five-year trend.
‡Other expenditures include income tax and other miscellaneous purchases other than merchandise.
§There was carry-over surplus of $1,000 from the previous year.

Table 19–3. Monthly Cash Budget

Day	Budget Balance	Purchases	Expenses	Other Expenditures	Total Cash Expenditures
1	$29,000	$ 1,246	$ 150	—	$ 1,396
2	$27,604	$ 4,200	$2,415	$ 55	$ 6,670
3	$20,934	$ 3,160	$1,240	—	$ 4,400
31	(558)	$18,525	$8,978	$2,055	$29,558

the budgeted amounts. The actual cash income and expenditures are entered in the chart at the end of each month and provide the basis for preparing the next year's budget.

In addition to the overall budgetary control mechanism, the monthly budget (Table 19–3) should be constructed as a means of further controlling expenditures.

To provide even more accuracy, each category of cash expenditure can be controlled by applying appropriate procedures. Individual items of expense in all categories should be periodically compared to standards or averages for

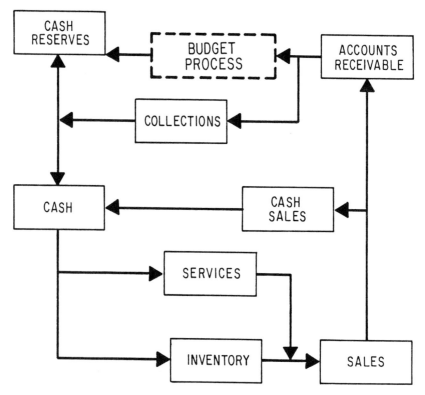

Figure 19–3. Cash flow cycle. (From Smith, H.A.: Financial analysis and control. In *Effective Pharmacy Management*. Kansas City: Marion Laboratories, Inc., 1979.)

similar pharmacies. Every effort should then be made to keep these items at or below the standards.

Budgeting Depreciation

Depreciation is a significant and unique expense. It is unique in that the expense is not a cash outlay, but rather a deduction allowed by the Internal Revenue Service (IRS) for the depreciation of fixed capital investments. Because of its unique features, and the various formulas of depreciation permitted by IRS, this topic will be discussed in considerable detail. However, changes in the income tax code have altered the manner of depreciation in recent years, but Table 19–4 provides a wide range of potential depreciations.

BASIS FOR DEPRECIATION

There are basically *three reasons* for allowing depreciation of an asset. *First,* the asset may be subject to *physical wear* with use and time, or depletion in the case of natural resources such as coal, oil, and gas. *Second* the asset may become *obsolete* because of changing technology and other changes. *Third,* depreciation of fixed capital investment *encourages investment and economic growth.* This is the basic reason double allowances and other fast write-off procedures for the first year's depreciation are allowed, especially during a period of economic recession or depression.

DEPRECIATION CRITERIA

The nature of the property determines: (1) whether an asset qualifies for depreciation, and (2) the duration of the period of depreciation. There are *three* criteria that the asset must meet to be eligible for depreciation. *First,* The life of the property must be definite and exceed one year. Thus, *real property* (land) cannot be depreciated.

Second, the property must be used in the enterprise for the production of income, but *inventory* held for sale cannot be depreciated. However, this does not mean that deteriorated or unsalable inventory may not be written off at the end of the fiscal period.

Third, intangible property can be depreciated *only* under certain conditions. The cost incurred in obtaining an intangible asset, such as a copyright or a covenant not to compete, may be depreciated at uniform rates over a period of time negotiated with the IRS. The value of goodwill, trade names, or trademarks is not eligible for depreciation.

COMPONENTS OF DEPRECIATION

The fundamental steps in setting up a depreciation schedule are: (1) determining the value basis for depreciation; (2) determining the useful life of the asset; (3) determining the salvage value of the asset; and (4) determining the maximum deduction allowed.

Value Base. The cost of the property ordinarily is the basis for determining the *value base* for computation of the depreciation. If a nonbusiness property is converted to business use, for example, a used personal automobile, the fair market value (blue-book value in this instance) would be used as the value base for calculating depreciation from the date of conversion to business use. If a pharmacist purchases a building in which he operates his practice, a valuation of both land and the building must be made since the land may not be depreciated. In those cases in which a pharmacist leases a building and improves the value of the building through remodeling, he may depreciate the cost of the remodeling over the established life of the improvements.

Useful Life. The Internal Revenue Service maintains a Table of Useful Lives of Depreciable Property. An abbreviated version is available as "IRS Bulletin F" from the Superintendent of Public Documents in Washington. Most fixtures and furnishings have a useful life of ten years. Refrigerators, for example, have a useful life of twenty years. Some equipment lasts only about five years. If a pharmacist's experience indicates a useful life other than the standard life, he can have this established for the particular fixture or equipment in his pharmacy by appropriate documentation of his prior experience with the particular property. The estimated useful life of a given asset may be modified at the end of a tax year, if the pharmacist can produce convincing evidence as a basis for changing the length of the useful life.

Salvage Value. The salvage value of an asset is the estimated value or sale value of the asset at the end of its useful life. This estimation is made at the time the asset is purchased or acquired, and it is indicated in the depreciation schedule on the next income tax return. This value depends on the nature of the property and the length of the useful life, which is affected, in part, by the replacement policy for the asset. If the pharmacist intends to keep the asset for its full inherent useful life and indicates this in the depreciation schedule, the pharmacist may deduct from the salvage value the cost of removing and transporting the property to a junk dealer.

Maximum Depreciation. The maximum depreciation allowance is the value base minus the salvage value. It is also the aggregate of annual deductions. A pharmacist should deduct the allowable depreciation each year; otherwise, he will lose it. A depreciation allowance cannot be carried over to future years. However, it is possible to get variable depreciation by selecting from among several methods of calculating depreciation.

DEPRECIATION METHODS

Four different methods for calculating depreciation are accepted by the IRS. In addition, there are some modifications allowed through negotiations.

In fact, the IRS states that any reasonable method of depreciation is permitted if negotiated and applied consistently. One frequently used modification is the additional first-year depreciation allowance, that is, allowing twice the normal deduction above the regular amount. This extra depreciation allowance is not a permanent rule, but it is used to encourage investment and expansion during economic recessions.

Straight-Line Method. The simplest method of calculating depreciation is the straight-line method. The salvage value is subtracted from the cost of the asset (or the value base) and the difference is divided by the number of years of the asset's useful life.

Declining Balance Method. This method is a little more complicated than the straight line method. With it, the salvage value is *not deducted* from the cost before the depreciation is calculated; however, the pharmacist cannot deduct depreciation below the salvage value. With this method, the amount of depreciation allowed is deducted from the cost, and the balance is used as the basis for computing the next year's depreciation allowance. Thus each year the basis for calculating the deduction is the declining balance, and hence, the name of the method. The rate of deduction is usually twice the straight-line rate and remains the same for the life of the asset. Under certain conditions, $1\frac{1}{2}$ to 2 times the straight-line rate of deduction is allowed. To qualify for this method, the asset must have a useful life of three years or more and be acquired, constructed, or renovated after December 31, 1953.

Sum-of-the-Years-Digits Method. The principle of this method is the application of a progressively smaller fraction (ratio) to the cost or other value base after subtracting the salvage value. This method can be applied to an individual asset or to a group of assets with the same useful life. The denominator of the fraction is determined by adding all the digits representing the years of the useful life of the asset(s). For example, a useful life of ten years would give a denominator of 55 ($10 + 9 + 8 + 7 + 6 + 5 + 4 + 3 + 2 + 1 = 55$). The denominator can also be computed by the formula of $\dfrac{n^2 + n}{2}$, where n = years of useful life $\left(\dfrac{10^2 + 10}{2} = \dfrac{100 + 10}{2} = 55\right)$. The numerator is simply the number of years of useful life remaining at the beginning of the year for which the deduction is being computed.

Remaining Life Plan. The fourth method of calculating depreciation is the remaining life plan, which is a modification of the sum-of-the-years-digits method. The fraction increases each year, while the base for computing the deduction decreases in a manner similar to the declining balance method. This method incorporates concepts from the declining balance and the sum-of-the-years-digits methods, but the results are the same as the latter. The purpose of this method is to permit a fast rate of depreciation of assets with different useful lives. Each asset with a different useful life remaining is computed separately.

The denominator of the fraction is the sum of the digits of the remaining years of useful life, while the numerator is the number of years of remaining useful life. For example, if an asset has five more years of useful life, the denominator is 15 and the numerator is 5, providing the fraction five fifteenths. This fraction is multiplied by the balance or unrecovered cost of the asset. A comparison of these four methods is shown in Table 19–4.

CHOOSING THE BEST METHOD

The choice of the method of depreciation depends primarily on the projected total income (net profit plus proprietor's salary for proprietorship or partnership). During the early years of a pharmacy, various conditions may exist that would cause a pharmacist to select a particular method of depreciation. First, let us assume the pharmacist's location analysis indicated a good potential for the location with rapid growth, yielding some net profit the first year and a significant net profit during the second year. If the pharmacist has a minimum amount of capital, he would need to generate as much cash as possible to meet his obligations. He will want to deduct the maximum depreciation during the early years to minimize the income tax liability. This will provide additional funds to meet either short- or long-term liabilities. The pharmacist should select the declining balance method of depreciation, since this method provides the fastest rate of depreciation. The slight penalty of unrecovered cost is a small price to pay for the advantage.

On the other hand, if the pharmacist has adequate capital and the location analysis indicates a slower but steady rate of growth with a significant amount of net profit in about the third or fourth year, the pharmacist would benefit most by the slower but steady depreciation rate of the straight-line method.

If the status of a pharmacy falls between these two extremes, the pharmacist should select the sum-of-the-years-digits or the remaining life plan. However, these latter two methods provide a much faster rate of depreciation than the straight-line method. Thus, by selecting the most appropriate depreciation method, the pharmacist can control one of his most significant fixed costs to his greatest advantage.

Summary

Management controls can take many forms, both budgetary (financial) and nonfinancial, indirect budgetary controls. Many of the controls are inherent in the total management system, especially if management by objectives is the basic method used. In addition, many of the controls have their roots in other phases of management—location analysis, capital planning, accounting systems, financial analysis, purchasing and inventory control, organization

Table 19–4. Comparison of Four Methods of Depreciation

	Straight-Line Method				Declining Balance Method			
Year	Base*	Rate	Depreciation	Accumulated Depreciation	Base*	Rate	Depreciation	Accumulated Depreciation
1976	$10,000.00	10%	$1,000.00	$1,000.00	$11,000.00	20%	$2,200.00	$2,200.00
1977	10,000.00	10%	1,000.00	2,000.00	8,800.00	20%	1,760.00	3,960.00
1978	10,000.00	10%	1,000.00	3,000.00	7,040.00	20%	1,408.00	5,368.00
1979	10,000.00	10%	1,000.00	4,000.00	5,632.00	20%	1,126.40	6,494.40
1980	10,000.00	10%	1,000.00	5,000.00	4,505.60	20%	901.12	7,395.52
1981	10,000.00	10%	1,000.00	6,000.00	3,604.48	20%	720.90	8,116.42
1982	10,000.00	10%	1,000.00	7,000.00	2,883.58	20%	576.72	8,693.14
1983	10,000.00	10%	1,000.00	8,000.00	2,306.86	20%	461.37	9,154.51
1984	10,000.00	10%	1,000.00	9,000.00	1,845.49	20%	369.10	9,523.61
1985	10,000.00	10%	1,000.00	10,000.00	1,476.39	20%	295.28	9,818.89†

	Sum-of-the-Years-Digits Method				Remaining Life Plan			
Year	Base*	Rate	Depreciation	Accumulated Depreciation	Base*	Rate	Depreciation	Accumulated Depreciation
1976	$10,000.00	10/55	$1,818.18	$1,818.18	$10,000.00	10/55	$1,818.18	$1,818.18
1977	10,000.00	9/55	1,636.36	3,454.54	8,181.82	9/45 (1/5)	1,636.36	3,454.54
1978	10,000.00	8/55	1,454.55	4,909.09	6,545.46	8/36 (2/9)	1,454.44	4,908.98
1979	10,000.00	7/55	1,272.73	6,181.82	5,908.98	7/28 (1/4)	1,272.78	6,181.76
1980	10,000.00	6/55	1,090.91	7,272.73	3,818.24	6/21 (2/7)	1,090.92	7,272.68
1981	10,000.00	5/55	909.09	8,181.82	2,727.27	5/15 (1/3)	909.09	8,818.77
1982	10,000.00	4/55	727.27	8,909.09	1,818.23	4/10 (2/5)	727.30	8,909.07
1983	10,000.00	3/55	545.45	9,454.54	1,090.93	3/6 (1/2)	545.47	9,454.54
1984	10,000.00	2/55	363.64	9,818.18	545.46	2/3	363.64	9,818.18
1985	10,000.00	1/55	181.82	10,000.00	181.82	1/1	181.82	10,000.00

*The base is the cost less salvage value or the declining balance depending on the method used.
†This method allows a maximum depreciation of $9,818.89, and an unrecovered cost of $181.11 above salvage value.

form and structure, personnel administration, and the philosophy and policies of management.

Controls are accomplished through four primary mechanisms—management objectives with measurable criteria for each, a well-designed accounting system, a computer system, and a two-way communication system based on openness, fairness, and integrity. As stated in previous chapters, a firm that utilizes MBO and good personnel policies will have little problem in controlling a pharmacy.

REFERENCES

1. Lauer, J.E., Aust, K.M., and King, A.S.: *Computers for Pharmacy.* Washington, D.C.: American Pharmaceutical Association, 1978.
2. Schwarting, A.E.: Presentation made to American Association of Colleges of Pharmacy, April, 1971.
3. Seidl, L.G., Thornton, G.F., and Smith, J.W.: Studies on the epidemiology of adverse drug reactions III: reactions in patients on a general medical service. *Bull. Johns Hopkins Hosp., 119*:229–315, 1966.
4. Schimmel, E.M.: The hazards of hospitalization. *Ann. Intern. Med., 60*:100–110, 1960.
5. Gardner, P., and Leighton, L.E.: The epidemiology of adverse drug reactions—a review and perspective. *Johns Hopkins Med. J., 126*:77–87, 1970.
6. Huffman, D.C., Jr.: Managerial aspects of patient medication record systems. Paper presented at the American Pharmaceutical Association Academy of General Practice of Pharmacy in Boston, Massachusetts, July 26, 1973.
7. Smith, H.A.: Application of cost-effectiveness analysis to patient record systems. *J. Am. Pharm. Assoc., NS13*:13, 14, 1972.
8. Billups, N.F., and Glascock, L.M.: Personal communications.
9. Solomon, D.K., et al.: Use of medication profiles to detect potential therapeutic problems in ambulatory patients. *Am. J. Hosp. Pharm., 31*:348–354, 1974.
10. Smith, H.A., et al.: Few pharmacists use cash registers fully. *Am. Druggist,* p. 55, May 24, 1965.
11. Doerr, D.W., and Evanson, R.V.: Consumer credit practices in pharmacies. Paper presented to the Section on General Pharmacy Practice, American Pharmaceutical Association, New York, 1964.
12. Kelly, P.C., and Lawyer, K.: *How To Organize and Operate a Small Business.* 3rd ed. Englewood Cliffs: Prentice-Hall, Inc., 1961, p. 501.
13. Chagaris, C.A.: *The Lilly Digest.* Indianapolis: Eli Lilly and Co., 1964, p. 5.
14. Steinmetz, L.L., Kline, J.B., and Stegall, D.P.: *Managing the Small Business.* Homewood: Richard D. Irwin, Inc., 1968, p. 559.
15. Mudd, F.P.: Director of Pharmacy Operations, Begley Drug Co., personal communication.
16. Steinmetz, et al., *op. cit.,* p. 249.
17. Deiner, C.H.: *The Lilly Digest.* Indianapolis: Eli Lilly and Co.
18. Pearson, F.A., and Bennett, K.K.: *Statistical Methods.* New York: John Wiley & Sons, Inc., 1945, p. 79.

REVIEW

1. Explain the concept and the mechanisms of total control.

2. Discuss the importance of the computer to a pharmacy practice and business in general.

3. Describe each of the functions, components, and elements of the computer.

4. Distinguish between hardware and software of the computer.

5. What is CRT?

6. Distinguish between the "batch" and "on-line" approach to data processing.

7. Discuss how the computer assists in managerial control functions, both business and professional.

8. Describe the steps of selecting a computer system.

9. Discuss the methods of control of professional activities.

10. Discuss credit control procedures and explain each specific mechanism.

11. Describe how the four types of charge accounts, credit cards, and lay-away plans operate.

12. Describe the process of investigation of credit applicants.

13. Discuss the monitoring of charge accounts, including the necessary calculations of the two basic techniques for monitoring accounts.

14. Describe efficient collection procedures fully.

15. Explain why forced collection of debts improves patrons' relations in many instances.

16. Explain the necessity of a good accounting system to budgetary control.

17. What are the objectives of a good accounting system?

18. Explain the influence of internal and external variables on the revenue portion of a budget.

19. Given an appropriate set of data, construct a budget including: (1) income section, projected with the least-squares method; (2) variable expense section, determined by using the average variable expense ratio of a typical pharmacy; and (3) fixed expense section, determined from data given.

20. Trace the flow of cash in pharmacy practice.

21. Discuss and explain how you would develop and monitor cash flow in a pharmacy practice.

22. What are the necessary criteria for an asset to qualify for depreciation?

23. What are the three reasons given for allowing depreciation deductions?

24. Explain the four methods of computing depreciation, list the four steps necessary for setting up a depreciation schedule, and compute a depreciation schedule by each of the methods when given the basic data.

25. Explain the basis for selecting the various methods of depreciation.

Glossary

Access Time. The time interval between the instant at which information is called from storage and the instant at which delivery is completed. The time interval between the instant at which data are ready for storage and the instant at which storage is completed.

Address. A unique identification (name, label, or number) for a register's location in storage, or other data source of destination.

Alpha (or alphabetic). Using only letters of the alphabet and the special characters of punctuation (period, comma, asterisk, for example).

Alpha-Numeric. The characters that include letters of the alphabet, numerals, and other symbols, such as punctuation or mathematic symbols.

Application. The system or problem to which a computer is addressed.

Assembly Language. A type of systems software that converts one line of human-generated programming code into one line of object code. Assembly languages are usually machine-dependent, i.e., developed for one brand of computer and often restricted to certain models within that product line.

Assembler. A computer program specifically used to convert a source program written in assembly language to a machine-coded or object program.

Backup. The term used to refer either to equipment, systems files, or the technique to maintain or to restart operations, in case malfunction or other problem affects normal computer processing.

Backup Equipment. Equipment maintained either at the user's site or within a reasonable distance from the user's site, to use in case of malfunction of equipment.

Backup Files. Files maintained to recreate current data files in case the files are destroyed. They may be machine-readable or manual.

Backup Procedures. The procedures, such as copying current files onto other storage media, normally used at the end of each day's processing, to provide good backup files.

Backup Systems. Alternate procedures, usually manual, that must be used or referred to when the computer system is inoperable for a significant length of time.

Batch Processing. An approach to processing in which similar types of data are collected and processed in one machine run. Example: inventory depletions are recorded and accumulated; at the end of the day, all information is fed into the computer to process updated inventory levels.

Binary. The number system that a computer uses; counting by twos. See "Decimal."

Bit. Derived by BInary digiT. The smallest information unit with which a computer works. See "Byte."

Bug. A mistake in program, data, or system.

Byte. A series of eight adjacent bits. Forms a single character, either a letter of the alphabet, a numeral, or a punctuation mark.

Cartridge Disc. Removable hard disc in plastic case.

Character. A human-readable letter, numeral, or punctuation mark; or, a special form of byte, using only six bits.

Compiler. A computer program specifically used to convert a source program written in a compiler language to a machine-coded, or object program.

Compiler Language. A type of systems software that converts one line of human-generated programming code into many lines of object code. Compiler languages are usually machine-independent and can be used on many brands of equipment. Examples of compiler languages are: BASIC, RPG, COBOL, FORTRAN.

Computer. The device that carries out calculations under the control of a program.

Computer System. The combined hardware and software that perform prescribed functions of accepting information, processing it according to instructions, and supplying the results.

CPU (Central Processing Unit). The part of the computer that performs the calculations. Identical to "Processor" and "Mainframe."

CRT (Cathode Ray Tube). A video display screen, much like a television screen. Also used to designate a terminal that uses a cathode ray tube screen in conjunction with a typewriter keyboard.

Data Storage. Media, such as discs and tape, in which the computer stores information for later use.

Debugging. The process of removing errors (bugs) from a system.

Decimal. The number system we use. Counting by tens. See "Binary."

Digital. Information expressed in discrete, numeric form. A computer that handles data in numeric (binary) form.

Disc Drive. The physical unit on which discs are mounted. Similar to a phonograph. The disc rotates on the disc drive while information is read/written on it.

Disc Storage. A method of storing information in code on magnetic discs, and of having it quickly accessible.

Display. Information presented to the system user on a video screen in human-readable form.

Down Time. The time during which a computer is not functioning, or is functioning improperly, because of machine or program malfunction.

Edit. To rearrange information for machine input or output, i.e., to delete, select, or insert any needed data, symbols, or characters. Also implies checking data for completeness, accuracy, and reasonableness.

Encode. Any process in which one form of data is changed to a different form, such as using a keyboard to transcribe information onto magnetic tape.

File. A collection of related records. For example, in inventory control in one line of an invoice is an item; a complete invoice is a record; and the complete set of invoices is a file.

Floppy Disc. Data storage medium made of Mylar with a magnetized surface. Smaller, with less storage capacity than hard discs.

Hard Copy. Computer output printed on paper.

Hard Disc. Data storage medium made of metal and coated with a magnetic surface. They are larger, more expensive, and hold more data than floppy discs.

Hardware. The actual mechanical, magnetic, electrical, and electronic equipment that makes up a computer system. See "Software."

In-House. Any computer that is entirely contained on the user's premises.

Input. The data or questions fed into the computer for processing.

I/O (Input/Output). The electronic and mechanical devices connected to the computer (keyboard, printer, CRT) that allow for entry and receipt of data. Also used to describe the function of entering or removing data.

K is 1,024 bytes.

Languages. Set of symbols, in which programs are written, that can be converted to machine-readable code. See "Compiler Language."

Leased Line. A telephone line strictly for the computer. Connects remote I/O devices or small computers to a centrally located mainframe or other computers.

Magnetic Card. A data storage medium based on reusable cards with magnetic-coated surfaces. Small storage capacity.

Magnetic Tape. A data storage medium based on large reels of half-inch wide magnetized tape, or smaller cassette-type tape.

Mainframe. The processing equipment in a computer facility. Technically identical to "CPU."

Megabyte. A unit of memory storage consisting of one million bytes.

Memory. The internal storage in the computer. The two main categories of memory are: (1) main memory, which is an integral part of the computer; and (2) ancillary memory, such as disc or tape storage. The second type of memory is generally referred to as peripheral or on-line storage, rather than as memory.

Microcomputer. The smallest type of computer system currently available. Usually uses floppy discs, but can be adapted to hard disc.

Microsecond. One-millionth of a second.

Millisecond. One-thousandth of a second.

Minicomputer. A small computer, usually employing hard disc storage. Larger than a microcomputer.

Modem. A hardware device used to translate computer signals into signals that can be transmitted over telephone lines. An acronym for MOdulator/ DEModulator.

Module. Segment of a program. A major program can be broken down into a number of modules. These modules can be written and tested separately, and then put together to form the complete program.

Off-Line. Not being directly connected to the computer. Certain types of records that are not needed immediately for processing would likely be stored off-line.

On-Line. A term applied to any storage or terminal device connected directly to the mainframe.

On-line Processing. Processing characterized by the user's entering of data directly into a computer through a terminal device connected on-line to the mainframe. The term does not necessarily mean immediate updating of the master files; it does imply, however, that certain master files are immediately available for on-line inquiry.

Output. The computer's answer, or result of instruction. Can be in the form of CRT display or a printed report.

Peripherals. Any devices external to the processer. Refers to I/O devices, such as CRTs, printers, keyboards, and storage devices (discs or tapes, for example).

Printer. The machine that prints computer output onto paper in human-readable form. Three types are "character" printers, which print one character at a time (slow); "line" printers, which print one line at a time (fast); and "page" printers, which print an entire page at a time (extremely fast).

Processor. The equipment that manipulates information inside the computer. See 'CPU'' and "Mainframe."

Program. The set of instructions that tells the computer how to perform specific functions. See "Software."

Random Access. A technique for storing and retrieving data that requires neither a strict sequential storage of the data nor a sequential search of an entire file to find a specific record. A record can be addressed directly at its location in the file.

Reference File. A set of semipermanent data maintained in the computer system as a frequent source of reference by the regular processing programs. Often called the "data base."

Removable Disc. Any disc that is not permanently mounted on the disc drive and can be removed for backup or other reasons. Usually used to store master and transactions files. Often in small systems, each distinct application has its own dedicated disc, i.e., the payroll files are on one disc, whereas the accounts payable files are on another.

Response Time. The amount of time that elapses between the initiation of an inquiry or other entry into a system and the receipt of a response. Response time may vary, depending on how many terminals are being used at once and on other technical design considerations.

Real Time. Refers to processing in which the master file is updated immediately on the entry of a transaction and thus is always in "real" condition.

Run Time. The total length of time required to process a specific collection of data in accordance with a program.

Sequential Access. A storage medium in which records are available only in a fixed, sequential order. See "Random Access."

Shared Service. Computer services characterized by many, often remote, users sharing the facilities of a central data center or computer. Users share both the time of processing and the applications programs.

Shared Time. The time, during which the mainframe is operating, that must be divided among all the users of a shared service.

Soft Copy. Output that is displayed on a video screen.

Software. The programs written for the computer.

Sort (noun). A utility program that organizes data stored on disc or tape into a prescribed arrangement.

Storage. Retaining information, either within or outside the system, from which it can be retrieved at a later time. Specifically, storage can refer to three concepts: Main Memory (obsolete "core storage"), which is the data stored internally in the CPU; On-Line storage, or the information filed on discs or tapes, which the computer can have access to directly; and Off-Line storage, which consists of punched cards or other media that the computer cannot work with unless the information is converted manually to another form.

System. A series of tasks, operations, or processes that change an identifiable set of inputs into a unique set of outputs.

Tape Drive. The physical unit on which tapes are mounted.

Terminal. An I/O device connected to the computer via a communications circuit. May be located either near the CPU, as with an in-house system, or at a remote site (e.g., individual pharmacy) in shared services.

Time Sharing. See ''Shared Time.''

Turnkey. A system that consists of functionally oriented programs designed to operate on equipment so standardized that it may be installed and operated by the ''turn of a key.''

Up Time. Time the computer is working.

20 | Risk Management and Insurance

The purpose of this chapter is twofold. The *first objective* is to acquaint the student with the basic nature of risk and insurance mechanisms and to discuss logical approaches to the management of risk. The *second objective* is to introduce the basic coverages available that may be needed in a particular situation.

Risk Management

TYPES OF RISK

A pharmacist invests his time (including his education), effort, and capital into his private practice in the hope of producing a reasonable salary and net profit. Obviously, there are risks involved when such a venture is undertaken. Risks arise from the uncertainty of the future and are of two basic types.

The first type is *market risk,* sometimes referred to as *dynamic risk* because of its changing character with changing market or economic conditions. The degree of market risk varies from ordinary risk, which is associated with most business enterprises, to high risk. The former is called *entrepreneur* risk; the latter is called *speculative* risk. Market risk was discussed in detail in Chapter 5. The second type is called *exogenous* or *static* risk because the risk arises outside the market or economic environment and is difficult, if not impossible, to control or prevent in many instances. Fires and windstorms are examples of this type of risk.

A pharmacy with a favorable location analysis, adequate capital, and a well-educated and experienced manager certainly would be classified as an ordinary entrepreneur risk. Even so, the pharmacist needs to take precautions to minimize both the market and the exogenous risks. Consistent with this objective, it is vitally important that he maintain adequate insurance coverage to provide protection against an unpredictable financial loss, which could seriously jeopardize the future success of his firm. For example, fire hazard is an ever-present danger that demands attention. Furthermore, liability coverage is also necessary to avoid losses evolving out of third-party claims against the business. Such claims can arise in cases of patrons injured on the premises, negligent employees, or use of the pharmacy's product or service. Attention should also be given to such perils as business interruption, theft, the death of key personnel, and a host of others.

APPROACHES TO RISK MANAGEMENT

It is appropriate at this point to discuss the various methods of handling the risk of financial loss in a pharmacy.

Risk Avoidance. First of all, it is possible that risk may be avoided. However, such a situation is most unusual in the case of market risk, since such risk can only be avoided before the choice to enter business is made. Hence, avoiding risk is simply avoiding the exposure.

Risk Assumption. Certain risk can be assumed or is assumed. For example, a lack of funds to purchase insurance may force the individual to assume the risk. On the other hand, risk may be assumed out of ignorance or the stubborn unreasonableness of the individual. An example is the case of a businessman who, recognizing his need for fire insurance, fails to realize that the standard fire contract, without the extended coverage endorsement, provides inadequate coverage.

It is possible that the decision to assume risk is the best decision, especially in cases of overinsurance. In other words, it is possible for the firm to become insurance-poor by simply having so much coverage that the total amount of premiums puts a strain on the financial position of the business. Another method for assuming risk is to self-insure. Self-insurance involves the establishment of a fund within the business to handle the possibilities of financial loss in relation to a particular peril or hazard. For example, many pension funds that offer both retirement and death benefits may actually be handled through a fund set up by management to meet the various types of liabilities as they arise. Finally, it may be necessary for the businessman to assume risk simply because the insurer will not write coverage for the particular situation. For example, credit insurance is not available at the retail level; hence all risk in regard to poor accounts and bad debts must be assumed by the businessman himself.

Reduction of Hazards. A third method of handling risk involves reducing the hazard of the risk. This approach to risk management involves an awareness on the part of the pharmacist as well as his employees that proper safety precautions are beneficial to all parties concerned. Loss prevention programs and a general recognition of proper safety precautions are important in the proper management of risk, for in many cases, the insurance company recognizes the value of such action and reduces insurance premiums.

All small businessmen should recognize also that losses can be reduced or minimized, should accident occur, by such measures as fire extinguishers, fire escapes, and an efficiently operating sprinkler system.

Shifting the Risk. The pharmacist may be in a position to shift risk by such arrangements as subcontracting, the use of surety bonds, and simply adopting the corporate form of organization. For example, through subcontracting, the person or persons contracted to perform a particular task will be responsible for adequate performance. In the case of surety bonds, the surety or the bonding company simply guarantees that a particular individual will perform in a prescribed manner. The corporate form of organization represents a risk shift situation in that it offers the limited liability feature.

Risk Reduction Through Insurance. Finally, the pharmacist must recognize that risk can be reduced. The principal means of reducing risk is through an insurance contract. Since insurance is the primary way to reduce risk, it would be enlightening to contrast insurance with gambling, an example of a risk that can be avoided. Insurance and gambling have the opposite effects in economic terms. The economic difference between gambling and insurance is based on the theory of marginal utility. The theory, in simple terms, rests on the concept that each additional unit of any economic good has a decreasing value with the accumulation of that good. Thus, $100 is less valuable to a person if he has $600 than if he has only $500. For example, if two people have $500 each and gamble $100 on a fair and even bet, the person who loses $100 experiences a greater economic loss in contrast to the $100 economic gain. The marginal utility of $100 in relation to the $600 of the winner is less than the marginal utility of $100 in relation to the $400 of the loser. The overall net effect of a gamble is a reduction in marginal utility. Insurance works to reduce risk and increases the overall marginal utility. The theoretical basis of insurance is explained in more detail in Marshall's economic treatise entitled *Principles of Economics.*[1]

Insurance Principles

DEFINITIONS OF INSURANCE

When financial loss involves the negligence of another party, the loss is shifted by society through the common law to the person responsible. When the loss evolves out of an act of God, the burden of loss must be assumed by the injured party. Regardless of the shift in the burden of loss or the assumption of the burden of loss, the loss is likely to cause someone serious financial difficulty. The insurance mechanism represents an effective solution to this problem by providing a private contractual arrangement allocating the burden of individual losses to members of a group who are exposed to similar losses. The insurance mechanism does not merely represent an accumulation of funds to meet uncertain losses, but, by virtue of the insurance contract, also spreads the risk.

The insurance mechanism is able to operate efficiently through the application of the law of large numbers. In other words, the greater the number of exposures, the more nearly will the actual experience approach the probable results expected. As the number of exposure units increases, events that occur by chance, or randomly, occur with amazing predictability. Thus the law of large numbers, the law of probability, provides the basis for the social benefit of the insurance mechanism.

Economic Definition. The insurance contract is defined as an economic device for reducing risk by combining a sufficient number of exposure units in such a manner as to make their individual losses predictable collectively but not individually. The predictable loss is then shared by all group members, and this simply means that certain small "losses" in the form of insurance premiums are exchanged for the possibility of a large loss that any given individual in the group may experience. The insurance company is in business to indemnify the injured party, that is, to compensate for the loss or injury sustained. Thus, the function of the insurance company is to determine whether a financial loss has occurred, and if so, to place the injured party in the same position as he was prior to the loss.

Legal Definition. In addition to the aforementioned socioeconomic definition of insurance, there is the legal definition of insurance. In legal parlance, insurance is a contract whereby a company or group undertakes to indemnify a person or firm against loss, damage, or liability arising out of an unexpected or uncontrollable event or contingency.

Accounting Definition. The accounting definition may be stated in the following terms. Insurance is a technique whereby a person or firm substitutes a small, fixed, and regularly occurring cost for a larger and uncertain cost.

REQUISITES OF INSURABLE RISK

For the insurance mechanism to operate effectively, there are certain requisites of an insurable risk.

Common Peril. First of all, there must be a large group of "homogeneous" units exposed to the same peril. This condition is necessary for the application of the law of large numbers and to provide a situation in which the probable deviation of actual loss from predicted loss is small enough to be offset by reasonble premium additions.

Definite Loss. The loss must be definite. This means the loss must be difficult to counterfeit, and it must be subject to value determination. Insurance companies have run into some difficulty in this respect in writing sickness insurance, disability insurance, and burglary insurance because in these areas the company is somewhat susceptible to fraudulent claims.

Substantial Loss. A large loss must be possible. This requisite is based on the assumption that pharmacists and other people find it feasible to assume small losses.

Accidental Event. The loss must be of an accidental nature. This simply means that such losses as the depreciation of capital assets, shoplifing, ex-pected bad debts, or other forms of market risk are not insurable.

Feasibility. The insurable risk must involve an economically feasible cost. In other words, the chance of loss must be small enough to permit assessment of a reasonable premium level. Efforts by insurance companies to satisfy this requirement of a feasible cost are evident in the widespread use of deductibles. This requisite is also the reason for the slow development of prescription coverage under private insurance policies. Younger and healthier individuals do not need the coverage, and therefore the premiums for the older and less healthy people would have to be high. Drugs and pharmaceutical coverage have been included in major health insurance policies, union negotiated in-surance coverages, and certain government programs in recent years because such policies cover a broad spectrum of people. These pharmaceutical cov-erages came about to meet the special needs of certain groups of people and because of the realization of the positive cost-effectiveness ratio of drugs and pharmaceutical services in relation to other categories of health care services.

Loss Dispersion. The risk must be such that it is unlikely to produce a financial loss to the majority of the exposed units simultaneously. Insurance companies protect against this possibility by distributing their underwriting efforts geographically and by prescribing certain minimum standards of con-formity for exposure units. When the risks are great, insurance companies spread the risk with cross or shared insurance by underwriting only a portion of the total risk. In other words, the primary insurer reinsures a portion of the risk with several other companies. Insurance companies also protect them-selves against this possibility through the use of certain clauses in the insurance contract. For example, the standard fire policy contains the war exclusion clause, which suspends coverage under conditions of war, insurrection, re-bellion, revolution, or action taken by the government to stem the possibility of such activity.

Actuarial Soundness. A seventh requisite of an insurable risk is the re-quirement that the chance of loss be determinable. This means that statistical information and data must be available in adequate quantities to permit the application of the law of probability, which in turn will yield reliable estimates of expected losses. The mathematical technique of calculating the pure pre-mium rate (exclusive of administrative costs and profits) for a given risk is based on the statistical probabilities derived from historic data related to the frequency of the incidence and costs of the losses. This special technique is known as actuarial science.

FORMULATING THE INSURANCE PROGRAM

The pharmacist typically is ill-equipped to formulate his own insurance program and should resort to the help of a competent insurance agent or insurance broker. The agent or broker approaches the problem by considering the nature of risk in the particular situation as it relates to the type of pharmacy, the location of the firm, the personnel involved, the market situation, and the general characteristics of the physical properties. A sound program of insurance coverage encompasses both *required* and *optional* types of coverage. For example, certain types of coverage, such as workmen's compensation and auto insurance, represent required coverages, whereas business interruption or burglary insurance may be considered optional.

Hall et al. made a survey of the use of insurance by owners of pharmacies in the Southwest.[2] The survey indicated that the majority of pharmacists were well covered in the traditional areas of fire, extended coverage, and liability, but inadequately covered by insurance for employees and business life insurance.

In selecting those types of coverage that are optional, the insurance broker or agent is extremely helpful in eliminating or avoiding unnecessary types of coverage. From an analytical point of view, the decision to provide a particular coverage is based on the relationship between the cost of insurance and the probability of loss. It is safe to assume that in the majority of cases the pharmacist would be unable to make this type of analysis. Furthermore, the insurance agent or broker can be helpful in recognizing situations that require actions that will minimize the cost of insurance or the loss. For example, the use of a deductible would be of benefit in terms of the cost of the insurance when applied to certain types of coverage. On the other hand, certain changes in the physical property, such as the installation of a sprinkler system or improvement in the construction, may have a significant influence on premium rates.

The questions of how much insurance is enough, what types of coverge are required, and how much coverage is adequate all demand the careful attention of an experienced, competent insurance agent or broker. The pharmacist cannot afford to use his good judgment alone. The pharmacist should select an agent he can trust, provide him with all the information necessary to arrive at proper advice, and give all his insurance business to him. Not only will this encourage him to give the best advice, but it is also economical. The pharmacist should give the agent the necessary time and keep him informed of any significant change in the value of the pharmacy's assets, especially inventory. This, of course, requires complete and accurate accounting records. In case of a loss, the agent should be notified promptly. The pharmacist should review his insurance coverage with his agent at least annually. For this reason it is better if there is a single all-encompassing policy, or a common expiration date if there is more than one policy.

Types of Insurance Coverage

The major types of insurance coverage available to the pharmacist are described only briefly. A basic knowledge of the coverages available will enable the pharmacist to communicate more intelligently with his agent or broker.

FIRE INSURANCE

A type of coverage that certainly should be required in every case is the standard fire insurance policy, which covers direct loss to all physical property, including leasehold improvements, resulting from fire or lightning and the removal from the premises of goods endangered by the perils of fire and lightning. The basic fire policy of and by itself, however, is grossly inadequate and requires the endorsement of additional forms of coverage. These forms fall into two basic categories: (1) forms covering additional perils and (2) forms covering additional losses.

Extended Coverage. Coverage under the standard fire policy can be considerably enhanced by the addition of the extended coverage endorsement. This endorsement extends the coverage of the basic policy to include direct loss to physical goods resulting from the perils of windstorm, hail, explosion, civil commotion, damage by aircraft or other vehicle, and smoke and smudge damage. The extended coverage endorsement has two distinct advantages. First, by including these additional perils within one policy, the cost is considerably lower than it would be if each of the additional perils had to be added separately. Second, the extended coverage endorsement tends to avoid or eliminate any disagreement as to the particular cause of loss. For example, assume that as a result of fire an explosion takes place. Without the extended coverage endorsement, the problem would be to determine the amount of loss resulting from the fire and the amount of loss resulting from the explosion. Obviously, with the extended coverage endorsement there would be no question as to the amount of loss resulting from the individual perils, since both fire and explosion are covered.

In addition to the extended coverage endorsement, there are a number of other allied endorsements that fire insurance companies are permitted to write that may or may not be appropriate in a particular case. Among the additional coverages available are building collapse, earthquake, flood and rain (under certain conditions and places), sprinkler leakage, and fire legal liability insurance.

CONSEQUENTIAL COVERAGE

As previously noted, the standard fire policy only covers direct loss, and yet in many cases the pharmacist finds himself exposed to indirect or consequential loss situations. The following forms are available to cover such additional loss situations and may be endorsed to the standard fire policy.

Business Interruption. This coverage is available to cover loss of profits as well as to cover fixed costs, which continue to be assessed despite the fact that the pharmacy is forced to discontinue operations as a result of a fire loss or a direct loss resulting from some other covered peril.

Profits and Commissions Insurance. This endorsement is available to cover a situation in which, although the business operations are not entirely suspended, a loss of profit occurs. For example, if a fire in early December destroys a lot of Christmas merchandise, a loss of profit would be apparent despite the fact that the business may not be entirely suspended. It is important to note at this point that the business interruption form only covers loss of profit and fixed charges in a situation in which operations are entirely suspended; hence the profit and commissions form would be necessary to cover a partial loss situation that does not totally suspend operations.

Extra Expense Coverage. Insurance is available to cover a situation in which additional costs are incurred as a result of doing business under unfavorable conditions. In other words, as a result of a loss, it may be necessary for the business to incur additional costs in avoiding suspension of operations. For example, if a pharmacy suffers a fire loss that forces them to rent or lease a building and additional equipment temporarily to avoid the suspension of business, the extra expense form would cover the added cost.

Rental Endorsements. Additional insurance may be endorsed to the standard fire policy if the pharmacist has rental or leased properties, for example, offices above the pharmacy. With the first endorsement, the rental insurance forms indemnify the insured for rent revenues that are not forthcoming because of a fire loss. With the second endorsement the insurance would protect the pharmacist who is forced to continue lease payments despite the fact that a fire loss has temporarily interrupted business operations. Obviously the rental insurance endorsements are valuable additions to the standard fire policy in a situation in which the business involves the renting of rooms or apartments.

Demolition Insurance. This form of endorsement is available to cover the situation in which an expensive fire loss occurs and a building or buildings must be totally reconstructed. In such a case, demolition insurance is the answer because it can be written to cover not only the cost of tearing down the remains of the destroyed building, but also the increased costs of reconstruction resulting from certain city ordinances or requirements that call for a particular type of construction.

Indirect Damage Insurance. This type of insurance covers consequential loss from damage to physical properties that indirectly results from a fire or other perils covered under the standard fire policy and the extended coverage endorsement. Consequential loss insurance is available in two basic forms. One form covers damage to goods resulting from temperature change or a change in other physical conditions. For example, it may well be that a fire loss results in the deterioration of drugs or a malfunction of a refrigeration unit which in turn results in damage to perishable items that require refrigeration. The other form covers damage to one of a set of items. For example, it may be that a combination of three products which was sold and used as a unit would suffer an indirect financial loss because fire damaged one part of the combination set, and the remainder of the set would certainly not maintain its proportional value if the entire set was not available.

Replacement Cost Insurance. Replacement cost insurance covers the actual cost of replacing damaged property without deduction for depreciation. In other words, the replacement cost endorsement actually violates the principle of indemnity, which states that the function of insurance is to place the insured party in the same relative position that he maintained prior to the loss. Replacement cost insurance provides a valuable and desirable type of coverage, because ordinary indemnification on the original cost less depreciation normally does not provide the insured party with adequate funds for replacement. For example, assume that a pharmacy has fixtures that are 10 years old and based on an original cost less depreciation, they have a present value of $3,000. Assume further that the fixtures are totally destroyed by fire and that under the standard fire policy indemnification only $3,000 will be paid. It is safe to assume that the $3,000 would be grossly inadequate in providing comparable fixtures. In such a situation the replacement cost form would be a valuable addition to the standard fire policy.

In summary, the standard fire policy, of and by itself, only provides coverage for direct loss resulting from fire and lightning, and hence must be supplemented by various forms that tend to broaden the coverage. First, the standard fire policy can be extended to include additional perils, either in a package form through the use of the extended coverage endorsement or on a peril by peril basis. Second, the standard fire policy can be endorsed to cover various types of indirect loss situations or consequential coverage.

CASUALTY INSURANCE

It is necessary for the pharmacist to use certain insurance policies written by casualty insurance companies. This category includes third-party liability, employer's liability, and other types of liability insurance. Third-party liability insurance protects the insured party against monetary penalties arising out of his negligence. Coverage is available to pay claims from court action, the cost of defense and investigation, and also first-aid and medical expenses. It is important to note that liability insurance does not in any way protect the insured against injury to himself, his partner or partners, his employees or any person or persons engaged in maintenance or alteration work on the premises. These are covered by other types of insurance. The usual forms available in the professional and/or business liability area are briefly described below.

Owners, Landlords, and Tenant's Liability Insurance. The owners, landlords, and tenants liability form covers bodily injury or property damage sustained in or about the building or business premises. The policy covers negligence or alleged negligence of the insured party. It also covers medical payments. The owners, landlords, and tenants policy does not cover elevator, professional or product liability, or liability arising out of alterations, new repairs, or demolition activity at the place of business.

Elevator Liability. Elevator liability insurance is optional and can be endorsed to either the owners, landlords, and tenant's policy or a contractor's liability policy, or it may be acquired separately. This policy includes any liability of the insured party resulting from the operation of elevators, escalators, or hoists, and it covers bodily injury, property damage, collision coverage, and medical payments. The pharmacist may have little use for this type of coverage unless he owns the building, but he should be sure his landlord has the coverage in order to preclude any possibility that he may be held responsible. This is especially important to a pharmacy or apothecary located above or below the ground floor, in which case elevators may be used to enter the pharmacy.

Contractual Liability. Often the leasing or rental of business properties creates a situation in which contractual liability exists. For example, the tenants of an office building are liable for accidents that may occur in the hallways or on the stairways of the building. Also, a pharmacist may be held liable for accidents that occur on the sidewalk in front of a pharmacy. Therefore, the pharmacist should determine whether his landlord's insurance covers injuries occurring on the sidewalk or in the vicinity of the building, and if not, it would be advisable to have this extra protection. The reality of this type of liability is illustrated by the following case. A pharmacist, the lessee of the building, was held liable for the injuries sustained by a person who was walking in front of the pharmacy when the front plate glass window suddenly exploded. Many city ordinances require the owners of buildings to keep the sidewalks in front of their buildings safe, and this liability devolves to the person leasing the building.

Contractor's Protective Liability Insurance. According to the law, a general contractor is liable for the actions of subcontractors, and similarly any individual hiring another person as an independent contractor to work on the premises is liable for the actions of the independent contractor. The obligation of the owner to protect the public cannot be shifted. Hence, there are situations in which the owner of a building can become liable to the public for the actions of independent or subcontractors. The owners and contractors protective liability insurance policy is intended to meet this need by providing the same basic coverages as the owners, landlords, and tenants policy. This type of situation could involve the subleasing and subcontracting of the operation of a department in a pharmacy, such as a fountain or some special skills department.

Product Liability Insurance. An important area of liability insurance that demands the pharmacist's attention is product liability. Product liability insurance in intended to cover liability for injuries sustained by any person or damage to any property caused by accident and arising out of the handling or use of goods or products manufactured, sold, handled, or distributed by the insured. The product liability form only covers the use and consumption of products off the premises; therefore it excludes fountains in a pharmacy. Where there is consumption of products on the premises, such as fountains, a special endorsement to the policy is available.

The pharmacist should understand the basis of product liability, its importance, and its relationship to professional liability. Product liability arises out of a contractual relationship between a pharmacist and his client. When a pharmacist sells a product to his patron, he gives a guarantee or warranty, either expressed or implied, that the product is suitable for its intended purpose, if it is for human consumption. If the pharmacist either expressly states, or implies by his actions, that a product (and this is especially true in the case of a drug) has particular beneficial characteristics or values, he may be held legally liable if an injury is sustained by the person who used the product while relying on the pharmacist's judgment. If the injury results from a faulty or inadequate product, the complaint normally is based on the breach of warranty associated with the sales contract.

Professional Liability Insurance. Professional liability insurance is of great concern to the pharmacist because it offers protection to the professional man in connection with services rendered or services that should have been rendered but were not. The insurance covers the cost of defense as well as damages. All pharmacists, both proprietors and employees, should carry the necessary professional liabiliity insurance to complement the pharmacy's product liability clause, which is commonly referred to as the "druggist's liability policy." The two types of coverage are analogous to the situation of damage resulting from either a fire or an explosion or both—the pharmacist is covered in either instance.

Professional liability insurance is especially useful for a pharmacist who consults with a hospital or nursing home, works in several pharmacies as a "relief" pharmacist, works as a hospital pharmacist, or is an employed pharmacist in a pharmacy that may have inadequate coverage for the employed pharmacist under the pharmacy's regular product liability or "druggist's liability insurance." A pharmacist can purchase professional liability insurance through the American Pharmaceutical Association group policy, which covers $200,000 per claim and up to $600,000 per year. The American Druggists' Insurance Co. now offers and actively promotes professional liability insurance.

Pharmacists and students should not view the problem of professional liability in a negative or passive manner. The modern pharmacist has a positive duty to perform professional services as a result of the expanding roles of the pharmacist and the increasing expectations the public has of pharmacists. With physicians becoming more pressed to use their time wisely because of an increasing patient load, the pharmacist is expected to fill some of the resulting void in patient consultation. For example, it is rapidly becoming the standard of pharmacy practice, if indeed it is not already, that the pharmacist should warn the patient against driving or manipulating heavy machinery while taking an antihistamine or a sedative purchased either on a prescription or over-the-counter. The same is true of nasal rebound from overuse of a nasal decongestant, the proper use of laxatives, and drug interactions. All of these situations place a positive duty on the pharmacist to provide the necessary professional consultation when dispensing these drugs. Injuries resulting from a failure to perform a professional service that is considered to be a standard of practice are subject to liability suits just as readily as those resulting from the dispensing of an incorrect drug.

"All-Risk" Liability Insurance. For small pharmacies, there is a comprehensive general liability policy available that can be used in lieu of either the owners, landlords, and tenants policy or the contractors policy. The comprehensive general liability form provides an all-risk type of coverage for small businesses in that it covers bodily injury and property damage at specific locations as well as at operations not specifically mentioned. In addition, product liability, professional liability, and contractual liability can be endorsed to the comprehensive general liability form.

SPECIAL TYPES OF COVERAGE

There are several special types of insurance that every pharmacist-proprietor should consider and, in most instances, purchase.

Automobile Insurance. The pharmacist undoubtedly needs automobile insurance coverage. Automobile or vehicular insurance involves elements of casualty or liability insurance as well as insurance against damage to the vehicle itself. There are sufficiently unique features in this type of insurance to warrant its separate treatment.

For the pharmacist who uses his private passenger car for business purposes, the insurance companies provide liability coverage in addition to collision insurance for both private and business use. The basic policy usually covers accidental body injury and property damage arising from the ownership or use of the vehicle, and it also protects the insured's vehicle either for specified perils or on an all-risk basis. The legal liability section protects the insured in any vehicle driven by him or his agent for business purposes, covering such items as first-aid and medical expenses, cost of bail bond, cost of defense, cost of judgments, and court costs. The policy may also cover those situations in which another vehicle is temporarily used because of breakdown, service, theft, or total destruction of the original vehicle. If the vehicle is stolen, a daily compensation is provided for necessary transportation.

Glass Insurance. If the pharmacist has a great deal of glass in the pharmacy building, he will find that the standard fire policy provides inadequate coverage, and comprehensive glass coverage is recommended. Glass insurance can be written to cover not only the loss of the glass itself, but also the frames, and the cost of removal and repair. Also, injury resulting from broken glass may be covered. This type of coverage is relatively expensive, and it should be cautiously considered as an endorsement.

Crime Insurance. Protection against burglary, robbery, and theft of merchandise, fixtures, or other equipment owned or held by the insured is available through the mercantile open-stock burglary policy. This policy is available to pharmacists to cover direct losses or damage when the pharmacy is not open. The mercantile interior robbery policy provides the same coverage for the same premises while the pharmacy is open. For insurance purposes, the distinction between robbery and burglary is a simple one. Burglary involves forced entry, and thus could only take place when the pharmacy is closed. Robbery, on the other hand, does not involve forced entry, and thus it occurs when the pharmacy is open. In addition to the burglary and robbery coverage, the pharmacist may have need for the mercantile safe burglary policy, which covers the forced entry into a safe. Other forms that may be required in particular situations are exterior messenger robbery policy which covers the insured or the insured's representative if robbery takes place while he is away from the pharmacy, and provides protection for money, securities, or other properties outside the premises. The money and securities broad form policy gives a much more complete coverage, on or off the premises, for securities or money for deposit, records, and accounts, which are either limited in coverage or omitted completely from the standard mercantile burglary and robbery forms.

The owner of a small pharmacy may satisfy his needs with the storekeepers burglary and robber policy, which is an "all-risk" type of coverage. This form covers inside robbery, outside robbery, safe burglary, the loss of money and securities in limited amounts, mercantile open stock, and finally, damage that results from actual or attempted robbery or burglary. This type of coverage, sold in units of $250, would be feasible only in the case of small pharmacies.

INSURANCE FOR EMPLOYEES

Workmen's Compensation. The laws of the several states and territories of the United States require that an employee is entitled, without consideration of personal fault, to indemnification for all economic loss due to accident or disease resulting from his employment. Thus, the pharmacist as an employer is required to have workmen's compensation insurance. The basic benefits under workmen's compensation include disability pay, medical and surgical benefits, rehabilitation and re-education benefits, and death benefits. It is customary, if not required, that the employer insure his liability under the workmen's compensation law with a private insurance company.

Bonding. A bond is a written contract under which one party binds himself financially for the performance or honesty of another. The three parties to a bonding arrangement are the principal who will perform, the surety who guarantees that the first party will fulfill his obligation, and the obligee, to whom the promise is made. If the principal does not perform, the surety must pay the obligee. The surety is a type of insurance company.

There are two basic types of bond—the *fidelity bond,* which guarantees the honesty of the principal, and the *surety bond,* which guarantees the performance of the principal of an agreed task or obligation.

Fidelity bonds, which guarantee the honesty of the employees, are available on an individual or a blanket bond for all employees. They can be made to cover a particular person by name, a group of people by name, a particular position in the firm, or group of positions in the firm. For example, a pharmacist could bond the position of accountant, without specifying the particular individual performing the duties of the accountant, or he may bond the particular individual regardless of what functions this individual performed in the business.

Pharmacists have little need for surety bonds; however, a general knowledge may prove to be useful, especially if he should have a building constructed for his use. The latter type of bond does not apply to employees in the usual sense. Surety bonds, which guarantee the performance of the principal, can also be purchased on an individual or blanket basis by position or name. The types of surety bond which the pharmacist may find useful include the supply bond, the construction bond, and the completion bond, which are all forms of the basic contract bond that guarantees fulfillment of an obligation.

Employee Group Insurance. If a pharmacist hires several employees, he may want to develop an employee group insurance plan. Group plans are available for life insurance, accident, accidental death, dismemberment, hospitalization, medical care coverage, and annuities. The benefits of employee group plans should be apparent. First of all, such plans enable employees to secure insurance that would otherwise be available at a high cost. Also, such plans offer employees insurance coverage that otherwise might not be insurable on an individual basis. This is true because the insurance company is only concerned with the average results of the group and not individual results. Each group of employees has its own eligibility rules, usually based on period of service, occupation, and wages. These group insurance plans can be set up on a contributory or noncontributory basis, and membership can be optional. Pharmacists who are members of state or national organizations may become part of a large group insurance plan, often at greatly reduced rates. This is one of many advantages of joining pharmaceutical organizations. There is a potential feature of group insurance policies through associations that has not been fully exploited for the mutual benefit of all concerned. This feature is the extension of insurance coverage to all employees who have been employed in a member pharmacy for a designated number of years, with the privilege of reciprocity among member employers thereafter.

MINIMUM COVERAGE

As a minimum, the pharmacist-proprietor should carry the following types of insurance: Fire insurance with extended coverage; business interruption; owners, landlords, and tenants liability (casualty); product liability; professional liability; automobile, and workmen's compensation insurance. If the pharmacist-proprietor employs several persons (ten or more), he should consider employee group insurance.

CO-INSURANCE

Broadly speaking, any type of deductible is a form of co-insurance. Deductibles may take one of several forms: (1) the insured pays a designated amount referred to as "first dollars" or a corridor deductible before the insurance covers the loss; (2) the insured pays a designated percentage of the loss, for example 20 percent; (3) the insured pays a fixed amount of a recurrence of each incidence of a loss, for example, $1.00 each time a prescription is dispensed; and (4) sometimes the deductible takes the form of a combination of (1) and (2) or (1) and (3).

In a more restricted sense, co-insurance clauses are attached to fire and extended coverage insurance policies commonly encountered in the practice of pharmacy. The policyholder, in consideration of a reduced rate, agrees to carry insurance equal to a certain percentage of the *actual value* of the property insured—usually 80 percent or more. If the insured fails to carry the designated amount of insurance, he becomes a co-insurer, and he can collect only that proportion of his loss which the amount he carries bears to the amount required. For example, if the value of the property is $50,000 and the insured agrees to carry at least 80 percent insurance, the amount of insurance required to comply with the co-insurance clause is $40,000. If, however, the policyholder carries only $30,000 worth of insurance and has a partial loss, he is a co-insurer and can collect only three-fourths of the loss because he is carrying only three-fourths of the amount required to comply with the clause. If the loss is $20,000, the insured will collect $15,000 and will have to bear the $5,000 loss himself. If the policyholder carries the required amount of insurance, he collects the full amount of his loss up to the amount of the policy. If there is a complete loss in the above example, the insured collects $40,000, the full value of the insurance policy.

Since most fires and related or extended damages seldom cause a complete loss of the property insured, the pharmacist should seriously consider the co-insurance clause.

The formula below is used to calculate the insurance company's liability under a co-insurance clause.

$$Li = \frac{C}{R} \times L$$

where: C = the amount of insurance carried;
     R = the amount required under the co-insurance clause;
     L = the loss sustained; and
    Li = the insurance company's liability.

Business Life Insurance

BASIC INFORMATION

Nature of Business Life Insurance. Business life insurance is life insurance used to protect a business, or the family of a businessman, from the financial loss that results from the death of someone associated with the business, usually the proprietor. Many billions of dollars worth of protection is now in force, giving assurance of business continuity to the firms and full value of the business equity to the family of the deceased. There is no basic difference between business life insurance and regular life insurance used for personal and family needs. Both provide insurance on the lives of individuals. But the protection set up by business firms does involve many more complex details to meet legal, financial, tax, and technical problems.

Implementation. A pharmacist contemplating the establishment of a business life insurance plan faces technical problems that require advice. He should consult *four experts* who can make certain that every aspect of the firm's interests is being safeguarded. These experts include the firm's *attorney, accountant, trust officer* of its bank, and *life insurance agent.* The insurance agent provides the technical advice concerning the arrangement of policies, while the others provide additional essential information on which the plan is based. They will double-check the plan when completed and assume the responsibility for carrying out the legal and banking details. Many life insurance agents who specialize in business life insurance are familiar with the whole range of problems, but they prefer to have their client's lawyer, banker, and accountant included in the consultation. The owner of a pharmacy, devoting his energies to make his practice a success, is not usually in a position to analyze his insurance needs or prescribe the correct policies or policy arrangements to meet those needs. Such a prescription calls for the highly specialized knowledge and technical advice of experts.

Tax Factors. Taxes, both income and estate, are involved in many business life insurance arrangements. These should be taken into consideration in order that the plan will not involve unnecessary additional taxes. On the other hand, too much weight should not be given to the tax angles, as they are constantly changing, and a plan set up today on the basis of a certain tax advantage may prove to be disadvantageous next year.

Reserves for Emergencies. Most business life insurance plans utilize life insurance that has cash value that grows over the years. This cash value provides the firm with a valuable reserve for emergencies in the event of any sharp dislocation in business conditions. When necessary, the cash value of the policy can be used as the basis for loans. When, for one reason or another, this type of policy is not possible, term life insurance may be used.

TYPES OF BUSINESS LIFE INSURANCE

Key-Man Insurance. Almost every pharmacy has one or more persons upon whom it depends heavily for its major success. Frequently it is the proprietor or manager. It may be the employed pharmacist, upon whose shoulders rests a major responsibility of the pharmacy and whose technical efforts are vital to the firm's success. It may be any employee whose death would be a considerable loss to the business. Key-man insurance is indicated for anyone whose death would cripple the business, or at least cause a setback until a replacement is secured. Such insurance provides insurance benefits at the death of this vital employee in order that the firm will have resources with which to employ and train a successor in the competitive market and to cushion the loss of profits in the meantime.

Proprietorship Insurance. Life insurance protection for the sole proprietor provides his dependents or heirs with cash representing the sound valuation of the business at his death and ensures continuity of the pharmacy. This is *as yet an undeveloped and widely neglected area of protection,* probably because the need is considered to be in the province of personal life insurance. Even in sole proprietorships, there are special considerations that should be recognized when writing the business life insurance policy. Adequate and specific provisions must be made to meet the conditions of a will or trust agreement concerning sales or liquidation of the business when such is desired. These include the selection of the beneficiary to fit the particular situation, and the question of who is to pay the premiums for a particular plan.

There is no set pattern; each case has to be determined on its own merits. One plan may call for sale of the pharmacy to specified employees, with the purchase money provided by the insurance. Another plan may provide that the pharmacy be run by the executor or the heirs, and in still another case, a trust company may be named as beneficiary and management control may be established. Many a small pharmacy has foundered after the death of the sole owner merely because he did not take the proper steps while alive to ensure its continuance. Numerically, pharmacies of the individual proprietor type no longer predominate, comprising approximately 30 percent of all units engaged in the practice of pharmacy. The sole proprietor who is interested in selling his pharmacy to one or more of his employees should consult with an attorney and a life insurance underwriter about the advantages of combining a pension or profit-sharing plan with a purchase agreement, funded by life insurance on the life of the pharmacy owner.

Partnership Insurance. In the absence of legal safeguards to avoid dissolution, a partnership automatically dissolves at the death of any of its partners. This results in cessation of normal partnership activities, and the surviving partners become what is known as "liquidating trustees." They cannot do any new business, but must confine themselves to winding up the affairs of the partnership. If they continue the business, they may become personally liable for any losses incurred should the assets not cover such losses. There are several ways to avoid these difficulties, one of which is an adequately financed *buy-and-sell agreement* providing for the purchase at a pre-arranged valuation of the deceased partner's interest. An attorney will draw up the necessary papers carrying out the wishes of the partners. After a buy-and-sell agreement has been executed, the next step is to fund the arrangement, which can be done effectively through business insurance. It enables the surviving partners to reorganize at once and continue in business; it liquidates the interest of the deceased partner without loss; it enables the beneficiaries of the deceased partner to secure full, fair value for his interest in the firm at once and with a minimum of trouble; and it lends support to the credit standing of the firm.

Corporation Insurance. A corporation is not as directly and immediately affected by the death of a shareholder as is the partnership by the death of a partner, but unfortunate consequences are a distinct hazard. Unlike the partnership, the corporation is not terminated at the death of an owner. However, with the transfer of the deceased stockholder's shares, new stockholders, new to management and possibly an unknown element, may enter the picture. The death of a principal stockholder may deal a severe blow to the firm's credit. There are several ways to handle the problem, one of which is an *adequately financed stock sale and purchase agreement,* drawn up by the firm's attorney. This too may be funded by insurance. An adequate corporation insurance program on the lives of its principal shareholders provides retirement of their interest at death. It gives the deceased shareholder's heirs full value for his interest at once and reduces the shock of changes in ownership. This is of special concern to the small corporation with a few shareholders whose interests keep them close to the management of the business. Frequently, ownership and management are one and the same. The great bulk of the country's corporations are in this category. Large numbers of them are small, closely held businesses which adopted the corporate form primarily for its legal, tax, and continuity advantages. By so doing, however, these owners have not escaped the death hazards that affect any business organization. Life insurance can provide the corporation with funds to purchase the interest of a stockholder at his death.

Periodic Analysis and Evaluation of Program

Once established, the business life insurance plan should receive a careful periodic evaluation by experts. Financial conditions change, tax laws vary in their effects, valuations of the interests of the owners are never constant—just to mention but a few of the changing conditions that can affect the plan. It is important that the details of the plan be kept up to date at all times. Reevaluations should be made whenever necessary in connection with buy-and-sell agreements and partnership and corporation policies. Every new revenue act suggests a need for a special checkup to make certain the tax angles are still adequately covered. At least once each year, the plan should go through a careful screening by the life insurance agent.

Since each state regulates insurance through its insurance statutes and regulations, the insurance agent, properly licensed, should be utilized at least annually for an analysis and evaluation of the insurance program.

Summary

Providing for appropriate and adequate insurance coverage must be of primary concern to the pharmacist. Failure to recognize the various needs for insurance protection leaves the pharmacist susceptible to conditions in which one unpredictable, accidental event can cause financial disaster and wipe out the benefits of many years of hard work.

The pharmacist is advised to deal with an independent insurance agent or broker because he has available a wider range of insurance policies and endorsements by dealing with a number of different companies. There are two types of insurance companies, mutual companies and stock companies. In the mutual company, the policyholders are the owners and the "profits," if any, are returned to the policyholders as dividends, rebates, or reductions in the cost of the premiums. A stock company is owned by the stockholders and is operated for the benefit of the stockholders just like any other stock company. Most of the life insurance in the United States is written by mutual companies, whereas about 80 percent of the business insurance is written by stock companies. One of the most active stock companies in the pharmaceutical profession is The American Druggists' Insurance Co. The majority of the shares of this company are held by pharmacists. The pharmacist's insurance package should be custom-tailored in consultation with his agent.

CITED REFERENCES

1. Marshall, A.: *Principles of Economics.* 8th ed. New York: The Macmillan Co., 1920, footnote p. 135.
2. Hall, E.J.W., Owen, H.T., and Daniel, B.: The uses of insurance by owners of pharmacies— a survey. *Texas J. Pharm. 1*:90–98, 1960.

GENERAL REFERENCES

1. Memorandum to Small Business No. 1—*Group Life Insurance for Employees.**
2. Memorandum to Small Business No. 2—*The Insured Pension Plan for Employees.**
3. Memorandum to Small Business No. 3—*Group Accidental and Sickness Insurance.**
4. BSB No. 33—*Sole Proprietorship Life Insurance.*†
5. BSB No. 35—*Corporation Life Insurance.*†

---

*All three of these pamphlets are published by the Institute of Life Insurance, 277 Park Ave., New York, N.Y. 10017.
†All four of the publications may be ordered from the Department of Commerce, Washington, D.C., or from any of its field offices.

6. BSB No. 36—*Partnership Life Insurance*.†
7. BSB No. 125—*Building an Insurance Plan for Your Business*.†
8. Duncan, D.J., and Phillips, C.F.: *Retailing Principles and Methods*. 6th ed. Homewood, Ill.: Richard D. Irwin, Inc., 1963, Chapter 26, pp. 715–739.
9. Steinmetz, L.L., Kline, J.B., and Stegall, D.P.: *Managing the Small Business*. Homewood, Ill.: Richard D. Irwin, Inc., 1968, Chapter 16, pp. 319–336.
10. Greene, M.R.: *Insurance and Risk Management for Small Business*. Washington: Small Business Administration (S.B.A. Management Series No. 30), 1963.
11. Brochure for pharmacy graduates, published by The American Druggists' Insurance Co., Amer. Bldg., Cincinnati, Ohio 45202.
12. Williams, A.C., and Hedges, B.: *Risk Management and Insurance*. Part II, New York: McGraw-Hill Book Co., Inc., 1964.

REVIEW

1. What are the two basic types of risk and which is insurable?

2. Differentiate between entrepreneur and speculative risks.

3. Discuss the five approaches to risk management.

4. Define insurance as a social device in socioeconomic terms, as a legal instrument in legal terms, and as an accountancy instrument in accounting terms.

5. Discuss the law of large numbers and how it forms the basis of insurance.

6. Identify and describe the seven criteria or requisites of insurable risk.

7. Describe the methods insurance companies have to mitigate the effects of a very large number of losses in a given period of time.

8. Describe the two basic forms or types of *extended coverage endorsements*.

9. Describe seven types of consequential endorsements to the standard fire policy.

10. Describe casualty insurance and the seven types of coverages included under this type of insurance.

11. Discuss what should be included in a comprehensive automobile or vehicular insurance policy.

12. Describe glass and crime insurance.

13. Discuss employee insurance including bonding, workmen's compensation, and employee group insurance.

14. What is the difference between fidelity and surety bonds?

15. Define co-insurance in the restricted sense and calculate the company's liability when given the appropriate data.

16. Discuss the general purpose of business life insurance and list six specific purposes.

17. Discuss the procedure in setting up a business life insurance program and identify the four experts the pharmacist should consult.

18. Discuss key-man, partnership, corporation, and individual proprietorship business life insurance in terms of purposes and coverage.

Index

Page numbers in italics indicate illustrations. Those followed by t indicate tables.

466   *Index*